ERP and EEG Markers of Brain Visual Attentional Processing

ERP and EEG Markers of Brain Visual Attentional Processing

Editor

Alberto Zani

MDPI • Basel • Beijing • Wuhan • Barcelona • Belgrade • Manchester • Tokyo • Cluj • Tianjin

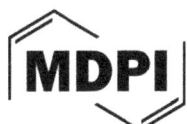

Editor
Alberto Zani
School of Psychology
Vita Salute San Raffaele University
Italy

Editorial Office
MDPI
St. Alban-Anlage 66
4052 Basel, Switzerland

This is a reprint of articles from the Special Issue published online in the open access journal *Brain Sciences* (ISSN 2076-3425) (available at: https://www.mdpi.com/journal/brainsci/special_issues/Brain_Visual_Attentional_Processing).

For citation purposes, cite each article independently as indicated on the article page online and as indicated below:

LastName, A.A.; LastName, B.B.; LastName, C.C. Article Title. *Journal Name* **Year**, *Article Number*, Page Range.

ISBN 978-3-03936-752-8 (Hbk)
ISBN 978-3-03936-753-5 (PDF)

© 2020 by the authors. Articles in this book are Open Access and distributed under the Creative Commons Attribution (CC BY) license, which allows users to download, copy and build upon published articles, as long as the author and publisher are properly credited, which ensures maximum dissemination and a wider impact of our publications.

The book as a whole is distributed by MDPI under the terms and conditions of the Creative Commons license CC BY-NC-ND.

Contents

About the Editor vii

Alberto Zani
From Correlational Signs to Markers. Current Trends in Neuroelectric Research on Visual Attentional Processing
Reprinted from: *Brain Sciences* 2020, *10*, 350, doi:10.3390/brainsci10060350 1

Alberto Zani, Clara Tumminelli and Alice Mado Proverbio
Electroencephalogram (EEG) Alpha Power as a Marker of Visuospatial Attention Orienting and Suppression in Normoxia and Hypoxia. An Exploratory Study
Reprinted from: *Brain Sciences* 2020, *10*, 140, doi:10.3390/brainsci10030140 11

Emmanuelle Tognoli
More than Meets the Mind's Eye? Preliminary Observations Hint at Heterogeneous Alpha Neuromarkers for Visual Attention
Reprinted from: *Brain Sciences* 2019, *9*, 307, doi:10.3390/brainsci9110307 35

Claudio de'Sperati
Cortical Resonance to Visible and Invisible Visual Rhythms
Reprinted from: *Brain Sciences* 2020, *10*, 37, doi:10.3390/brainsci10010037 45

Tugba Kapanci, Sarah Merks, Thomas H. Rammsayer and Stefan J. Troche
On the Relationship between P3 Latency and Mental Ability as a Function of Increasing Demands in a Selective Attention Task
Reprinted from: *Brain Sciences* 2019, *9*, 28, doi:10.3390/brainsci9020028 53

Rolf Verleger, Kamila Śmigasiewicz, Lars Michael, Laura Heikaus and Michael Niedeggen
Get Set or Get Distracted? Disentangling Content-Priming and Attention-Catching Effects of Background Lure Stimuli on Identifying Targets in Two Simultaneously Presented Series
Reprinted from: *Brain Sciences* 2019, *9*, 365, doi:10.3390/brainsci9120365 65

Manon E. Jaquerod, Sarah K. Mesrobian, Alessandro E. P. Villa, Michel Bader and Alessandra Lintas
Early Attentional Modulation by Working Memory Training in Young Adult ADHD Patients during a Risky Decision-Making Task
Reprinted from: *Brain Sciences* 2020, *10*, 38, doi:10.3390/brainsci10010038 89

Yanni Liu, Gregory L. Hanna, Barbara S. Hanna, Haley E. Rough, Paul D. Arnold and William J. Gehring
Behavioral and Electrophysiological Correlates of Performance Monitoring and Development in Children and Adolescents with Attention-Deficit/Hyperactivity Disorder
Reprinted from: *Brain Sciences* 2020, *10*, 79, doi:10.3390/brainsci10020079 109

Julie Bolduc-Teasdale, Pierre Jolicoeur and Michelle McKerral
Electrophysiological Markers of Visuospatial Attention Recovery after Mild Traumatic Brain Injury
Reprinted from: *Brain Sciences* 2019, *9*, 343, doi:10.3390/brainsci9120343 123

Amedeo D'Angiulli, Dao Anh Thu Pham, Gerry Leisman and Gary Goldfield
Evaluating Preschool Visual Attentional Selective-Set: Preliminary ERP Modeling and Simulation of Target Enhancement Homology
Reprinted from: *Brain Sciences* 2020, *10*, 124, doi:10.3390/brainsci10020124 137

Andrea Orlandi and Alice Mado Proverbio
Left-Hemispheric Asymmetry for Object-Based Attention: an ERP Study
Reprinted from: *Brain Sciences* **2019**, *9*, 315, doi:10.3390/brainsci9110315 . . . . **159**

Kyle K. Morgan, Dagmar Zeithamova, Phan Luu and Don Tucker
Spatiotemporal Dynamics of Multiple Memory Systems during Category Learning
Reprinted from: *Brain Sciences* **2020**, *10*, 224, doi:10.3390/brainsci10040224 . . . . **181**

About the Editor

Alberto Zani (https://orcid.org/0000-0002-3906-7988) (Full Professor at the School of Psychology of Vita Salute San Raffaele University), while being a plurennial research fellow in "Electrophysiological Techniques: Early Diagnosis and Prevention of Neurosensory Diseases" of the Italian National Research Council (CNR), has also been a Visiting Researcher at the Institute(s) of Physiology and Psychology of University of Leiden, Holland, and the Center for Mind and Brain, Uni-CA at Davis, USA. Additionally, he has been a Scholar in various institutes of CNR, where he directed the "Electro-Functional Brain Imaging Unit" investigating the relationships between mind and brain. Since 2012, he has been the Editor-in-Chief of the International Journal of Brain and Cognitive Sciences, CA, USA, and, since 2019, he has been a member of the Editorial Board of Brain Sciences. In addition to his various research articles, among his relevant publications there are Zani A & Proverbio AM, "The Cognitive Electrophysiology of Mind and Brain", Academic Press, 2003, and Proverbio AM and Zani A, "Instrumental Research Methods in Cognitive Neuroscience, EEG and ERP", Aracne Publisher, 2013 (in Italian). For exhaustive biographical info, see: https://erplabcnr.wordpress.com/alberto-zani/.

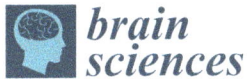

Editorial

From Correlational Signs to Markers. Current Trends in Neuroelectric Research on Visual Attentional Processing

Alberto Zani

School of Psychology, Vita Salute San Raffaele University, 20132 Milan, Italy; zani.alberto@hsr.it

Received: 31 May 2020; Accepted: 3 June 2020; Published: 6 June 2020

Abstract: Traditionally, electroencephalographic (EEG) and event-related brain potentials (ERPs) research on visual attentional processing attempted to account for mental processes in conceptual terms without reference to the way in which they were physically realized by the anatomical structures and physiological processes of the human brain. The brain science level of analysis, in contrast, attempted to explain the brain as an information processing system and to explain mental events in terms of brain processes. Somehow overcoming the separation between the two abovementioned levels of analysis, the cognitive neuroscience level considered how information was represented and processed in the brain. Neurofunctional processing takes place in a fraction of a second. Hence, the very high time resolution and the reliable sensitivity of EEG and ERPs in detecting fast functional changes in brain activity provided advantages over hemodynamic imaging techniques such as positron emission tomography (PET) or functional magnetic resonance imaging (fMRI), as well as over behavioral measures. However, volume conduction and lack of three-dimensionality limited applications of EEG and ERPs per se more than hemodynamic techniques for revealing locations in which brain processing occurs. These limits could only be overcome by subtraction methods for isolating attentional effects that might endure over time in EEG and may be riding even over several different ERP components, and by intracerebral single and distributed electric source analyses as well as the combining of these signals with high-spatial resolution hemodynamic signals (fMRI), both in healthy individuals and clinical patients. In my view, the articles of the Special Issue concerned with "ERP and EEG Markers of Brain Visual Attentional Processing" of the present journal Brain Sciences provide very good examples of all these levels of analysis.

Keywords: EEG; ERPs; brain visual attentional processing; neural markers; intracerebral single and distributed electric source localization analyses; hemodynamic imaging; psychological sciences; cognitive neurosciences

1. Introduction

During the call for papers for the Special Issue concerned with "ERP and EEG Markers of Brain Visual Attentional Processing" of the present journal, I found myself compelled to move from the Institute of Molecular Bioimaging and Physiology (IBFM), where I spent about twenty years, to the Institute for the History of Philosophical and Scientific Thought in Modern Age (ISPF) of the Italian National Research Council (CNR), for a series of reasons that would be too long to explain here.

On my first days at the CNR-ISPF, some of my new theoretical philosopher colleagues asked me reasonable but at the same time "thorny" questions about my electrophysiological experimental research.

They asked me to characterize my electroencephalographic (EEG) and event-related brain potentials (ERPs) research as a "research program", not from the perspective of a series of isolated studies but as a body of work which, over a period of ten or twenty years, has made definite progress in theory and methodology. What was my research program? What questions was I asking? What techniques were available to answer these questions? Could these techniques, in principle, provide the answers?

Fortunately, I had already dealt with such matters in the past in my editorial endeavors, e.g., [1,2]. Therefore, taking those questions as a challenge to myself, I tried to answer them later on explicitly during a presentation seminar, after some meditations to update and focus my thoughts on these matters.

I started my presentation by telling them that, for me, the truly big questions concerned human mental processes—among them, most specifically, visual selective attention processing e.g., [1,3–6], which I have particularly fancied over many years of my career—and their relationships to overt behavior. I also told them that, historically, these questions had been addressed at three different levels of analysis, which I referred to as the mind (psychological or cognitive sciences), the brain (brain science), and the cognitive neuroscience levels of analysis, very much aware that I might be somehow violating the common usage of these terms.

I went on to explain that, traditionally, the mind level attempted to account for mental processes in conceptual terms without reference to the way in which they were physically realized by the anatomical structures and physiological processes of the human brain [1,7–9]. Psychological theories in this sense did not use terms such as "superior parietal cortex" or "temporo-parietal junction" of the brain in relation to visuospatial attention orienting processes. Rather, they used other constructs, such as "visuospatial endogenous attention orienting" and/or "visuospatial exogenous attention orienting", which, traditionally, did not imply any specific physical realization.

The brain science level of analysis, in contrast, attempted to explain the brain as an information processing system and to explain mental events in terms of brain processes. As such, it allowed the development of particular explanations, such as "visuospatial attention orienting consists of computational processes of neuronal circuits located in fronto-parietal and occipito-temporo-parietal structures of the brain having properties of engagement, disengagement of attention orienting and selection of relevant in comparison to irrelevant information [10–12]."

Somehow overcoming the separation between the two abovementioned levels of analysis, the cognitive neuroscience level—which I explained I had enthusiastically embraced for my endeavors for quite some time—considered how information was represented and processed in the brain, i.e., the mental/psychological level. At the same time, an analysis at the cognitive neuroscience level allowed one to pursue the exploration of underlying functional organization of distributed but often overlapping brain networks involved as a set of algorithms in mental functions in general and in visuospatial attentional functions in particular, i.e., the brain/neuropsychological level of analysis. From this perspective, every statement about mind/psychology was a statement about brain function [12–14].

Now, where did EEG and ERP research fit into this characterization? EEG and ERP are continuous, multidimensional electrical signal waveforms reflecting brain voltage fluctuations in time. These waveforms consist of a series of positive and negative electrical voltage deflections relative to baseline activity [1,2,7,9,15–20]. Only those voltage deflections varying as a function of the changes in the flow of information during cognitive processing are indicated as intervening EEG spectra or ERPs "components"—or "scalp manifestations"—of the abovementioned changes [1,2,7,17].

Neurofunctional processing takes place in a fraction of a second. Hence, the very high time resolution—in the order of milliseconds—and the reliable sensitivity of EEG and ERP in detecting functional changes in brain activity as well as the noninvasiveness of these techniques provided advantages [15–19] over hemodynamic imaging techniques such as positron emission tomography (PET) or functional magnetic resonance imaging (fMRI), as well as over behavioral measures [12,13], for investigating details of brain functional organization and the timing of the activation of regional areas of anatomically distributed processing systems involved in cognitive functions [1,2].

It is true that volume conduction and the lack of three-dimensionality limit applications of EEG and ERPs per se more than hemodynamic techniques for revealing locations in which brain processing occurs [1,2,7,9,14]. A limitation much less attributable to magnetoencephalography (MEG), the complementary magnetic signals that simultaneously accompany EEG and ERP signals, which should be interpreted together whenever possible [21,22]. However, simply knowing the neural locus of a given functional activation can in no way explain the mechanisms of a cognitive domain, such as how we direct our attention to objects and the surrounding space [1,23–26].

I worked to explain that at the cognitive neuroscience level of analysis, the neural localization of mental domains was considered only as good as the unveiling of the mechanisms underlying the different mental domains [23–26], such as visuospatial attention processing [1,2,20].

Therefore, while relating variations in EEG and ERPs to changes in psychological processes is important for adding knowledge of the mechanisms governing mental domains, it cannot by itself contribute to knowledge at the brain localization level [1,2,7,9,17]. As a consequence, to cope with the spatiotemporal overlap in the scalp-recorded bioelectrical manifestations of underlying single brain structure activation and with problems in determining their neurophysiological generators, cognitive electrophysiologists identify the portions of the recorded waveforms that can be independently changed by different cognitive conditions as true components of activity in specific cerebral structures. These components can only be identified by subtraction methods for isolating effects that might endure over time and may be riding even over several different components. Importantly, these subtraction methods can be applied to investigate attention effects (i.e., the differential brain response to items that are attended with respect to those that are not) [1,2,7,17].

With the theoretical backing of modern cognitive neuroscience, high-time resolution EEG and ERP research has been augmented by new developments at a dizzying speed over recent years. This occurred thanks to the introduction of new techniques, e.g., Morlet's wavelet (the time-related EEG band power-spectra computation [2,16,23]) and algorithms for intracerebral single source analyses such as Brain Electrical Source Analysis (BESA) [1,2,14,27], and, later on, for distributed intracerebral source localization analyses such as Low Resolution Tomography (LORETA) [28]. In its upgraded versions, i.e., exact LORETA (eLORETA) or sLORETA and (swLORETA), the algorithm assumes that extended segments of the brain cortex can be active simultaneously while allowing the contribution of single areas to vary over time [1,2,29,30]. Indeed, thanks to the introduction of these new techniques and of the constrained "combining" with hemodynamic methods (e.g., MRI, fMRI), EEG and ERPs have contributed, as a research tool, to both cognitive and brain sciences, putting together new knowledge about humans as integrated sociobiological individuals [1,2,11,12,17,20,31,32].

These contributions also occurred thanks to the application of EEG and ERPs in the evaluation of psychological and psychiatric as well as neurological patients and to reciprocal relationships between the clinic and the experimental laboratory in the framework of an interdisciplinary integration of neurofunctional concepts and cognitive protocols and models, such as those proposed in cognitive neuroscience [33–35]. With hindsight, I indicated to my new colleagues these contributions and relationships as being specially relevant for EEG and ERP research, although, in my entire career, I rather rarely worked with patients and/or clinical populations (e.g., see the "References" section for my sober "contributions" to the literature [36,37]). These studies, in fact, not only allow the probing of brain processing when the system is impaired but also the involvement of localized brain districts in cognitive domains, as is done by traditional clinical neuropsychology for the benefits of patients. Most importantly, they shed some light on neural sources of ERP components possibly involved in cognitive processing [1,2,33], as directly pursued in the past by means of intracerebral microelectrode recordings during surgery in human patients [38] and brain lesional studies in animals to the detriment of fair ethical judgments.

I concluded my presentation by stating that I believed that cognitive electrophysiology had at present laid the groundwork for the use of EEG and ERPs, in combination with other available techniques and analysis methods, as quantifiable "markers" of integrated cognitive and affective processing of the brain. I added that, using these markers, during my career, I had been humbly able, together with my colleague Alice Mado Proverbio and our coworkers, to make some contributions to the testing of existing general theories on the mind and brain, especially with respect to visuospatial attentional processing [1,2,10], and, perhaps, to advancing fresher and more heuristic ones [39–41]. I also outlined that to be successful in this endeavor of exploring how visual attention processing arose from specific brain structures, I had worked in the context of interdisciplinary cognitive and brain functional theories as well as with sophisticated methodologies.

I have used these reflections to guide my work when, unexpectedly, after a few months spent at the CNR-ISPF, I was, for better or for worse, hired as a full professor of general and experimental psychology from the School of Psychology of Vita-Salute San Raffaele University. Indeed, it is also in the framework of the theoretical assumptions and "research program" discussed above that I gave my final evaluations of the reviewing process as a guest editor on the influential papers published in the Special Issue, out of the several others submitted.

2. The "ERP and EEG Markers of Brain Visual Attentional Processing" Special Issue—Overview

The research articles of this Special Issue—published by a panel of authoritative international cognitive neuroscientists and electrophysiologists—present state-of-the art developments in the knowledge of the relationships between visuospatial attentional processing and the brain as investigated by means of EEG and ERPs in the framework of theoretical orientations of cognitive science and neuroscience. All the articles compare overt behavioral data obtained in universally renowned visual selective attention protocols with the electrophysiological data obtained in these same protocols aimed at investigating different facets of visuospatial attentional processing. The articles have been published by the *Brain Sciences* journal at different dates during the call for papers for the Special Issue. Rather than following their publication order, I thought that it was appropriate to organize their presentation into relative theoretical and methodological as well as "thematic sections" in order to guarantee to each of them the deserved regards in the framework of a systematic discussion.

For the cognitive/psychological level of analysis of brain function "EEG markers" section, the article by Alberto Zani, Clara Tumminelli, and Alice Mado Proverbio [42] robustly proved that EEG alpha power computed during both a typical normoxia and an atypical oxygenation condition (hypoxia) in the brain might usefully serve as a marker of visuospatial attention orienting or suppression. Alpha power was lowest during the exogenous orienting of spatial attention, highest during alerting, and intermediate during the endogenous orienting of attention, regardless of brain oxygenation levels. The data also indicated that the dramatic increase in alpha power found in hypoxia over the right-sided lateral occipito-parietal scalp areas, independent of attention cueing and conflict conditions, possibly marked an overall suppression or impairment of separate visual attention network functionality.

Most interestingly, Emmanuelle Tognoli's paper [43] also considered how EEG brainwaves within the 10 Hz band governed brain visuospatial attentional processing. At the same time, the author discussed theoretically the salient power distribution and privileged timescale of these waves for cognition and behavior, hinting positively at the intriguing possibility that a number of other 10 Hz neuromarkers had function and topography clearly distinct from alpha power, such as an activity measurement named xi (χ), recorded over the left centroparietal scalp regions when subjects held their attention to spatially peripheral locations while maintaining their gaze centrally. The author challengingly outlines several potential functions for xi (χ) activity as a putative neuromarker of covert attention distinct from alpha power.

Both of the abovementioned papers provide the foremost constraints for further probing the functions of these 10 Hz brainwaves in close relation to brain neuroanatomy as searched by combining these brainwaves with hemodynamic and/or single and distributed source modeling data.

Still at the cognitive/psychological level of analysis, Claudio de'Sperati's paper [44] measured steady-state visual evoked potentials (SSVEPs) to video speed modulations in a group of observers and found a clear perceptual sensitivity increase and a moderate SSVEP amplitude increase with increasing speed modulation strength. Importantly, cortical responses also appeared with weak, overtly undetected speed modulations. Overall, these preliminary ERP findings suggest that the brain cortex responds selectively to periodic stimulus speed modulations, even when observers are not aware of them, thus hinting at an entrainment mechanism that may be the basis of a perceptual automatic resonance to the rhythms of the external visual world.

Further contributing to the cognitive/psychological level of study of brain functions, Tugba Kapanci's, Sarah Merks's, Thomas H. Rammsayer's, and Stefan J. Troche's study [45] illustrated how latency measurements of ERP P3 recorded in an increasing demand selective attention task administered to a sizeable sample of participants allowed them to settle the inconsistency in the literature of findings on the chronometric speed of information processing as a function of mental ability (MA), with higher speed in individuals with higher MA vs. the speed of those with lower MA. Indeed, using this increasing demand task, the authors were able to show that, in agreement with overt behavioral data (RTs) increases, MA and P3 latency negatively correlated in the standard condition of a continuous performance test (CPT), and this negative relationship increased systematically from the higher to the highest task demand conditions (CPT1 vs. CPT2) but was absent in the lowest demand (CPT0) condition.

To test how the brain visual attentional processing system dealt with changes in the relevance of stimulus features in time and space, Rolf Verleger, Kamila Śmigasiewicz, Lars Michael, Laura Heikaus, and Michael Niedeggen [46] used a task with rapid serial presentation of two stimulus streams where two targets ("T1" and "T2") had to be distinguished from background stimuli and where the difficult T2 distinction was impeded by background stimuli presented before T1 that resembled T2 ("lures"). A blue digit among black letters was used as T2, and lures resembled T2 either by alphanumeric category (black digits) or by salience stimuli (blue letters). Same-category lures were expected to prime T2 identification, whereas salient lures would impede T2 identification. Behavioral results confirmed these predictions, yet the precise pattern of results did not fully fit the authors' conceptual framework. Selection mechanisms were additionally probed by measuring ERPs. Consistent with the assumption that color lures attracted more attention, they induced larger N2pc than digit lures and affected the ensuing T1-related N2pc. T2-evoked N2pc was indistinguishably reduced by all kinds of preceding lures. A lure-related enhancement of mesio-frontal negativity from the first lure to the third lure both with digit and color lures also hinted at an increase in expectancy for T1.

Most interestingly, three articles gathered in a "clinical section" of the simultaneous psychological and brain levels of analysis provide new insights on the use of ERPs in both psychological and neurological clinical settings and into the fruitful, reciprocal relationships between the clinic and the experimental laboratory, thanks to the addition of cognitive neuroscience complex protocols to the traditional clinical ones.

The study by Manon E. Jaquerod, Sarah K. Mesrobian, Alessandro E. P. Villa, Michel Bader, and Alessandra Lintas [47] provided robust data showing that Working Memory training (WMT) with a high cognitive load affected the top-down modulation of brain visual attentional processing in a probabilistic gambling task in young Attention Deficit Hyperactivity Disorder (ADHD) adults compared with matched controls. ERPs elicited by the choice of the amount wagered in a gambling task were recorded before and after WMT in a dual n-back task in these two groups. In ADHD, the P1 wave component was selectively affected at frontal sites, and its shape was recovered close to that of controls only after adaptive WMT. Based on these findings, they propose that modified frontal site activities might constitute a neural marker of this effect in a gambling task. In controls, conversely, an increase in late parietal negativity might rather be a marker of an increase in transfer effects to fluid intelligence.

Yanni Liu, Gregory L. Hanna, Barbara S. Hanna, Haley E. Rough, Paul D. Arnold, and William J. Gehring [48] provided behavioral and ERP component data positively contributing to closing the gap in knowledge concerning the developmental trajectory of brain visual attentional processing underlying performance deficits in children and adolescent youths with ADHD. Compared with healthy controls (HCs), participants with ADHD obtained slower and more variable reaction times (RT), as well as reduced post-error slowing, in a congruent–incongruent arrow flankers task; they also exhibited reduced error-related negativity (ERN) and error positivity effects and reduced N2 and P3 congruency effects. Most importantly, developmental effects were observed across groups: with increasing age, participants responded faster, with less variability, and with increased post-error slowing. They also exhibited increased ERN effects and increased N2 and P3 congruency effects. Increased variability in RTs and reduced P3 amplitudes in incongruent trials were associated with increased ADHD Problems Scale scores on the Child Behavior Checklist across groups.

The study by Julie Bolduc-Teasdale, Pierre Jolicoeur, and Michelle McKerral [49] adds original findings on different forms of mild traumatic brain injury (mTBI) compared to uninjured controls by means of a novel and sensitive as well as rigorous ERP task implemented at the diagnostic and follow-up levels. Thanks to this task, the authors were able to show that both earlier VEPs (P1, N1) and visuospatial-attention orienting-related N2pc as well as encoding in visual short-term memory (vSTM), at later stages of brain processing, were as a whole comparable between mTBI and controls. However, there appeared to be a disruption in the spatiotemporal dynamics of attention (N2pc-Ptc, P2) in subacute mTBI that recovered within six months. This pattern was also reflected in altered neuropsychological performance (information processing speed, attentional shifting). Most interestingly, the orientation of attention (P3a) and working memory processes (P3b) were also affected and remained as such in the chronic postmTBI period, in cooccurrence with persisting post-concussion symptomatology.

Last but not least, a small collection of three additional papers also directly assessed ERP manifestations of visual attentional processing with their brain area localizations either with both single dipole (e.g., D'Angiulli et al.) [50] and distributed swLORETA source modeling (e.g., Orlandi and Proverbio) [51] or with hemodynamic fMRI data (e.g., Morgan et al.) [52].

The study by Amedeo D'Angiulli, Dao Anh Thu Pham, Gerry Leisman, and Gary Goldfield [50] sought to examine enhanced brain responses to targets during visual sustained selective-set attention in preschool children. Notably, the study indicated conceivable novel directions for further tests and falsifiable hypotheses on the origins and development of visual selective attention brain networks and their ERP manifestations. ERPs concurrent with target presentation were, in fact, enhanced relative to distractors, without manual response confounds. Triangulation of peak analysis, ERP-based adaptive control of thought–rational (ACT–R) modeling, and simulation for the entire ERP epochs up to the moment of manual response (~700 ms, on average) suggested converging evidence of distinct but interacting processes of enhancement and planning for response release/inhibition, respectively. The latter involved functions and structures consistent with adult ERP activity, which might correspond to a large-scale network involving dorsal and ventral attention networks, corticostriatal loops, and subcortical hubs connected to prefrontal cortex top-down working memory executive control.

Further emphasizing ERP-related research on brain networks subserving visual attention, the study by Andrea Orlandi and Alice Mado Proverbio [51] provided evidence on the time course and activity in the left hemisphere of the brain underlying object-based attention. They recorded both the behavioral and ERP responses to 3D graphic images falling into different object categories (e.g., wooden dummies, chairs, structures of cubes) posing alternatively as targets and nontargets in separate runs of a selection task. Nontarget stimuli elicited a larger anterior N2 component, which was likely associated with motor inhibition. Conversely, target selection resulted in an enhanced selection negativity (SN) response lateralized over the left occipito-temporal regions, followed by a larger centro-parietal P300 response. These potentials were interpreted as indexing attentional selection and categorization processes, respectively. The left-sided generators of SN were also supported by distributed standardized-weighted low-resolution electromagnetic tomography (swLORETA) source reconstruction, which indicated a fronto-temporo-limbic network as a system directly involved in object-based visual attention.

Importantly, the multi-experiment study by Kyle K. Morgan, Dagmar Zeithamova, Phan Luu, and Don Tucker [52] used both fMRI and ERP measures to determine whether multiple memory systems are involved in a categorization task and to evaluate the time course under which these systems are recruited. Their findings robustly showed that once the participants acquired the task, clear differences in the left lateral inferior anterior negativity (LIAN), medial frontal negativity (MFN), and P3b components were seen between visually similar and visually distinct category conditions. A region-based fMRI multivoxel pattern analysis (MVPA) also showed that the lateral frontal and parietal regions provided the most reliable classification between the visual categories, consistent with previous findings that rule-based categorization requires a higher degree of attentional resources. Additionally, based on the correspondence of MFN latency with the initial orienting of attention in a visuomotor association task, the authors propose that the MFN is indexing the controlled attention allocated to select the memory system best suited for categorizing the perceived stimulus.

As a concluding remark, I would add that, in my view, this Special Issue represents a further step in the disclosure of "the principles to which brain areas are assigned to functions and get assembled into circuits [20]" as well as in networks, whose dynamic activations during visual selective processing may be directly and robustly reflected by EEG and ERP signals, as well as their MEG counterpart.

Funding: This research did not receive external funding.

Conflicts of Interest: The author declares no conflict of interest.

References

1. Zani, A.; Proverbio, A.M. Cognitive electrophysiology of mind and Brain. In *The Cognitive Electrophysiology of Mind and Brain*; Zani, A., Proverbio, A.M., Eds.; Academic Press: Amsterdam, The Netherlands; London, UK; New York, NY, USA, 2003; pp. 3–12.
2. Proverbio, A.M.; Zani, A. (Eds.) *Instrumental Methods in Cognitive Neuroscience; EEG and ERP*; Aracne Publisher: Rome, Italy, 2015. (In Italian)
3. Proverbio, A.M.; Zani, A. ERP studies of selective attention to non-spatial features. In *Neurobiology of Attention*; Itti, L., Rees, G., Tsotsos, J., Eds.; Academic Press: San Diego, CA, USA, 2005; pp. 514–519.
4. Proverbio, A.M.; Del Zotto, M.; Zani, A. Electrical neuroimaging evidence that spatial frequency-based selective attention affects V1 activity as early as 40–60 ms in humans. *BMC Neurosci.* **2010**, *11*, 59. [CrossRef] [PubMed]
5. Zani, A.; Proverbio, A.M. Endogenous attention to object features modulates the ERP C1 component. *Cogn. Neurosci.* **2017**. [CrossRef] [PubMed]
6. Zani, A.; Proverbio, A.M. How voluntary orienting of attention and alerting modulate costs of conflict processing. *Sci. Rep.* **2017**, *7*, 46701. [CrossRef] [PubMed]
7. Donchin, E. *Cognitive Psychophysiology: Event-Related Potentials and the Study of Cognition*; Erlbaum: Hillsdale, MI, USA; London, UK, 1984.
8. Kutas, M.; Hillyard, S.A. Reading senseless sentences: Brain potentials reflect semantic incongruity. *Science* **1980**, *207*, 203–205. [CrossRef]
9. Rugg, M.D.; Coles, M.G.H. (Eds.) *Electrophysiology of Mind*; Oxford University Press: Oxford, UK, 1996.
10. Posner, M.I.; Petersen, S.E. The attention system of the human brain. *Ann. Rev. Neurosci.* **1990**, *13*, 25–42. [CrossRef] [PubMed]
11. Reiman, E.M.; Lane, R.D.; VanPetten, C.; Bandettini, P.A. Positron emission tomography and Functional magnetic resonance imaging. In *Handbook of Psychophysiology*; Cacioppo, J.T., Tassinary, L.G., Bernston, G.C., Eds.; Cambridge University Press: Cambridge, UK, 2000; pp. 85–118.
12. Bandettini, P.A. Functional magnetic resonance imaging. In *Methods in mind*; Senior, C., Russel, T., Gazzaniga, M.S., Eds.; The MIT Press: London, UK; Cambridge, MA, USA, 2006; pp. 193–236.
13. Federmeier, K.D.; Kluender, R.; Kutas, M. Aligning linguistic and brain views on language comprehension. In *The Cognitive Electrophysiology of Mind and BRAIN*; Zani, A., Proverbio, A.M., Eds.; Academic Press: Amsterdam, The Netherlands; London, UK; New York, NY, USA, 2003; pp. 143–168.
14. Scherg, M. Functional imaging and localization of electromagnetic brain activity. *Brain Topogr.* **1992**, *5*, 103–111. [CrossRef]
15. Regan, D. *Human Brain Electrophysiology. Evoked Potentials and Evoked Magnetic Fields in Science and Medicine*; Elsevier: New York, NY, USA, 1989.
16. Davidson, R.J.; Daren, C.J.; Larson, C.L. Human Electroencephalography. In *Handbook of Psychophysiology*; Cacioppo, J.T., Tassinary, L.G., Bernston, G.C., Eds.; Cambridge University Press: Cambridge, UK, 2000; pp. 27–52.
17. Fabiani, M.; Gratton, G.; Coles, M.G.H. Event-related potentials. Methods, theory, and applications. In *Handbook of Psychophysiology*; Cacioppo, J.T., Tassinary, L.G., Bernston, G.C., Eds.; Cambridge University Press: Cambridge, UK, 2000; pp. 53–84.
18. Picton, T.; Cohen, J. Event-related potentials: Whence? Where? Wither. In *Brain and Information: Event-related Potentials*; Karrer, R., Cohen, J., Tueting, P., Eds.; The New York Academy of Sciences: New York, NY, USA, 1984; pp. 753–765.

19. Zani, A. Evoked and event-related potentials. In *Encyclopedia of Sciences and Religions*; Runehov, A.L.C., Oviedo, L., Eds.; Springer: New York, NY, USA, 2013; pp. 787–792.
20. Posner, M.I. Electrical probes of mind and brain. In *The Cognitive Electrophysiology of Mind and Brain*; Zani, A., Proverbio, A.M., Eds.; Academic Press: Amsterdam, The Netherlands; London, UK; New York, NY, USA, 2003; pp. XV–XVII.
21. Aine, G.J.; Stephen, J.M. MEG Studies of visual processing. In *The Cognitive Electrophysiology of Mind and Brain*; Zani, A., Proverbio, A.M., Eds.; Academic Press: Amsterdam, The Netherlands; London, UK; New York, NY, USA, 2003; pp. 93–142.
22. Hari, R.; Baillet, S.; Barnes, G.; Burgess, R.; Forss, N.; Gross, J.; Hamalainen, M.; Jensen, O.; Kakigi, R.; Maugiere, F.; et al. IFCN-endorsed practical guidelines for clinical magnetoencephalography (MEG). *Clin. Neurophysiol.* **2018**, *129*, 1720–1747. [CrossRef]
23. Cohen, M.X. The Future of Cognitive Electrophysiology (Chp. 38). In *Analyzing Neural Time Series Data: Theory and Practice*; Cohen, M.X., Ed.; The MIT Press: Cambridge, MA, USA; London, UK, 2014.
24. Michel, C.M.; Koenig, T.; Brandeis, D.; Gianotti, L.R.R.; Wackermann, J. (Eds.) *Electrical Neuroimaging*; Cambridge University Press (Medicine): Cambridge, UK, 2009.
25. Nidal, K.; Jatoi, M.A. *Brain Source Localization Using EEG Signal Analysis*; CRC Press (Taylor & Francis): London, UK, 2017.
26. Cavanagh, J.F. Electrophysiology as a theoretical and methodological hub for the neural sciences. *Psychophysiology* **2019**, *56*, e13314. [CrossRef]
27. Scherg, M.; Picton, T.W. Separation and identification of event-related potential components brain electric source analysis. In *Event-Related Brain Research*; EEG and Clin. Neurophysiol (Suppl. 42); Brunia, C.H.M., Mulder, G., Verbaten, M.N., Eds.; Elsevier: Amsterdam, The Netherlands; London, UK; New York, NY, USA; Tokyo, Japan, 1991; pp. 24–37.
28. Pasqual-Marqui, R.D.; Michel, C.M.; Lehmann, D. Low resolution electromagnetic tomography: A new method for localizing electrical activity in the brain. *J. Psychophysiol.* **1994**, *18*, 49–65. [CrossRef]
29. Palmero-Soler, E.; Dolan, K.; Hadamschek, V.; Tass, P.A. swLORETA: A novel approach to robust source localization and synchronization tomography. *Phys. Med. Biol.* **2007**, *52*, 1783–1800.
30. Zanow, F.; Knösche, T.R. ASA-Advanced Source Analysis of Continuous and Event-Related EEG/MEG Signals. *Brain Top* **2004**, *16*, 287. [CrossRef] [PubMed]
31. Horwitz, B.; Poeppel, D. How can EEG/MEG and fMRI/PET data be combined? *Hum. Brain Mapp.* **2002**, *17*, 1–3. [CrossRef] [PubMed]
32. Vitacco, D.; Brandeis, D.; Pascual-Marqui, R.; Martin, E. Correspondence of event-related potential tomography and functional magnetic resonance imaging during language processing. *Hum. Brain Mapp.* **2002**, *17*, 4–12. [CrossRef] [PubMed]
33. Verleger, R. Event-related potential research in neurological patients. In *The Cognitive Electrophysiology of Mind and Brain*; Zani, A., Proverbio, A.M., Eds.; Academic Press: Amsterdam, The Netherlands; London, UK; New York, NY, USA, 2003; pp. 309–341.
34. McLoughlin, G.; Makeig, S.; Tsuang, M.T. In search of biomarkers in psychiatry: EEG-based measures of brain function. *Am. J. Med. Genet. B Neuropsychiatr. Genet.* **2014**, *165B*, 111–121. [CrossRef] [PubMed]
35. Newson, J.J.; Thiagarajan, T.C. EEG frequency bands in psychiatric disorders: A review of resting state studies. *Front. Hum. Neurosci.* **2019**, *12*, 521. [CrossRef]
36. Proverbio, A.M.; Zani, A.; Gazzaniga, M.S.; Mangun, G.R. ERP and RT signs of a rightward bias for spatial orienting in a split-brain patient. *NeuroReport* **1994**, *5*, 2457–2461. [CrossRef]
37. Proverbio, A.M.; Zani, A. Interhemispheric transfer of visuomotor inputs in a split-brain patient: Electrophysiological and behavioral indexes. In *The Parallel Brain. The Cognitive Neuroscience of the Corpus Callosum*; Zaidel, E., Iacoboni, M., Eds.; The MIT Press: Cambridge, MA, USA; London, UK, 2003; pp. 296–300.
38. Goff, W.R.; Allison, T. The functional neuroanatomy of event related potentials. In *Event-Related Brain Potentials in Man*; Callaway, E., Tueting, P., Koslow, S.H., Eds.; Academic Press: New York, NY, USA; San Francisco, CA, USA; London, UK, 1979; pp. 1–91.
39. Zani, A. Mind and Brain in developmental and educational processes. In *Mind, Learning and Knowledge in Educational Contexts. Research Perspectives in Bioeducational Sciences*; Frauenfelder, E., Santoianni, F., Eds.; Cambridge Scholars Press: Cambridge, UK, 2003; pp. 48–67.

40. Zani, A.; Proverbio, A.M. The timing of attentional modulation of visual processing as indexed by ERPs. In *Neurobiology of Attention*; Itti, L., Rees, G., Tsotsos, J., Eds.; Academic Press: San Diego, CA, USA, 2005; pp. 496–501.
41. Proverbio, A.M.; Zani, A. Developmental changes in the linguistic brain after puberty (Invited Research Focus paper). *Trends Cogn. Sci.* **2005**, *9*, 164–167. [CrossRef]
42. Zani, A.; Tumminelli, C.; Proverbio, A.M. Electroencephalogram (EEG) Alpha Power as a Marker of Visuospatial Attention Orienting and Suppression in Normoxia and Hypoxia. An Exploratory Study. *Brain Sci.* **2020**, *10*, 140. [CrossRef]
43. Tognoli, E. More than Meets the Mind's Eye? Preliminary Observations Hint at Heterogeneous Alpha Neuromarkers for Visual Attention. *Brain Sci.* **2019**, *9*, 307. [CrossRef]
44. de'Sperati, C. Cortical Resonance to Visible and Invisible Visual Rhythms. *Brain Sci.* **2020**, *10*, 37. [CrossRef]
45. Kapanci, T.; Merks, S.; Rammsayer, T.H.; Troche, S.J. On the Relationship between P3 Latency and Mental Ability as a Function of Increasing Demands in a Selective Attention Task. *Brain Sci.* **2019**, *9*, 28. [CrossRef] [PubMed]
46. Verleger, R.; Śmigasiewicz, K.; Michael, L.; Heikaus, L.; Niedeggen, M. Get Set or Get Distracted? Disentangling Content-Priming and Attention-Catching Effects of Background Lure Stimuli on Identifying Targets in Two Simultaneously Presented Series. *Brain Sci.* **2019**, *9*, 365. [CrossRef] [PubMed]
47. Jaquerod, M.E.; Mesrobian, S.K.; Villa, A.E.P.; Bader, M.; Lintas, A. Early Attentional Modulation by Working Memory Training in Young Adult ADHD Patients during a Risky Decision-Making Task. *Brain Sci.* **2020**, *10*, 38. [CrossRef] [PubMed]
48. Liu, Y.; Hanna, G.L.; Hanna, B.S.; Rough, H.E.; Arnold, P.D.; Gehring, W.J. Behavioral and Electrophysiological Correlates of Performance Monitoring and Development in Children and Adolescents with Attention-Deficit/Hyperactivity Disorder. *Brain Sci.* **2020**, *10*, 79. [CrossRef]
49. Bolduc-Teasdale, J.; Jolicoeur, P.; McKerral, M. Electrophysiological Markers of Visuospatial Attention Recovery after Mild Traumatic Brain Injury. *Brain Sci.* **2019**, *9*, 343. [CrossRef]
50. D'Angiulli, A.; Pham, D.A.T.; Leisman, G.; Goldfield, G. Evaluating Preschool Visual Attentional Selective-Set: Preliminary ERP Modeling and Simulation of Target Enhancement Homology. *Brain Sci.* **2020**, *10*, 124. [CrossRef]
51. Orlandi, A.; Proverbio, A.M. Left-Hemispheric Asymmetry for Object-Based Attention: An ERP Study. *Brain Sci.* **2019**, *9*, 315. [CrossRef]
52. Morgan, K.K.; Zeithamova, D.; Luu, P.; Tucker, D. Spatiotemporal Dynamics of Multiple Memory Systems During Category Learning. *Brain Sci.* **2020**, *10*, 224. [CrossRef]

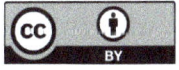

© 2020 by the author. Licensee MDPI, Basel, Switzerland. This article is an open access article distributed under the terms and conditions of the Creative Commons Attribution (CC BY) license (http://creativecommons.org/licenses/by/4.0/).

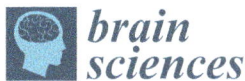

Article

Electroencephalogram (EEG) Alpha Power as a Marker of Visuospatial Attention Orienting and Suppression in Normoxia and Hypoxia. An Exploratory Study

Alberto Zani [1,2,*], Clara Tumminelli [3] and Alice Mado Proverbio [3]

[1] School of Psychology, Vita e Salute San Raffaele University, 20132 Milan, Italy
[2] Institute of Molecular Bioimaging and Physiology (IBFM), National Research Council (CNR), 20090 Milan, Italy
[3] Dept. of Psychology, University of Milano-Bicocca, 20126 Milan, Italy; c.tumminelli@campus.unimib.it (C.T.); mado.proverbio@unimib.it (A.M.P.)
* Correspondence: zani.alberto@hsr.it

Received: 23 January 2020; Accepted: 27 February 2020; Published: 2 March 2020

Abstract: While electroencephalogram (EEG) alpha desynchronization has been related to anticipatory orienting of visuospatial attention, an increase in alpha power has been associated to its inhibition. A separate line of findings indicated that alpha is affected by a deficient oxygenation of the brain or hypoxia, although leaving unclear whether the latter increases or decreases alpha synchronization. Here, we carried out an exploratory study on these issues by monitoring attention alerting, orienting, and control networks functionality by means of EEG recorded both in normoxia and hypoxia in college students engaged in four attentional cue-target conditions induced by a redesigned Attention Network Test. Alpha power was computed through Fast Fourier Transform. Regardless of brain oxygenation condition, alpha desynchronization was the highest during exogenous, uncued orienting of spatial attention, the lowest during alerting but spatially unpredictable, cued exogenous orienting of attention, and of intermediate level during validly cued endogenous orienting of attention, no matter the motor response workload demanded by the latter, especially over the left hemisphere. Hypoxia induced an increase in alpha power over the right-sided occipital and parietal scalp areas independent of attention cueing and conflict conditions. All in all, these findings prove that attention orienting is undergirded by alpha desynchronization and that alpha right-sided synchronization in hypoxia might sub-serve either the effort to sustain attention over time or an overall suppression of attention networks functionality.

Keywords: EEG; FFT; alpha desynchronization; attention orienting; alerting; attention inhibition; neurocognitive perceptual and motor workload; hypoxia; overt motor responses; hemispheric lateralization

1. Introduction

The human brain continuously receives sensory and cognitive inputs, including even unimportant and unnecessary information for thriving and survival. Therefore, our attentional system must carry out a selection of the most relevant information to be thoroughly processed. Two different neural systems are involved in carrying out this selective function: An endogenous or voluntary system and an exogenous or automatic system [1,2]. Both hemodynamic and event-related potential (ERP) source neuroimaging studies identified in the frontal and in the temporo-parietal lobes the visual-spatial attentional endogenous and exogenous control areas [3,4], respectively. Corbetta and Shulman [3] and Shulman et al. [5] identified the endogenous attention system in the dorsal frontal-parietal areas.

Indeed, both processes would primarily engage higher-level cortical circuits including, for endogenous orienting, frontal, parietal and temporal regions, and particularly the frontal eye fields (FEF) and the intraparietal sulcus (IPS) [6,7], and, for exogenous orienting, the right temporo-parietal junction (TPJ) [5,8]. Interestingly, the left frontal areas were more active than the parietal areas, but only during endogenous attention. In alerting tasks, endogenous and exogenous attention interact, and there is an increase both in global perceptual sensitivity and in the perception of exogenous spatial cues. Recently, Han and coworkers [9] showed that anterior insula (AI) is the key structure in endogenously reorienting of attention after reflexive attention is captured by a salient distractor. In tasks in which the participants know that a target will appear after a cue, brain responses will be optimized, and endogenous attention will be deployed [10]. There is an increased activation of the dorsal system when a stimulus appears at the same point in space of the cue. Top-down signals originate in the dorsal system and modulate sensory areas activity, detecting the current position of the presented stimuli [11]. Stimuli presented outside the attentional focus automatically catch attention and activate exogenous attention control in consequence of which ventral parietal areas and frontal cortex are activated. These stimuli activate the right-sided TPJ and the left-sided inferior frontal gyrus (IFG) [5]. Compared to exogenous spatial cues, vigilance tasks induce changes in endogenous and exogenous attention interactions and perceptual sensitivity. The sensitivity is reduced when stimulus onset is predicted, because an exogenous cue and the prediction time prepare participants to take over next stimulus [9]. Neurocognitive attentional processes related to the environmental input generate brain waves and electrical potentials with specific frequencies and amplitudes. In attentional processes, alpha band frequency, ranging between 7–14 Hz, plays a dominant role. Alpha electroencephalogram (EEG) activity is renown, like a typical response of the brain during relaxed wakefulness, for example, when the eyes are closed and/or attention is not heeded to any incoming information. Overall, this EEG frequency band has an occipito-parietal scalp distribution. It has been proposed that alpha oscillations provide pulsed inhibition for gamma activity and thereby dynamically route cortical information flow [12]. Kelly and colleagues [13,14] showed that alpha band activity was synchronized during visual selective or sustained attention tasks based on the presentation of visuospatial cues. The increase of this activity showed to be related to the inhibition of active processing of irrelevant and unexpected stimuli and contributed to the sustaining of top-down attentional control. Magnetoencephalography (MEG) studies (e.g., [15]) on visual attention perception also showed a pre-stimulus alpha activity. Most interestingly, a synchronization of alpha power in the parietal-occipital sulcus showed to be related to a functional modulation of information discrimination ability as undergirded by an overall inhibition of both the posterior occipital areas and the dorsal visual stream. This inhibition blocked out irrelevant information and avoided interference in working memory. Additionally, Foxe et al. [16] used an endogenous cueing task and found a different modulation of alpha rhythm at parietal-occipital areas. Furthermore, they also found that an alpha band desynchronization—or decrease—related to target information active processing possibly reflected a preparatory process [17], and that, during the valid visuospatial cueing task, an asymmetric, contralateral alpha deactivation in visual areas optimized orienting of visuospatial attention [18]. When a cue appeared prior of a target and the task required a greater attentional effort, Foxe and coauthors [16] also showed that alpha activity inhibited part of the visual space field in which interfering flankers were presented. Interestingly, alpha could be localized to the occipital-parietal areas of both hemispheres, and was active before the presentation of a stimulus, as if it had a role in the attentional preparatory mechanisms [18]. Indeed, while occipital-parietal areas integrate cue-related sensory information from multiple sensory modalities for programing the next engagement of visual attention, the inferior parietal cortex (IPC) would take care of maintaining attention orienting.

Experimental evidences have been provided showing task-related changes both in alpha power and scalp hemispheric lateralization or dominance. Indeed, a decrease in alpha power (i.e., alpha desynchronization) was found at occipital-parietal areas in attention orienting tasks, while an increase in this index was found during sustaining of attention [19]. Moreover, Li et al. [20] also found that task difficulty and visual stimulus handling could change alpha band amplitudes in different ways and at different points in time during endogenous processing. The participants to the study had to decide whether an object was a car or a face; alpha activity showed a higher amplitude at the right-sided occipital-parietal regions when the decisional task was more difficult. Volberg et al. [21] studied changes in alpha oscillatory activity in tasks of visual attention globally or locally directed by a cue. In this experiment, the subjects were prompted with a sound associated to the appearance of the target at a certain point of the screen, and with different sounds associated to the presence of the stimulus at any point of the screen. They saw that, in a task demanding a certain speed of response and in which the target was presented at a certain point of the screen, the right occipital-parietal area was activated for processing of global information, and, consequently, the left homologous region had a greater presence of alpha band, being inhibited. Conversely, the left hemisphere became more active in response to a target stimulus fallen at a specific location and the processing of its features at local level, so that the right hemisphere was in this case inhibited. Interestingly, alpha band was prevalent before the presentation of the stimulus, as if it had a role in the attention preparatory mechanisms. Alpha rhythm power measured at frontal-parietal areas during top-down processing was functionally interpreted as if the brain dealt with participants' expectations towards the task. Most interestingly, alpha modulation in the posterior scalp areas is governed by the anterior, prefrontal areas, which have an important role in attentional selection: this might be a neural signature of executive control, in relation to which prefrontal and posterior occipital-parietal areas form an attention-related network. Wavelet-based EEG studies have also found an interaction between top-down and bottom-up processing hinting at the view that alpha activity preceding a stimulus would reflect a top-down preparatory mechanism modulating both the response timing and the performance in an attentional task [22].

In selective attention, alpha rhythm is higher on parietal-occipital sites. Furthermore, it has been proved that prefrontal cortex rules alpha power in posterior area during top-down processing. Wavelet Analysis studies also measured EEG oscillation bands in terms of spatio-temporal frequency. A desynchronization of alpha oscillations was related to a perceptual difficulty in identifying a visual target in a discrimination task (target/mask). Larger pre-stimulus desynchronizations showed to be closely related to a better performance and to anticipatory attention [23].

As far as brain frequency-specific oscillatory activity in relation to cognitive functions is concerned, it is an acknowledged assumption that alpha power is affected by its oxygen supply. Indeed, from an inadequate blood oxygen delivery to the brain, it may in fact derive hypoxia, which is a common feature in many clinical disorders, including severe anemia, respiratory diseases (e.g., serious asthma and sleep apnea), and ischemic brain lesions, with or without a coma. This condition often also occurs in healthy individuals faced with extreme operational environments, such as high-altitude (HA) and/or low air pressure milieus (e.g., acknowledged alpinists and climbers as well as HA natives), often in relation with very low temperatures.

Altered EEG recordings, considered by clinicians as indicators of cerebral metabolism and useful tools for evaluating hypoxia severity—i.e., hypoxia with or without ischemia—in individuals affected by such a condition (e.g., [24–26]), have generally been reported in many electrophysiological studies based on different types of both acute and chronic hypoxia. In human EEG studies of transient hypoxia, for instance, the latter was induced by low oxygen gas mixtures or hypoxic normobaric hypoxia (e.g., [27]), by simulated HA in hypobaric pressurized chambers (e.g., [28–31]), during rapid ascent to HA and lowland reoxygenation (e.g., [32–34]), and in HA natives [35]. Overall, a slowing activity of EEG in hypoxia with respect to normoxia has been generally advanced by all these studies.

As for the specific effects of acute hypoxia—regardless of the method of its induction—on spectral power density in the alpha frequency band, somehow inconsistent findings can be found in the literature. For example, 19 min of hypobaric hypoxia resulted in a significant decrease of alpha power (i.e., 8.9–11.8 Hz) in the spontaneous EEG of healthy volunteers as measured at the P_4-O_2 bipolar derivation [28]. Schellart and Reits [27] found that alpha content of brain spontaneous EEG during systemic hypoxia was strongly affected by the "eyes open/closed" volunteers' condition. In contrast to the eyes closed condition, a transient increase of alpha synchronization occurred during the eyes-open condition. An alpha (i.e., 10–11 Hz) spectral power selective desynchronization at a reduced air pressure of 3000 m, and a meaningful gradual desynchronization of this frequency with increasing altitude to 4000, 5000, and 6000 m, respectively, was found in the posterior scalp areas by Ozaki et al. [29], in volunteers who did not perform any active task during EEG recordings. Conversely, Papadelis and coauthors [30] showed an absolute significant increase of alpha power during acute hypoxia as induced by decreasing the pressure of a barometric chamber, compared to 100% oxygen condition, in right-handed volunteers who performed a simple computerized flight-simulation task in which participants had to keep a continuously moving aircraft-target as much closer to the center of a personal computer (PC) screen denoted by a rectangle, in order to avoid the drifting of the target towards the edges of the screen if no control was applied [30]. Additionally, a significant increase of alpha synchronization at posterior scalp sites after an HA chronic acclimatization of 30 days, but not after a sojourn of seven days only, with respect to previous HA EEG baseline, together with a cogent desynchronization after re-descending to lowland, have instead been described by Zhao and coworkers [34], in the spontaneous EEG of a group of young soldiers who did not perform any tasks during the recording sessions.

Inasmuch, both alpha oscillatory synchronization or desynchronization have been associated with attention, attention-orienting inhibition, long-range synchronization, memory performance, and inhibition of interfering visual memories (e.g., [36,37]); these inconsistencies represent a nuisance for a more specific definition of both the functional significance of this EEG oscillatory activity in relation to attentional functions and, most importantly, of their possible alterations with hypoxia.

However, because attention is not a unitary function, it is important to relate EEG alpha oscillatory activity to the three specialized networks sub-serving the human attentional system as originally conceptualized by Posner and Petersen [38]. After the reviewing of many neuroanatomical and neuropsychological studies, in fact, Posner's group [39], advanced the view that human attention system is undergirded by three different networks regulating different sub-processes, which is, alerting, orienting, and executive control. The alerting system would take care of achieving and maintaining an alert state; it would be focalized in frontal and parietal regions of the right hemisphere (RH). The orienting system, driving attentional focus on a specific point of space, would be localized in the frontal-parietal areas. Executive control, allowing to solve conflicting cognitive situations and psychomotor responses, would be associated with medial frontal regions and lateral prefrontal cortex.

To analyze the functional activation and interdependence/independence of these networks, Fan et al. [40] devised a so called Attention Network Test (ANT) based on the presentation of four different cueing conditions, that is, NC (no cue), CC (central cue), 2C (two vertically lateralized spatial cues at the same time above and below the fixation point), and LC (one vertically lateralized spatial cue above or below the fixation point). Each of these cueing conditions was randomly followed by directionally congruent and incongruent strings of five arrows, of which the central one, which might point either toward the left or to the right, posed as a target, and the peripheral ones as low-level (congruent condition) or high-level interfering (incongruent condition) flankers. A third target condition made up of a central arrow-target pointing either leftward or rightward surrounded by four simple straight-lines was originally included. Due to some inessential experimental findings and to the theoretical interpretation of the latter in several behavioral studies, Posner's group later hemodynamic (i.e., functional magnetic resonance imaging (fMRI) [41]) and electrophysiological imaging (i.e., EEG [42]) studies omitted the 2C cue type and the target-arrow-surrounded by straight-line flankers condition, and used three cueing types, namely the NC, CC, and LC conditions, and two target-arrow vs. flanker-arrows conditions only.

1.1. ANT and Functional Meaning of its Cueing Conditions

The ANT has shown to be a useful and simple measure of attentional efficiency so that it can be used with adults, children, monkeys and patients with various abnormalities of attention [40]. As the cueing conditions are concerned, both neutral (CC) and valid spatial cues (LC) serve as a form of alerting cue, but only the latter provides always valid, predictive spatial information that allows participants to begin orienting attention to the appropriate location before the target is presented. Conversely, the central cue (CC) tends to keep reflexive attention focused on one location, which is the central location at the fixation cross, before the target exogenously attract orienting of attention at its appearance location. Unlike for these cueing conditions, under NC, there are neither alerting nor spatial cues and participants see only the fixation cross and the sequence of randomly presented targets above or below it. According to Fan et al. [40], the NC condition is a relatively low-alertness tonic orienting condition in which attention tends to remain diffused across the two potential target locations.

Since the three sources of attention, alerting, orienting, and executive attention appear to engage separate brain mechanisms, Fan et al. [40] investigated the independence and/or interaction of these networks and concluded that the latter were relatively independent mechanisms. Indeed, while phasic alerting enhanced flanker interference costs, both LC and NC conditions reduced them. According to Fan et al. [40], this occurred, in the first case, because participants directed attention to the target ahead of time, and, in the second case, because the NC condition is a relatively low-alertness condition and resulted in longer RTs and relatively lower errors. Consistent behavioral and electrophysiological findings were more recently found by Zani and Proverbio [43], in that both RTs and mean latency measures of a so-called ERPs conflict negativity (CN) component showed a decreased flanker conflict interference for both NC and LC cueing conditions as compared to both CC and 2C conditions. Overall, these findings support the view that, far from being independent from each other, the attentional system networks somehow directly interact one another.

1.2. Rationale for the Present Study

Purpose of the present study was to identify the most prominent features of EEG alpha power in the classification of attention modes and response control as related to the ANT neural networks with the hope of providing alpha-based reliable markers of their functionality. Moreover, we wanted to assess the possible impact of respiratory hypoxia on these three attention networks because not yet investigated and renown up to now. More specifically, we wanted to tap possible differences in this impact between conditions of lower or greater motor and cognitive workload. To achieve these aims we used the afore-mentioned ANT-SR (ANT-Slightly Redesigned) version and measured the decrease and/or increase of alpha power synchronization as a function of the possibly independent and/or partly interdependent activation of the three attention networks. We wondered whether hypoxia would have affected the three attentional networks independently from one another or in interaction.

Considered that ANT paradigm is an extremely simple task so that "The instructions to the subjects only require they know how to press a left key for a leftward-pointing arrow and a right key for a rightward-pointing arrow [40]", we slightly redesigned it with the goal to carry out a behavioral and electrophysiological study aimed to find possible differences in the effects of hypoxia on a simple with respect to a difficult, psycho-motor overloaded attention orienting task. In details, we devised one cue-target condition in which a valid, spatially informative local cue preceded the delivery of one out of two different types of arrow-strings which had to be discriminated to provide a dual motor-choice overt response with the index or medium fingers of the left or right hand, depending on the type and direction of the arrowhead, no matter the congruency of the flankers. In this difficult motor variant, defined by us "LCmot", the participants had to use one out of four fingers to give their response. The goal was to investigate the mechanisms of visuospatial attention, and, more specifically, of attentional conflict control situations during the execution of a relatively difficult motor task. In order to compare the effects of hypoxia on this condition with those possibly occurring in a simple orienting of attention condition, besides on alerting and executive conditions, we added to our ANT-SR the no Cue (NC), the Central Cue (CC), and the Local Cue (LC) conditions used in the original version of the ANT paradigm by Fan and colleagues [40], and in Fan's et al. [41,42] later studies. However, to make the four cue conditions comparable from the stimulus-information point of view, the two types of arrows were also presented in the three afore-mentioned conditions despite the fact that the volunteers had not to discriminate between their types and gave an overt motor response using alternatively only the index fingers of the two hands depending on the target arrowhead orientation.

The ANT-SR [40] was used to investigate the effects of hypoxia on endogenous and exogenous visuospatial attention orienting modes. Capitalizing on the different set of alerting and attention-orienting cue-target conditions of the redesigned ANT-SR test [40,44], and assuming that an increase of alpha synchronization represented an inhibition of attention orienting, we hypothesized that:

1. an increase in alpha power would have been found for the spatially uninformative CC condition as compared to both the LC and NC conditions;
2. the addition of a perceptual and motor-choice workload (as in the LCmot condition) would have adversely affected overt motor responses and brain attention orienting capacity as reflected by an increase of alpha oscillations;
3. alpha power would have been affected differently by exogenous and endogenous attention orienting modes over the two hemispheres;
4. hypoxia would have resulted in a general increase in alpha power in both exogenous and endogenous attention orienting modes.

2. Materials and Methods

2.1. Study Compliance with Ethical Standards and Participants

The study was approved by the ethics committee of the Italian National Research Council (CNR) and was conducted in the Electro-Functional Brain Imaging unit (EFBIu) of the CNR-IBFM Institute in accordance with American Psychological Association (APA) ethical standards for the treatment of human experimental participants (APA, Monitor Staff, 2003, vol. 34, n. 1). Furthermore, the experiments were conducted with the understanding and the written consent of each participant in compliance with the indications of the 2018 Declaration of Helsinki ethical principles for medical research involving human subjects by the World Medical Association (WMA Declaration of Helsinki, 9 July, 2018, PDF file).

Ten (10) healthy volunteers (4 females and 6 males), with age ranging from 19 to 27 years (Mean = 24, SD = 2.7) were selected for participating in randomized order in two EEG recording sessions during which they breathed either ambient air (also indicated as "normoxia") or a 12.5% O_2-impoverished air mixture (also indicated as "hypoxia"). Besides suffering or having suffered of any neurological and psychological syndromes or the intake of any psychopharmacological substances, criteria of exclusion from the study were cigarettes smoking, arterial hypertension, and cardiovascular or respiratory diseases. In addition, to minimize confounding effects, no participant had to have sojourned at a higher altitude than 300–400 m in the 4 weeks preceding the study nor had to have been regularly and intensively engaged in any physical training program. Again, volunteers were required to refrain from any strenuous physical activity and from unlimited consumption of alcohol, caffeine, and theophylline containing beverages in the 24 h prior to the experimental sessions of the study. All selected participants had normal or corrected-to-normal vision and right-eye as well as right-hand dominance and none of them had any left-handed relatives as assessed by the Edinburgh Inventory. Unfortunately, the data of two volunteers had to be excluded from the statistical analyses either because of excessive eye—and body—movement artifacts during EEG recordings or for not completing the two recording sessions cycle.

Sample Size Limit

The small size of the sample here used introduced a risk of underpowered statistical computations in the study. However, we kept this risk under thorough control estimating the effect size for the statistically significant factors by means of partial eta squared values, i.e., η_p^2. Additionally, the alpha inflation due to multiple comparisons was also controlled by means of Greenhouse–Geisser epsilon (ε) correction.

2.2. Stimulus Materials and Experimental Conditions

Stimulus materials consisted of strings of five (5) contiguous arrows, serving as targets. Arrows were of two types: so-called "standard" and "star" arrows. While the former had a tip with a vertically linear rear side, the latter showed a slightly inward-bound and oblique rear-side at the starting of their shaft (see Figure 1a). The central arrow of each string consisted of the true target while the flanking two arrows on each side of the latter posed as potential distracters. Overall, each target-and-flankers-string subtended 8.7 degrees of visual angle along the horizontal meridian and 1.3 degrees along the vertical meridian. Regardless of the arrow-type, the tip of the central target arrow could point to the left or to the right side, whereas the flanking arrows could point toward the same (Congruent flankers) or the opposite direction (Incongruent flankers) as the target. All in all, then, there were eight (8) different target strings combinations (see Figure 1b for examples of the latter).

Prior the presentation of arrow-strings, stimulation also included the administration or the omission of white asterisks in different points in space of the stimulation PC monitor so to produce four different cue-target conditions. All these stimulus materials were presented on the blackened background of a 17"- cathode-ray tube (CRT) screen in front of the volunteers. The luminance of both the asterisk-cue and the two types of target-arrow-strings were measured in candela/m^2. The luminance of the asterisk amounted to 7.3 candela/m^2. Conversely, the luminance assessments for the standard-arrow- and star-arrow-strings were 27.81 and 26.96 candela/m^2, respectively, and were matched across arrow-pointing directions and target-flankers congruency.

Depending on the cue presentation positions (above or below the fixation cross (FC) or centered over it) or omission, as well as to target-related motor tasks to be performed, four (4) different attention alerting or valid spatial attention orienting sets were induced in the participants (Figure 1c). More in details, the latter had to deal with: (1) the sequential presentation at random of vertically eccentric (above or below the FC) target strings without being preceded by any cue aimed at eliciting a possibly tonic and unspecific alerting or sustained attention condition over time (No Cue, NC) as well as a target-related exogenous spatial orienting of attention to the point in space where the arrow-strings were contingently presented from trial-to-trial; (2) the presentation of a cue overimposed on the FC aimed at eliciting a phasic attention alerting but not an attention orienting response followed by the presentation of a target string above or below the FC so to elicit a target-related exogenous spatial orienting of attention to the point in space where the target-string was delivered (Central cue, CC); (3) the presentation of a vertically eccentric (above or below the FC) cue aimed at eliciting both a cue-related phasic attention alerting and an exogenous orienting of attention to the point in space indicated by the cue, later on followed by a further endogenous orienting onto the target at that same point because the focus of attention was already centered there (Local or Spatial cue condition, LC).

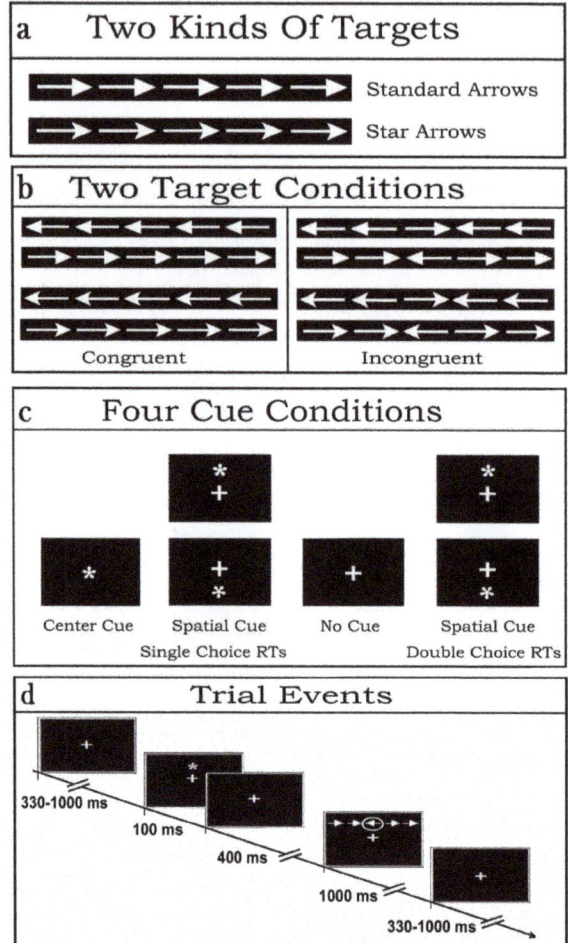

Figure 1. Graphical depiction of the stimulus materials, of cue-target conditions, and of trial events used in the present study (ANT-SR (Attention Network Test-Slightly Redesigned); modified and redrawn from Fan et al. [40] and Posner [44]). (**a**) Two kinds of white arrow-target strings were presented: "standard" and "star" arrows. (**b**) Congruent and incongruent central targets vs. flanker strings were presented. Based on the direction of the arrow tip (left or right), eight target-flanker conditions resulted. (**c**) Four different cue-target and motor-task experimental conditions were administered in randomized order: a no cue (NC) condition; a center, alerting but spatially unpredictable cue (Central Cue, CC), and a valid spatially informative cue (Local Cue, LC). In these three conditions, participants' motor response to targets depended on a single-choice reaction time (RT) button-press. In a fourth cueing condition, LCmot, volunteers had to discriminate both the target-arrow type and orientation in order to make a double-choice RTs button-press. (**d**) Schematic exemplification of cue–target stimulus-events and inter-stimulus interval (ISI) duration during a single trial of the LC condition as well as of the random inter-trial interval (ITI) length. See text for further details.

For each of these three cueing conditions of the original ANT, on each trial the participants had to discriminate the direction towards which the central target-arrow-tip of the five-arrows-string pointed, independent of the arrow type presented (i.e., standard or star arrow), and of the direction of the flanking-arrows (Congruent and Incongruent), and to perform a single-choice-RTs button-press with the index finger of the corresponding hand (right or left). Participants had also to deal with a fourth, newly introduced, cueing condition of the ANT-SR, defined LCmot. The latter was like LC but demanded a double-choice-RTs button-press according to the target-arrow type presented. Indeed, during the LCmot condition participants had to discriminate the type of target-arrows (i.e., standard- or star-target-arrow), besides the direction to which the latter were pointing to, in order to perform a double-choice button-press with the index or middle fingers, respectively, of the corresponding hand (right or left, respectively; See Figure 1b,c again).

No matter the cue-target condition considered, on each trial the cue was presented for 100 ms followed after 400 ms by the delivery of an arrows-string, which remained on the screen for 1000 ms before its offset in order to avoid any possibly baffling stimulus-offset, besides stimulus-onset, related ERP recordings. Inter-trial interval (ITI) randomly varied between 330 and 1000 ms (Figure 1d).

2.3. Procedure

The selected participants took part in randomized order in two 4 h lasting EEG recording sessions, one week apart from each other. During these two experimental sessions they breathed either ambient air (or normoxia) or a 12.5% O_2-impoverished air mixture (simulating respiration conditions at an high altitude of ~4200 m (~13,780 feet) at sea level), which may be assimilated to an acute bout of tolerable and far from pathogenic normobaric hypoxia while performing in four different cue-target visuo-spatial attention conditions taken and readapted from Fan's et al. [40] and Posner's [44] ANT.

Independent of the respiratory session with which the volunteers started their participation in the study, while being prepared for the EEG recording during their first report to the lab, they underwent a general psychophysiological screening that included the chronicling of their chronobiological daily habitual activity patterns (Morningness Eveningness Questionnaire—MEQ [45]). In addition, we also measured their subjective mood and alert levels by means of so-called paper-and-pencil psychophysiological Likert-like scales and three minutes speeded-up letter-cancellation tasks. As for the hypoxia session, just starting from their arrival to the laboratory the volunteers breathed a normobaric hypoxic mixture obtained removing a controlled amount of oxygen from air (i.e., 12.5% O_2) by means of a MAG-10 hypoxicator apparatus (Higher Peak LLC, Winchester, MA, USA). The mixture was delivered through a facemask at 30 L/min. Excess air flow was diverted outside the mask to prevent inspired oxygen pressure from increasing above 90 Torr (see Figure 2 for a visual exemplification).

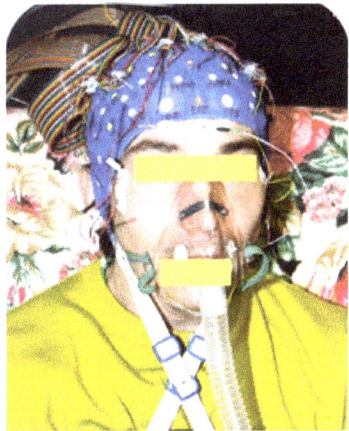

Figure 2. A picture of a participant wearing the mask connected to the hypoxicator apparatus which provided air impoverished of a 12.5% of oxygen during the electroencephalogram (EEG) recording session.

Since there are influential data in the physiological literature indicating that in humans the most relevant cardiorespiratory and blood plasmatic effects were found in between 2–4 h of serious hypoxic respiration (see, e.g., [46]), all our volunteers were systematically submitted to the EEG recording session starting after 2 h of such a respiratory condition, which was spent in the application and jellying of a 128 electrodes electrocap as well as in the filling of the mood and alert paper-and-pencil scales, besides in an alert letter-cancellation-based task. For experimental standardization and session comparison-sake, the volunteers started their tasks-related EEG recordings after 2 h during the normoxic session too, a span of time overall spent in the activities mentioned above besides the electrocap application.

At the end of the preparation time-span, participants were invited to take a seat in a comfortable easy chair with a high backrest within an electrically and magnetically shielded cubicle (Faraday cage) in front of a CRT screen with a small white fixation cross (FC) in the center of its black background placed at a distance of 114 cm (or 3.34 feet) from them. During the EEG recordings, sequences of the white arrow-strings were randomly presented above or below the fixation-cross at the center of the visual screen. The central target-arrow of each string fell just in correspondence of the fixation cross with a vertical eccentricity of ±1.25 degrees of visual angle from the latter. Apart for the NC condition, an asterisk-cue always preceded the arrow-strings in the CC, LC, and LC mot conditions.

To familiarize participants with the task to be performed in each cue-target condition, before recording was started volunteers read detailed written instructions and performed a practice run of 30 stimulus pairs. For each of the four cue-target condition, there were four separate blocks of trials, each containing 128 trials grouped in a differently randomized order and lasting approximately 3.5 min. To avoid any confounding and systematic interacting effects of practice, fatigue and hypoxia, we also randomized the order of administration of the respiratory conditions, of the cue-target conditions, of the type of target-arrows, of the falling of the target in the upper or lower visual field, and of blocks presentation across participants.

2.4. EEG Recording and Analysis

For EEG recordings we used scalp electrodes mounted in an ANT elastic Waveguard 128-electrodes electrocap. The electrodes were densely spaced all over the frontal, central, temporal, parietal, and occipital scalp-sites as proposed by the 5% system [47] devised for high-spatial resolution EEG/ERP recordings. Two electrodes placed below and above the right eye recorded vertical eye movements, whereas two further electrodes placed at the outer canthi of the eyes recorded horizontal eye movements. Linked ears served as the reference lead, whereas a frontal electrode served as a ground site. Electrode impedance was below 5 kΩ. Both EEG and electrooculogram (EOG) continuous signals were acquired using directional-current (DC) amplifiers and a digitization rate of 512 samples/s. Offline, automated rejection of electrical artifacts was performed before EEG averaging to discard epochs in which eye movements, blinks, or excessive body muscle potentials occurred. The artifact rejection criterion was a peak–to–peak amplitude exceeding ± 70 µV for EEG signal or ± 100 µV for EOG signal, and, in line with the trials stimulus events timing, went from 100 ms before the cue-type to 1500 ms after it for each trial in sequence, until the routine detected EEG values falling within the indicated window-values. Overall, the rejection rate was ~6.0 %. Although we used the indicated rejection method implemented in our EEG signals analysis applications package, we are aware that other independent component analyses would have quite efficiently worked [48,49]. Trials associated with missing (i.e., overt motor responses falling after 1000 ms from the target) were also discarded, which resulted in a rejection rate of less the 2%. Overall, then, a global 92% out of the 100% trials administered were accepted for averaging. Trials associated with motor-response errors (i.e., on the one hand, responses given with the wrong hand with respect to the left/right target-arrow pointing directions, no matter the arrow types, for the NC, CC, and LCmot conditions, and, on the other hand, the wrong finger with respect to the standard/star arrow types, besides with the wrong hand, for LCmot) were also computed separately as a function of respiratory conditions and discarded from EEG averaging. So, after rejection procedures and the due mean computations over the sample of participants, the mean percentages of correct trials averaged as a function of NC, CC, LC, and LCmot conditions in normoxia amounted to 98%, 99%, 99%, and 94% of the 100% of total trials administered, respectively, and to 98%, 95%, 94%, and 89%, respectively, in hypoxia. More specifically, in normoxia the percentages of congruent vs. incongruent trials averaged for the former congruency level of NC, CC, LC, and LCmot conditions were 50.41%, 49.79%, 50.69%, and 47.29% of the 100% total trials administered, respectively, and 48.35%, 48.83%, 49.15%, and 46.65%, respectively, for the latter congruency level. In hypoxia the percentages of congruent vs. incongruent trials averaged for the congruent target trials of the four cueing conditions were 49.90%, 48.61% 47.50%, and 45.54% of the 100% total trials administered, respectively, and 48.32%, 47.23%, 46.70%, and 43.42%, respectively, for the incongruent target trials.

Before selective averaging, accepted EEG signal chunks were digitally filtered with a half–amplitude band-pass of 0.016–70 Hz. As for the rejected epochs, accepted EEG epochs in the averages were synchronized with the onset of cue presentation (CC, LC, and LCmot conditions) or omission (NC condition) and went from 100 ms before the cue-type to 1500 ms after it, the target-related EEG being elicited 500 ms after cue-onset. In order to compare the averaged EEG epochs relative to the single-choice motor-workload conditions (i.e., NC, CC, and LC) with those generated in the double-choice motor-workload condition (LCmot), EEG responses to the different types of arrow-targets (i.e., standard and star arrows) were collapsed together in all cueing conditions. Furthermore, in order to increase the signal-to-noise ratio EEG trials related to targets delivered in the upper and lower visuospatial hemifields were also collapsed together in all cueing conditions.

Hence, for each subject distinct EEG average waveforms were obtained according to respiratory condition (i.e., ambient-air or hypoxia), cueing-task condition (CC, LC, NC, LCmot), and target-congruency (i.e., congruent, incongruent) condition. Besides average EEG waveforms for each single participant, grand-average EEG signals were also computed for the participants' sample.

2.5. Alpha Power Analysis

To obtain the alpha power as a function of the different experimental conditions, the Fast Fourier Transform (FFT; [50]) computation was used. The reference point for the FFT analysis or Start Time was the time of cue presentation, at 0 ms latency, while the End Time was the 1500 ms latency. The time span of the EEG waveforms was divided in three (i.e., 3) blocks, each with a length of 500 ms, with a sample count which had the power of two (i.e., 512 Hz). Alpha oscillations content and, more specifically, alpha amplitude in the range of 7.5–12.5 Hz was computed and averaged over the three blocks. To allow a better comparison of FFT results over experimental conditions, a normalization of the computed alpha power in the aforementioned band with respect to the summed power over all frequency values of the channels with the highest power was carried out, and, as a whole, reported in μV^2. Additionally, the baselines of the spectral analyses were corrected across conditions before FFT computation. These procedures were automatically applied to each site of the electrodes montage so to obtain a topographic distribution of the alpha power spectra over the scalp as a function of the experimental variables. Topographical voltage maps of alpha were obtained by plotting color-coded alpha power values derived by interpolating frequency content values between scalp electrodes as a function of respiratory and cueing conditions. Eye-balls inspection of the maps indicated that EEG alpha power reached higher amplitude values at posterior than anterior scalp regions regardless of respiratory and attention cueing conditions, and that the topographic distribution of alpha amplitude at posterior scalp regions changed as a function of experimental conditions considered. In order to test the statistical significance of these apparent data changes, taking into account previous EEG findings in the literature, alpha power amplitude was measured at four posteriorly-anteriorly distributed couples of homologous electrode sites: O_1 and O_2, mesial-occipital electrodes; PO_7 and PO_8, lateral parietal-occipital electrodes; TPP_{7h} and TPP_{8h}, temporo-parietal-parietal electrodes; and F_5 and F_6, pre-frontal lateralized electrodes.

3. Statistical Analyses

3.1. Statistical Analyses for Behavioral Data

Behavioral data, namely both motor response errors and speed (reaction times—RTs), underwent two separate 3-way repeated-measures ANOVAs whose factors of variability were: Respiratory conditions (2 levels: Air and Hypoxia), Cueing conditions (4 levels; NC, CC, LC and LCmot) and Target congruency (2 levels: Congruent, Incongruent). Before being submitted to the multifactorial repeated-measures ANOVA, error rate percentages were converted to arcsine values because percentage values do not exhibit homoscedasticity (e.g., [51], which is necessary for ANOVA. In fact, the distribution of percentages is binomial, whereas the arcsine transformation of the data makes the distribution normal [52].

3.2. Statistical Analyses for Electrophysiological Data

Alpha power measures were submitted to a five-way repeated–measures ANOVA with respiratory condition (R, 2 levels: Ambient-air and Hypoxia), attention cueing condition (AC, 4 levels: NC, CC, LC, and LCmot), arrows-target array congruency (C, 2 levels: Congruent and Incongruent), hemisphere (H, two levels: left hemisphere, LH, and right hemisphere, RH), and electrode (E, 4 levels; O_1–O_2, PO_7–PO_8, TPP_{7h}–TPP_{8h}, and F_5–F_6 electrode sites).

For both behavioral and electrophysiological data, the partial eta squared values (η_p^2) were systematically provided to estimate effect sizes [53,54]. Additionally, (ε) Greenhouse-Geisser correction was applied to compensate for possible violations of the sphericity assumption associated with factors which had more than two levels. The epsilon (ε) values and the corrected probability levels (in case of epsilon < 1) are reported. Post-hoc comparisons among means for significant factors with more than two levels were performed by means of Tukey HSD and/or Newman–Keuls tests.

4. Results

4.1. Behavioral Results

4.1.1. Error-Percentage Rates

The ANOVA carried out on motor response errors proved the significance of the main "respiratory condition" factor (F (1,7) = 7.276: $p < 0.025$)), indicating that in air participants showed a 2.51% of errors, while during hypoxia this rate increased on average to 6.12%. In addition, error percentage-rates for the various cueing conditions significantly changed as a function of the respiratory condition (F (2.63, 18.45) = 31.25; ε = 0.879; adjusted p value < 0.000024; η_p^2 = 0.61). Post-hoc comparisons indicated that, in air, error rates for NC were higher than for both CC ($p < 0.0001$) and LC ($p < 0.0001$), but lower than for LCmot ($p < 0.0002$). In turn, CC did not differ from LC, but it showed a lower errors rate than LCmot ($p < 0.0001$). Again, LC obtained a lower errors rate than LCmot ($p < 0.0001$; see Figure 3 for these findings.)

In hypoxia, instead, the post-hoc contrasts indicated that error percentage rates progressively and significantly increased from NC to LCmot cueing conditions: NC vs. CC, $p < 0.0002$; NC vs. LC, $p < 0.0001$; NC vs. LCmot, $p < 0.0001$, respectively. Moreover, CC was also different from LC ($p < 0.0002$) and from LCmot ($p < 0.00001$), and, in turn, LC was different from LCmot ($p < 0.0001$). Due to the aforementioned increases, with the exception of NC, the CC, LC and LCmot cueing conditions showed significantly higher error rates in hypoxia than in air (i.e., $p < 0.001$ for CC; $p < 0.0001$ for LC; $p < 0.000025$ for LCmot; see Figure 3 again).

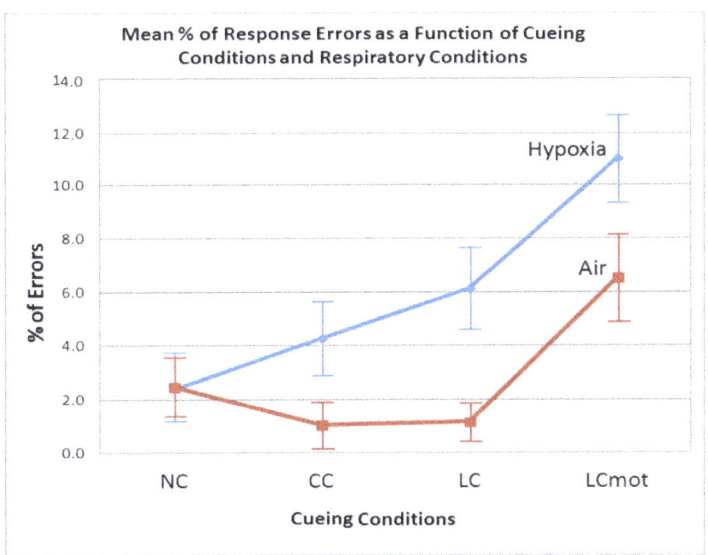

Figure 3. Mean percentages (along with standard errors (SE)) of errors committed by participants as a function of cueing condition and respiratory condition regardless of the target strings congruency.

4.1.2. Reaction Times (RTs)

The ANOVA carried out on mean RTs showed that the measures obtained for the two levels of the respiratory factor (i.e., Air: Mean = 458.60 ms, standard error (SE) = 13.68; Hypoxia: Mean = 474.21 ms, SE = 15.01) were significantly different (F (1,7) = 4.799; $\varepsilon = 1$; $p < 0.05$, $\eta_p^2 = 0.51$). The ANOVA also yielded significant effects of cue-type (F (2, 16; 15, 15) = 176.96; $\varepsilon = 0.72$; adjusted p value < 0.00001, $\eta_p^2 = 0.96$) and target flanker-type (F (1, 7) = 167.23; $p < 0.000004$) and a significant interaction between the two (F (2,58; 18,08) = 39.96; $\varepsilon = 0.86$; adjusted p value < 0.000002, $\eta_p^2 = 0.85$).

Post-hoc comparisons showed that, except for the LCmot cueing type, response times were much faster for all the other cueing conditions when target-strings were congruent than incongruent (i.e., NC ($p < 0.00002$), CC ($p < 0.0002$) and LC ($p < 0.0002$), respectively; see Figure 4). Post-hoc contrasts also indicated that RTs were slower for NC than for both CC (Cong: $p < 0.0002$; Incong: $p < 0.0002$) and LC (Cong: $p < 0.0002$; Incong: $p < 0.0002$), and in turn for CC than LC for both target flanker types (Cong: $p < 0.0002$; Incong: $p < 0.0002$). Further contrast analyses proved that LCmot obtained much slower RTs than the other three cueing conditions, namely NC, CC, and LC, for both target congruency conditions (Cong: LCmot vs. NC, $p < 0.0002$; LCmot vs. CC, $p < 0.0002$; LCmot vs LC, $p < 0.0002$; Incong: LCmot vs. NC, $p < 0002$; LCmot vs. CC, $p < 0.0002$; LCmot vs. LC, $p < 0.0002$; see Figure 4 again).

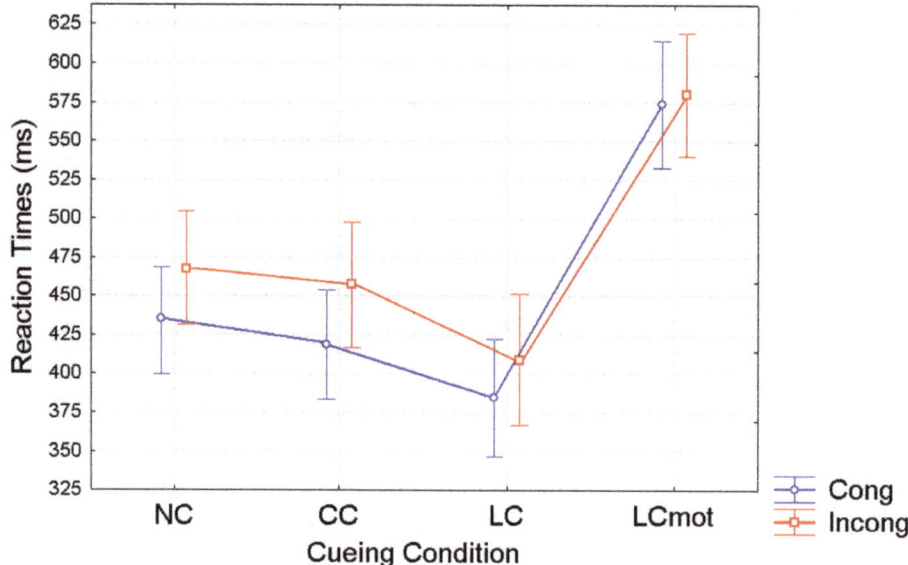

Figure 4. Mean RT and Standard Error (SE) values obtained as a function of the cueing condition and target congruency over the sample of participants. Note that RTs were measured starting from the target delivery time, that is 500 ms later than the cue omission or administration according to the cueing condition.

4.2. Electrophysiological Results

ANOVA showed the significant interaction of Cueing condition x Hemisphere ($F(2.17, 15.19) = 6.16$; $\varepsilon = 0.72$; adjusted p value < 0.00001). Effect size for this significant interaction was $\eta_p^2 = 0.47$. Post-hoc comparisons among means showed that alpha power was significantly stronger over the RH than LH for the LCmot condition only ($p < 0.000028$; for these effects see maps of Figure 5a–d as well as the mean and SE values drawn in Figure 6).

Further post-hoc contrasts between the alpha power values obtained for the different cueing conditions within the two hemispheres also indicated that alpha power was overall greater in the CC than NC condition over both hemispheres (i.e., $p < 0.00001$ for LH, and $p < 00001$ for RH, respectively). Alpha power was also greater in the LC than in the NC condition over both hemispheres. Conversely, alpha power was decreased in the LCmot compared to the CC condition ($p < 0.00001$ for LH, and $p < 0.0033$ for RH, respectively). Post-hoc tests also showed a difference between alpha power values for both the spatially informative conditions LC and LCmot over the LH ($p < 0.00001$), but not the RH. Again, alpha showed an enhanced power in the CC than in the LC condition over the LH ($p < 0.008$), but not the RH, despite an intriguing trend ($p < 0.062$).

The ANOVA also yielded a significant triple interaction of Respiratory condition, Hemisphere and Electrode factors ($F(1.74, 12.15) = 3.72$; $\varepsilon = 0.58$; adjusted p value < 0.05; effect size $\eta_p^2 = 0.35$) regardless of the cueing condition (For the topographic distribution across electrode sites and hemispheres in the two respiratory conditions see the maps drawn in Figure 7), while for the mean and SE values relative to the afore-mentioned findings see Figure 8). Post-hoc comparisons among means indicated that hypoxia significantly increased alpha power ($p < 0.0005$) determining a prominent alpha synchronization over the right-sided parieto-occipital scalp site (PO8), but not the left occipito-parietal (PO7) site. Furthermore, alpha power was greater over the right (PO8; $p < 0.004$) than the left occipito-parietal (PO7) site.

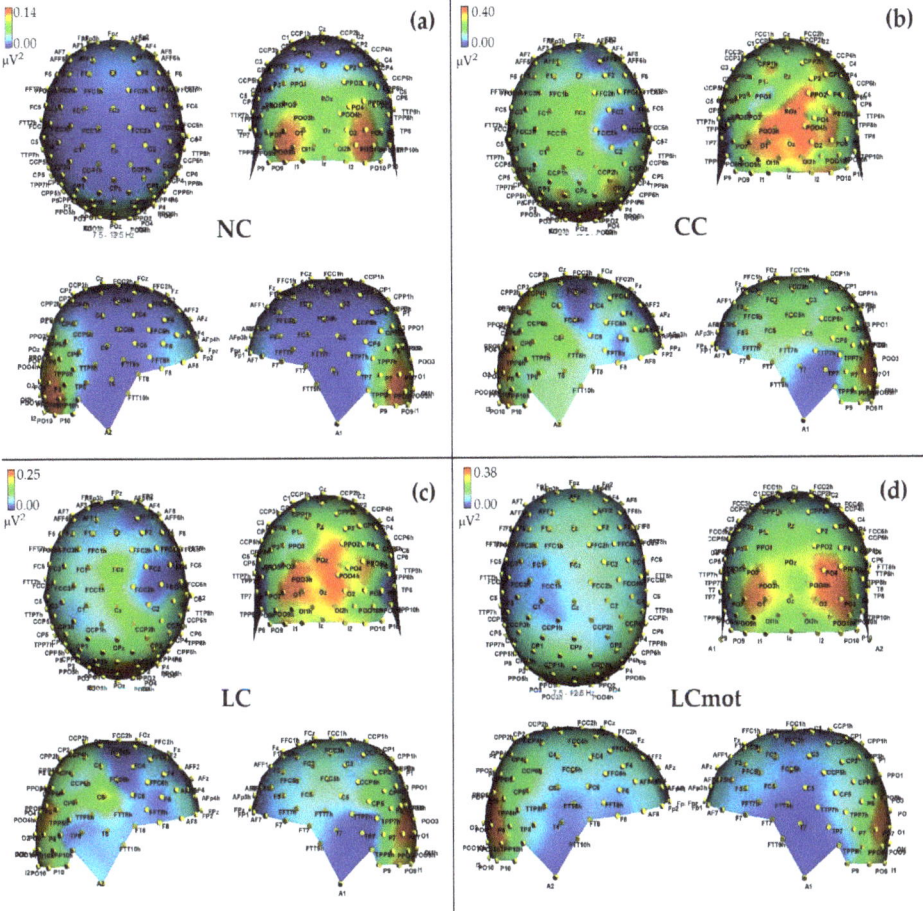

Figure 5. Three-dimensional (3D) maps of the topographical distribution of alpha power over the scalp as a function of the cueing-conditions grand-averaged over the respiratory conditions, and drawn from the top, the back, the right, and the left points of view, respectively. Time = 0 to 1500 ms, frequency = 7.5–12.5 Hz. (**a**): NC condition; (**b**): CC condition; (**c**): LC condition; (**d**): LCmot condition. Note that the scale of alpha power values (in μV^2) is unalike in the different attentional-cueing conditions. Note also that while the alerting but spatially unpredictable, exogenous-orienting of attention to target (CC) condition showed the highest alpha power, the fully uncued, exogenous-orienting of attention to target (NC) condition was characterized by the lowest alpha power.

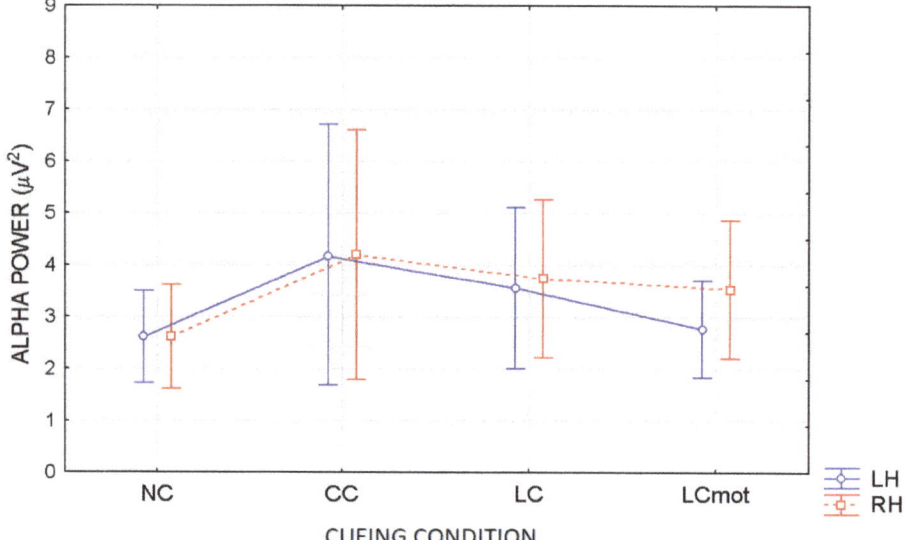

Figure 6. Mean and SE values of alpha power (in μV^2) as a function of cueing conditions and hemispheres collapsed across respiratory conditions. Note that for an easier readability, alpha power values were multiplied by 10 before being plotted.

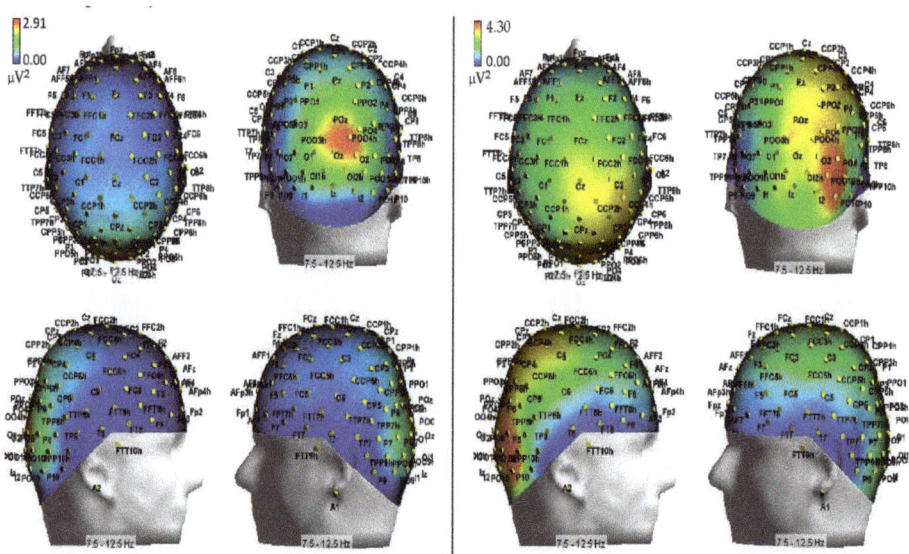

Figure 7. 3D topographical scalp maps of alpha power as a function of normoxia (left side) and hypoxia (right side) respiratory conditions grand-averaged across the attentional-cueing modes, and drawn from the top, the back, the right, and the left viewpoints, respectively. Worth of note is the prominent lateralization of alpha synchronization induced by hypoxia over the right-sided occipital and parietal scalp areas as compared to normoxia.

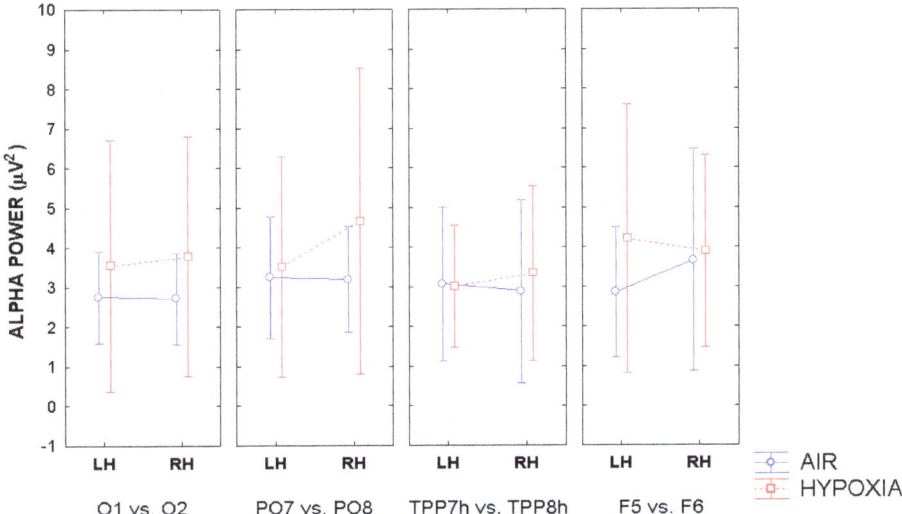

Figure 8. Mean and SE values of alpha power plotted as a function of respiratory mode, hemisphere, and electrode site. Note that also in this case alpha power values were multiplied by 10 before being plotted.

Additionally, hypoxia induced EEG alpha synchronization over the mesial-occipital areas of both the LH and RH ($p < 0.04$ and $p < 0.0072$, respectively). Hypoxia also induced stronger alpha synchronization than in ambient-air over the left-sided dorsolateral prefrontal scalp site ($p < 0.0011$) (see Figure 8 again for all these findings). Overall, however, at these anterior scalp regions EEG alpha synchronization was significantly stronger over the RH than the LH, but in air condition only ($p < 0.034$). Moreover, in hypoxia alpha synchronization showed to be much more prominent over the right parieto-occipital than over the temporo-parietal ($p < 0.001$) and the prefrontal ($p < 0.046$) scalp sites, while this topographical difference was much reduced in ambient-air condition and over the left hemisphere ($p < 0.0011$).

5. Discussion

The present study had the manifold aims of investigating the role of alpha synchronization and/or desynchronization in visuospatial attention orienting, and, more specifically, in the exogenous and endogenous modes of attention-orienting. Additionally, we aimed to investigate the relationships of alpha synchronization and desynchronization with the functional activation of brain alerting, orienting, and executive attentional neural networks. We wished to assess whether the separate attentional networks might have been independently or interactively affected by a reduced, non-pathogenic brain oxygenation state—or hypoxia—and, in case of interactions, which of them would have interacted. Last but not the least, we inquired into possible influences of induced hypoxia on overt motor performance.

From the behavioral point of view, our findings indicated that both error rates and RTs showed to be affected by hypoxia, in that, during this respiratory condition, the participants showed a tout court lower performance accuracy and speed than in air—or normoxia—regardless of cueing mode and target/flanker congruency.

However, error rate differences between cueing conditions also showed to be strongly affected by the respiratory factor regardless of target/flanker congruency. In normoxia, in fact, the lowest error rate was observed for both the spatially cued (LC) and the alerting but spatially unpredictable, centrally cued (CC) targets, without any difference between them (see Figure 3). A higher errors rate was obtained for uncued targets (NC), and a highest rate for spatially cued, motor-choice overloaded

(LCmot) targets. Conversely, with the exception of uncued targets (NC), hypoxia markedly affected performance accuracy in that the latter progressively decreased—i.e., participants committed a greater number of errors—as a function of both the alerting but spatially unpredictable, centrally cued (CC) and spatially cued targets, regardless of their demand of a single or a double-choice motor response (i.e., LC and LCmot). All in all, these overt motor-accuracy findings suggested that hypoxia affected the original ANT-related attention alerting, orienting, and conflict networks independently from one another. Moreover, our data suggested that hypoxia also strongly affected the motor-charged attention orienting cueing mode.

Unlike for error rates, overt responses (i.e., RTs) showed a distinct pattern of significant changes as a function of cueing conditions in close interaction with target/flanker conflict level, regardless of the respiratory condition. Shortest RTs were observed for validly spatially cued (LC) targets, intermediate RTs for the spatially unpredictable, centrally cued (CC) targets, longer RTs for uncued targets (NC) and longest RTs for spatially cued, motor double-choice demanding (LCmot) targets (see Figure 4). The relative benefits of original ANT alerting and orienting [40] amounted to about 25 ms and 50 ms, respectively, while for the motor double-choice-related orienting condition of our ANT-SR, a heavy cost of about 200 ms, rather than a benefit, was found. Response conflict due to target/flankers incongruency led to an increase of overt motor response latency with a greater mean RTs cost of about ~40 ms for the spatially unpredictable, centrally cued (CC) targets than for both the uncued (NC; ~30 ms) and the validly spatially cued targets (LC; ~20ms), and no cost for LCmot cueing condition.

At least for what concerned the behavioral findings in response to the original ANT-related cueing conditions in normoxia, the aforementioned pattern of results is in good accordance with those that were published originally by Fan et al. [40], Neuhaus et al. [55], and by our group (e.g., Zani and Proverbio [43]), in that the use of either a spatially informative cue (LC) or of a no-cueing condition (NC) reduced costs for incongruent vs. congruent targets processing as compared to both the 2C and CC cueing modes. According to Fan et al. [40], this occurred, in the first case, because participants directed attention to the target ahead of time, and, in the second case, because NC is a relatively low-alertness condition and resulted in longer RTs and relatively lower errors. In Fan's et al. [40] words, "it is possible that the longer time to produce a response due to low alertness can provide additional time for executive attention processes in the conflict condition, thus reducing executive costs." Following the above-mentioned lines of reasoning, it would seem highly plausible that these same neural mechanisms could be adopted for explaining the lack of any differences between the speed of motor response to the congruent and incongruent target/flanker patterns for the motor-charged, LCmot condition (see Figure 4 again).

Generally speaking, we believe that the consistency of our behavioral findings with those obtained by the studies quoted above strongly supports the views that, despite the relatively exiguous number of participants analyzed in the present study, the obtained data may be considered sound and reliable, besides being truly dependent on the manipulation of experimental variables.

As far as the electrophysiological data are concerned, our findings showed to be quite in accordance with those obtained for behavioral data. Indeed, alpha measures separately changed as a function of cueing condition and respiratory condition factors, either in interaction with the hemisphere and/or the hemisphere and electrode factors. Unlike behavioral data, however, electrophysiological data were not apparently affected by the executive neural processing, neither per se or in interaction with other factors.

It would seem rather plausible that this slight inconsistency between overt motor responses and covert alpha processing data depended on the fact that the former were timely closer to the executive conflict resolution processes than the latter because alpha power computed by FFT starting from the presentation of cue type, at time 0, up until 1500 ms after cue, with the target falling at 500 ms, included, according to the experimental conditions, time spans of either alpha synchrony or desynchrony occurring after the emission of the overt motor response. Due to this, it is somehow conceivable that alpha power processing occurring during these time spans may have been less closely related to the executive conflict resolution processes.

As for the specific trend of our electrophysiological data, it is worth of note that, notwithstanding the small size of our sample of participants, our findings are in line with those of previous studies, thus confirming the view that a bout of increased alpha amplitude or synchronization recorded at posterior occipito-parietal areas during a visuospatial attention task reflects an inhibition of attention orienting towards information presented at an irrelevant point in space [56]. Indeed, brain areas involved in the processing of task-irrelevant space may be actively inhibited during an increase of alpha-oscillations synchronization to refrain from processing of distracting information [19,57]. More in details, the data showed that alpha power changed not only as a function of endogenous and exogenous attention orienting modes, but also of the different informative content transmitted by the various cue-target combinations within the former and the latter modes of attention-orienting, regardless of brain oxygenation condition. They also indicated that attention-related alpha frequency desynchronization is more prominent in the LH than in the RH, thus suggesting asymmetries that might be regarded as a sign of cerebral lateralization or hemispheric dominance for this neurocognitive function.

In agreement with these viewpoints, alpha showed the lowest power (i.e., stronger desynchronization) during the no cue (NC) mode, in which, most likely, brain tonic alerting and utterly exogenous orienting of attention responses to targets sequentially presented in random order at one out of the two relevant space locations without being primed by any cue, took place (see EEG alpha-power maps drawn in Figure 5a, and Figure 6 for mean power values for this condition). At the opposite, alpha showed the highest synchronization in the ANT condition in which a spatially uninformative, but alerting cue was delivered to the center of the screen, followed later on by the presentation of a target at one out of the two spatially relevant locations (i.e., CC condition; see EEG alpha-power maps drawn in Figure 5b, and Figure 6 for mean power values for this condition). Very likely, this finding may have arisen because, in this condition, a phasic alerting together with a transient suppression of attention-orienting might have been elicited by the warning CC, followed by a reflexive orienting of attention to the stimulated space location as triggered by the target delivery.

As for the endogenous attention-orienting mode conditions, the alpha power recorded for LC task, where the cue was both alerting and validly informative of the spatial point at which the target would follow, showed to be somewhat lower than that elicited by CC condition over the LH, but not the RH, and, in general, pretty higher than that computed by FFT for the NC mode over both hemispheres. It seems highly plausible that alpha desynchronization found over the left hemisphere in response to LC condition may have undergirded a fast orienting of attention to the location indicated by the valid cue. A possibility strongly supported by Posner's theses [44] who considered the left lateralized processes as more likely involved with higher temporal (phasic) mechanisms, such as orienting of attention, and right lateralized processes often more involved with slower (tonic) alerting effects. Consistent with these views, LC showed a same alpha power as CC over the RH, but a significant higher desynchronization (i.e., a significant lower alpha power) over the LH (see EEG alpha-power maps drawn in Figure 5c, and Figure 6 for mean power values for this condition). Interestingly, a right sided asymmetry in alpha scalp distribution has been shown by several previous studies [21,58].

Most interestingly, the data also indicated that introducing a neurocognitive perceptual (e.g., a target-type discrimination) and psychomotor overload (e.g., a double-choice motor task) as in the LCmot condition further increased alpha desynchronization over the LH, but not the RH. This left-sided increase in alpha desynchronization in LCmot with respect to both CC and LC showed to be of such a degree that the alpha for this cueing mode did show any differences from that for the exogenous NC task over the LH as compared to the RH. Conversely, LCmot elicited a same alpha power level as LC over the RH. As a result of the afore-mentioned changes, a prominent right-sided hemispheric asymmetry of the alpha power occurred for this motor-charged cueing-mode only (see EEG alpha-power maps drawn in Figure 5d, and Figure 6 for mean power values for this condition).

As for the functional meaning of a left-sided asymmetry of alpha desynchronization and a right-sided asymmetry of alpha synchronization found for LCmot cueing condition, it might be possible that, in line with Posner's proposals [44], during this high-motor workload task the LH may have been engaged in the orienting of attention to the location indicated by the valid cue, as reflected by an increase of alpha desynchronization, but the demands of the target-type discrimination and of a decision relative to the double-choice overt response may have required to sustain alerting and/or attention over time, thus recruiting the slower, tonic processing by the RH, reflected at the scalp by an increase of alpha synchronization.

As far as hypoxia is concerned, our alpha measures indicated that this deficient-oxygenation condition mostly increased alpha power at right-sided brain posterior districts, and more in details striate and extrastriate occipital areas as well as parietal areas (Figure 7). However, some of our findings also indicated that hypoxia selectively enhanced alpha power at the left-sided anterior prefrontal areas (Figure 8). As for the effects of this respiratory condition on brain attentional processes, independent of brain areas involved, our results showed increases of alpha synchronization no matter the endogenous and exogenous nature of visuospatial attention orienting. Moreover, they also hinted at the view that hypoxia had diffused influences on all attentional processing networks (i.e., alerting, orienting and executive control networks), in that, no matter the network activated, hypoxia resulted in a general increase of alpha synchronization.

At least for the increase of alpha power in response to hypoxic hypoxia obtained at posterior occipital-parietal areas, our discoveries fully mesh with the findings reported by some previous studies (i.e., [27,30]). For truth sake, however, it must be said that these discoveries are only partially consistent with the results of another relatively recent study [32], and clearly in contrast with the results of some dated investigations (e.g., [28,29]). We believe that rather than to methodological and procedural differences in (1) the induction methods of hypoxia in neurologically healthy volunteers, (2) the different alpha frequency band ranges taken into account, and (3) the number of scalp sites at which the alpha power was computed, the different results obtained by the present investigation as compared to several previous studies (e.g., [28,29,34]) may be closely due to the participants' neurocognitive functional state during EEG recordings. Indeed, while the latter studies analyzed the alpha power in the spontaneous EEG of volunteers who were not submitted to any active psycho-motor or attentional tasks, the investigations showing fully consistent findings with our own (i.e., [27,30]) measured alpha power in EEG recorded either during a presumably more environmentally-aware or attentional-driven condition—though not directly analyzed or accounted for—such as the eyes-open state, compared to the eyes-closed one [27] or during a simple, though somehow effortful, computerized visuospatial attentional task in which participants had to keep a moving target as much closer to the center of a screen denoted by a rectangle, in order to avoid the drifting of the target towards the edges of the screen [30].

Despite the lack of any report of the participants' performance scores by these authors [30], it may be assumed that the aforementioned task might have been perceived as easier or less effortful in normoxia than in hypoxia, and that the generalized increases in alpha synchrony during the latter condition might have represented an alteration or, up-to a certain degree, a suppression of brain attentional orienting capacity. In support of this view, Zhao et al. [34] found changes of EEG during hypoxia/reoxygenation confined in posterior right cortices, with increased alpha synchrony related to hypoxia and increased beta desynchrony related to reoxygenation. Further support derived from our current data, which showed increased error rates and motor response times as well as of alpha power in hypoxia with respect to normoxia.

6. General Conclusions

All in all, the modulation of alpha power induced by the cueing conditions used in our study lends reliable and robust support to the view advanced by several previous studies e.g., [19,56,57] that the desynchronization versus the synchronization of this oscillatory-band reflects an active orienting versus an inhibition of visuospatial attention, respectively. Following this line of reasoning, the generalized right-sided alpha band synchronization observed in hypoxia as compared to normoxia would reflect the effort to sustain attention-alerting over time, as mediated by the RH, in order to cope with a transient impairment or, up to a certain degree, suppression of brain attention-orienting capacity, mediated by the LH. The lack of any effects of the different attentional cueing and executive conflict conditions on alpha synchronization induced by hypoxia may also indicate that this enhancement possibly reflected an overall transient alteration or tout-court suppression of attention alerting, orienting, and executive networks functionality independently from one another.

7. Study Limits and Wishes

A possible limitation of the present study was the relatively small sample size ($n = 8$.) The latter, in fact, was somewhat small and therefore conceivably statistically underpowered. However, the consistency of our general behavioral and electrophysiological findings with those of previous studies in the literature lends strong support to their soundness as also championed by partial eta squared values of computed size effects here provided. Furthermore, the sample size was large enough to assess the expected pattern of attentional effects predicted by available literature. Another edge for our data might be our use of parametric statistical tests which require the a-priori hypothesis of variables with normal distribution, here somehow not assured because of the lack of linearity of FFT values and of the small sample size. Nevertheless, because of the potential relevance of our findings, we think it is worth pursuing further research aimed at their sound replication by enlarging the sample size and the use of non-parametric statistical tests.

Author Contributions: A.Z. theoretically devised the study. A.Z., A.M.P., and C.T. collected the data. C.T. carried out computations of alpha power by means of the FFT for the single subjects' and the sample's grand-average EEG. A.Z., and A.M.P. wrote the manuscript. A.Z. and A.M.P. critically processed the final version of the latter and the theoretical interpretation and discussion of the experimental findings of the study. All authors have read and agreed to the published version of the manuscript.

Funding: This research was funded by CNR grants to A.Z. that were used for purchasing EEG recording supplies and materials required for data collection and analysis.

Conflicts of Interest: The authors declare no conflict of interest.

References

1. Cheal, M.L.; Lyon, D.R.; Habbard, D.C. Does attention have different effects on line orientation and line arrangement discrimination? *Quart. J. Exp. Psychol.* **2012**, *43*, 825–857. [CrossRef] [PubMed]
2. Pinto, Y.; van der Leij, A.R.; Sligte, I.G.; Lamme, V.A.F.; Scholte, H.S. Bottom-up and top-down attention are independent. *J. Vis.* **2013**, *13*, 1–14. [CrossRef] [PubMed]
3. Corbetta, M.; Shulman, G.L. Control of goal-directed and stimulus-driven attention in the brain. *Nat. Rev. Neurosci.* **2002**, *3*, 215. [CrossRef]
4. Patel, G.H.; Sestieri, C.; Corbetta, M. The evolution of the temporoparietal junction and posterior superior temporal sulcus. *Cortex* **2019**, *118*, 38–50. [CrossRef] [PubMed]
5. Shulman, G.L.; Pope, D.L.; Astafiev, S.V.; McAvoy, M.P.; Snyder, A.Z.; Corbetta, M. Right hemisphere dominance during spatial selective attention and target detection occurs outside the dorsal frontoparietal network. *J. Neurosci.* **2010**, *30*, 3640–3651. [CrossRef] [PubMed]
6. Mayer, A.R.; Dorflinger, J.M.; Rao, S.M.; Seidenberg, M. Neural networks underlying endogenous and exogenous visual–spatial orienting. *Neuroimage* **2004**, *23*, 534–541. [CrossRef]
7. Meyer, K.N.; Du, F.; Parks, E.; Hopfinger, J.B. Exogenous vs. endogenous attention: Shifting the balance of fronto-parietal activity. *Neuropsychology* **2018**, *111*, 307–316. [CrossRef]
8. Dugué, L.; Merriam, E.P.; Heeger, D.J.; Carrasco, M. Specific Visual Subregions of TPJ Mediate Reorienting of Spatial Attention. *Cereb. Cortex* **2018**, *1*, 2375–2390. [CrossRef]
9. Han, S.W.; Shin, H.; Jeong, D.; Jung, S.; Bae, E.; Kim, J.Y.; Baek, H.M.; Kim, K. Neural substrates of purely endogenous, self-regulatory control of attention. *Sci. Rep.* **2018**, *17*, 925. [CrossRef]

10. MacLean, K.A.; Aichele, S.R.; Bridwell, D.A.; Mangun, G.R.; Wojciulik, E.; Saron, C.S. Interactions between Endogenous and Exogenous Attention during Vigilance. *Attent. Percep. Psychophys.* **2009**, *71*, 1042–1058. [CrossRef]
11. Simpson, G.V.; Weber, D.L.; Dale, C.L.; Pantazis, D.; Bressler, S.L.; Leahy, R.M. Dynamic activation of frontal, parietal, and sensory regions underlying anticipatory visual spatial attention. *J. Neurosci.* **2011**, *31*, 13880–13889. [CrossRef] [PubMed]
12. Misselhorn, J.; Friese, U.; Engel, A.K. Frontal and parietal alpha oscillations reflect attentional modulation of cross-modal matching. *Sci. Rep.* **2019**, *22*, 5030. [CrossRef] [PubMed]
13. Kelly, S.P.; Lalor, E.C.; Reilly, R.B.; Foxe, J.J. Visual spatial attention tracking using high-density SSVEP data for independent brain-computer communication. *IEEE Transac. Neural Syst. Rehab. Eng.* **2005**, *13*, 172–178. [CrossRef] [PubMed]
14. Kelly, S.P.; Lalor, E.C.; Reilly, R.B.; Foxe, J.J. Increases in Alpha Oscillatory Power Reflect a Suppression during Sustained Visuospatial Attention Active Retinotopic Mechanism for Distracter. *J. Neurophysiol.* **2006**, *95*, 3844–3851. [CrossRef] [PubMed]
15. Van Dijk, H.; Schoffelen, J.M.; Oostenveld, R. Prestimulus Oscillatory Activity in the Alpha Band Predicts Visual Discrimination Ability. *J. Neurosci.* **2008**, *28*, 1816–1823. [CrossRef] [PubMed]
16. Foxe, J.; Simpson, G.V.; Ahlfors, S.P. Parieto-occipital approximately 10 Hz activity reflects anticipatory state of visual attention mechanisms. *Neuro Rep.* **1998**, *9*, 3929–3933.
17. Foxe, J.J.; Snyder, A.C. The role of alpha-band brain oscillations as a sensory suppression mechanism during selective attention. *Frnt. Hum. Neurosci.* **2011**, *2*, 154. [CrossRef]
18. Fu, K.M.G.; Foxe, J.J.; Murray, M.M.; Higgins, B.A.; Javitt, D.C.; Schroeder, C.E. Attention-dependent suppression of distracter visual input can be cross-modally cued as indexed by anticipatory parieto–occipital alpha-band oscillations. *Cogn. Brain Res.* **2001**, *12*, 145–152. [CrossRef]
19. Rihs, T.A.; Michael, C.M.; Thut, G. A bias for posterior α-band power suppression versus enhancement during shifting versus maintenance of spatial attention. *Neuroimage* **2009**, *44*, 190–199. [CrossRef]
20. Li, Y.; Lou, B.; Sajda, P. Post-stimulus endogenous and exogenous oscillations are differentially modulated by task difficulty. *Front. Hum. Neurosci.* **2013**, *7*, 9. [CrossRef]
21. Volberg, G.; Kliegl, K.; Hanslmayr, S.; Greenlee, M.W. EEG Alpha Oscillations in the Preparation for Global and Local Processing Predict Behavioral Performance. *Hum. Brain Mapp.* **2009**, *30*, 2173–2183. [CrossRef] [PubMed]
22. Min, B.K.; Herrmann, C.S. Prestimulus EEG alpha activity reflects prestimulus top-down processing. *Neurosci. Lett.* **2007**, *422*, 131–135. [CrossRef] [PubMed]
23. Klimesch, W. Alpha-band oscillations, attention, and controlled access to stored information. *Trend. Cogn. Sci.* **2012**, *16*, 606–617. [CrossRef] [PubMed]
24. Jonkman, E.J.; Van Dieren, A.; Veering, M.M.; Ponsen, L.; Lopes da Silva, F.H.; Tulleken, C.A. EEG and CBF in cerebral ischemia. Follow-up studies in humans and monkeys. *Prog. Brain Res.* **1984**, *62*, 147–171.
25. Jordan, K.G. Continuous EEG and evoked potential monitoring in the neuroscience intensive care unit. *J. Clin. Neurophysiol.* **1993**, *10*, 445–475. [CrossRef]
26. Geocadin, R.; Ghodadra, R.; Kimura, K.; Lei, H.; Sherman, D.L.; Hanley, D.F.; Thakor, N.V. A novel quantitative EEG injury measure of global cerebral ischemia. *Clin. Neurophysiol.* **2000**, *111*, 1779–1787. [CrossRef]
27. Schellart, N.A.; Reits, D. Transient and maintained changes of the spontaneous occipital EEG during acute systemic hypoxia. *Aviat. Space Environ. Med.* **2001**, *72*, 462–470.
28. Kraaier, V.; Van Huffelen, A.C.; Wieneke, G.H. Quantitative EEG changes due to hypobaric hypoxia in normal subjects. *Electroencephalogr. Clin. Neurophysiol.* **1988**, *69*, 303–312. [CrossRef]
29. Ozaki, H.; Watanabe, S.; Suzuki, H. Topographic EEG changes due to hypobaric hypoxia at simulated high altitude. *EEG Clin. Neurophysiol.* **1995**, *94*, 349–356. [CrossRef]
30. Papadelis, C.; Kourtidou-Papadeli, C.; Bamidis, P.D.; Maglaveras, N.; Pappas, K. The effect of hypobaric hypoxia on multichannel EEG signal complexity. *Clin. Neurophysiol.* **2007**, *118*, 31–52. [CrossRef]
31. Schneider, S.; Strüder, H.K. Monitoring effects of acute hypoxia on brain cortical activity by using electromagnetic tomography. *Behav. Brain Res.* **2009**, *197*, 476–480. [CrossRef] [PubMed]

32. Hota, S.K.; Sharma, V.K.; Hota, K.; Das, S.; Dhar, P.; Mahapatra, B.B.; Srivastava, R.B.; Singh, S.B. Multi-domain cognitive screening test for neuropsychological assessment for cognitive decline in acclimatized low landers staying at high altitude. *Indian J. Med. Res.* **2012**, *136*, 411–420. [PubMed]
33. Gritti, I.; Martignoni, M.; Calcaterra, R.; Sergio Roi, G. Electroencephalographic changes after a marathon at 4300m of altitude. *J. Behav. Brain Sci.* **2012**, *2*, 380–386. [CrossRef]
34. Zhao, J.-P.; Zhang, R.; Yu, Q.; Zhang, J.-X. Characteristics of EEG activity during high altitude hypoxia and lowland reoxygenation. *Brain Res.* **2016**, *1648*, 243–249. [CrossRef] [PubMed]
35. Richardson, C.; Hogan, A.M.; Bucks, R.S.; Baya, A.; Virues-Ortega, J.; Holloway, J.W.; Rose-Zerilli, M.; Palmer, L.J.; Webster, R.J.; Kirkham, F.J.; et al. Neurophysiological evidence for cognitive and brain functional adaptation in adolescents living at high altitude. *Clin. Neurophysiol.* **2011**, *122*, 1726–1734. [CrossRef]
36. Klimesch, W. EEG alpha and theta oscillations reflect cognitive and memory performance: A review and analysis. *Brain Res. Rev.* **1999**, *29*, 169–195. [CrossRef]
37. Uhlhaas, P.J.; Singer, W. High-frequency oscillations and the neurobiology of schizophrenia. *Dialog. Clin. Neurosci.* **2013**, *15*, 301–313.
38. Posner, M.I.; Petersen, S.E. The attention system of the human brain. *Annu. Rev. Neurosci.* **1990**, *13*, 25–42. [CrossRef]
39. Posner, M.J. Orienting of attention. *Quart. J. Exp. Psychol.* **1980**, *32*, 3–25. [CrossRef]
40. Fan, J.; McCandliss, B.D.; Sommer, T.; Raz, A.; Posner, M.I. Testing the efficiency and independence of attentional networks. *J. Cogn. Neurosci.* **2002**, *14*, 340–347. [CrossRef]
41. Fan, J.; Mc Candliss, B.D.; Fossella, J.; Flombaum, J.I.; Posner, M.I. The activation of attentional networks. *Neuroimage* **2005**, *26*, 471–479. [CrossRef] [PubMed]
42. Fan, J.; Byrne, J.; Worden, M.S.; Guise, K.G.; McCandliss, B.D.; Fossella, J.; Posner, M.I. The relationships of brain oscillations to attentional networks. *J. Neurosci.* **2007**, *27*, 6197–6206. [CrossRef] [PubMed]
43. Zani, A.; Proverbio, A.M. How voluntary orienting of attention and alerting modulate costs of conflict processing. *Sci. Rep. Nat.* **2017**, *7*, 46701. [CrossRef] [PubMed]
44. Posner, M.I. Measuring alertness. *Ann. N. Y. Acad. Sci.* **2008**, *1129*, 193–199. [CrossRef] [PubMed]
45. Mecacci, L.; Zani, A. Morningness-eveningness preferences and sleep-waking diary data of morning and evening types in student and worker samples. *Ergonomics* **1984**, *26*, 1147–1153. [CrossRef]
46. Colombo, E.; Marconi, C.; Taddeo, A.; Cappelletti, M.; Villa, M.L.; Marzorati, M.; Porcelli, S.; Vezzoli, A.; Della Bella, S. Fast reduction of peripheral blood endothelial progenitor cells in healthy humans exposed to acute systemic hypoxia. *J. Physiol.* **2012**, *590*, 519–532. [CrossRef]
47. Oostenveld, R.; Praamstra, P. The five percent electrode system for high-resolution EEG and ERP measurements. *Clin. Neurophysiol.* **2001**, *112*, 713–719. [CrossRef]
48. Urigüen, J.A.; Bengoña, G.-Z. EEG artifact removal—State-of-the-art and Guidelines. *J. Neural Eng.* **2015**, *12*, 031001. [CrossRef]
49. Di Fiumeri, G.; Aricó, P.; Borghini, G.; Colosimo, A.; Babiloni, F. A new regression-based method for the eye blinks artifacts correction in the EEG signal, without using any EOG channel. In Proceedings of the 38th Annual International Conference of the IEEE Engineering in Medicine and Biology Society (EMBC), Orlando, FL, USA, 16–20 August 2016; IEEE: Piscataway, NJ, USA, 2016.
50. Burrus, C.S. *Fast Fourier Transforms*; Rice University Publications: Houston, TX, USA, 2012.
51. Snedecor, G.W.; Cochran, W.G. *Statistical Methods*, 8th ed.; Iowa State University Press: Iowa City, IA, USA, 1989.
52. Lison, L. *Statistique Appliquée a la Biologie Experimentale. La Planification de L'expérience et L'analyse des Resultats*; Gauthier-Villars Éditeur-Imprimeur-Libraire: Paris, France, 1961.
53. Bakeman, R. Recommended effect size statistics for repeated measures designs. *Behav. Res. Methods* **2005**, *37*, 379–384. [CrossRef]
54. Thompson, B. *Foundations of Behavioral Statistics: An Insight-Based Approach*; Guilford: New York, NY, USA, 2006.
55. Neuhaus, A.H.; Urbanek, C.; Opgen-Rhein, C.; Hahn, E.; Tam Ta, T.T.; Koehler Gross, M.; Dettling, M. Event-related potential associated with Attention Network Test. *Int. J. Psychophysiol.* **2010**, *76*, 72–79. [CrossRef]
56. Poch, C.; Carretie, L.; Campo, P. A dual mechanism underlying alpha lateralization in attentional orienting to mental representation. *Biol. Psychol.* **2017**, *28*, 63–70. [CrossRef] [PubMed]

57. Rihs, T.A.; Michel, C.M.; Thut, G. Mechanisms of selective inhibition in visual spatial attention are indexed by alpha-band EEG synchronization. *Eur. J. Neurosci.* **2017**, *25*, 603–610.
58. Marshall, T.R.; Bergmann, T.O.; Jensen, O. Frontoparietal Structural Connectivity Mediates the Top-Down Control of Neuronal Synchronization Associated with Selective Attention. *PLoS Biol.* **2015**, *13*, e1002272. [CrossRef] [PubMed]

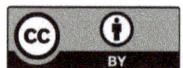

© 2020 by the authors. Licensee MDPI, Basel, Switzerland. This article is an open access article distributed under the terms and conditions of the Creative Commons Attribution (CC BY) license (http://creativecommons.org/licenses/by/4.0/).

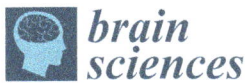

Communication

More than Meets the Mind's Eye? Preliminary Observations Hint at Heterogeneous Alpha Neuromarkers for Visual Attention

Emmanuelle Tognoli

Center for Complex Systems and Brain Sciences, Florida Atlantic University, 777 Glades Road, Boca Raton, FL 33431, USA; tognoli@ccs.fau.edu

Received: 1 October 2019; Accepted: 31 October 2019; Published: 2 November 2019

Abstract: With their salient power distribution and privileged timescale for cognition and behavior, brainwaves within the 10 Hz band are special in human waking electroencephalography (EEG). From the inception of electroencephalographic technology, the contribution of alpha rhythm to attention is well-known: Its amplitude increases when visual attention wanes or visual input is removed. However, alpha is not alone in the 10 Hz frequency band. A number of other 10 Hz neuromarkers have function and topography clearly distinct from alpha. In small pilot studies, an activity that we named xi was found over left centroparietal scalp regions when subjects held their attention to spatially peripheral locations while maintaining their gaze centrally ("looking from the corner of the eyes"). I outline several potential functions for xi as a putative neuromarker of covert attention distinct from alpha. I review methodological aids to test and validate their functional role. They emphasize high spectral resolution, sufficient spatial resolution to provide topographical separation, and an acute attention to dynamics that caters to neuromarkers' transiency.

Keywords: EEG; alpha; xi; Posner; covert attention

---

1. Introduction

A crucial set of experiments by Michael Posner and colleagues [1] buttressed the theory that minds are equipped with a covert visual orienting system to enhance detection of targets even as they lie out of the foveal center of the participant's overt visual attention. This is the notorious spotlight that had been postulated by James in 1890 [2], and evidenced by Helmoltz [3]—see also the reviews and controversies [4–8] and overviews of neuroanatomical bases [9–11] that lent credit to a view of multiple independent networks and processes for attention [9].

In a separate stream of research founded by Hans Berger in the 1920s [12,13], a rhythmic brain wave at about 10 Hz was shown to transpire from the scalp of human participants and reacted to such events as eye opening, involuntary attention to sudden startle from gunshot sound, other auditory, visual, olfactive, tactile, and pain stimuli, voluntary concentration, anesthesia, medications, and a variety of clinical conditions [12–17]. This brain wave is a dominant activity in human waking electroencephalogram (EEG) [18]. After the controversy of its cerebral origin was finally settled [15], what came to be known as the alpha wave [14] rose as one of the most studied electrophysiological phenomenon, with firmly established correlation to attentive processes [19–22].

Here, we restrict the name alpha to the 10 Hz phenomenon peaking in parieto-occipital regions when eyes are closed or attention and vigilance reduced. Alpha's anticorrelation with attentive behavior was noted from the start [12–14] and continued to be observed [23] after warning signals of target occurrence [24] and in relation with many tasks derived from Posner's cueing paradigm, consensually with a contralateral organization, that is, increase power opposite the stimulus side or decrease power ipsilateral to it [25–38] after target onset as well as during the cue period [26,39] and even in the absence of ultimate target [40]. Alpha is also modulated by temporal expectations [33] and abides to reverse causal inference that finds more omissions when background alpha is intrinsically larger [28,41], externally entrained [42] or perturbed [11].

The functional complexity of 10 Hz oscillations in posterior regions has also been noted [43,44]. First, a so-called paradoxical alpha response (increasing alpha during some exemplars of attentive behavior in violation of the otherwise strong record of alpha suppression during attention, see above) has led to a fervent debate [19,45–48] that appears to have been resolved with a distinction between endogenous and exogenous attention [21,46]: Internally-generated attentional processes are purported to increase alpha to actively inhibit sensory information. This hypothesis retained the idea of a unitary alpha that equally suppresses exogenous and endogenous distractors, but firm evidence of complete anatomical and dynamical equivalence remains unfulfilled. Second, studies of oscillatory power that paid close attention to the timing of oscillatory processes have suggested a complex temporal organization of posterior 10 Hz activities with different sub-bands of alpha playing a role at different moments [18,24,49–51], see also [31]. These studies beg for finer-grained models for the relation between local rhythmic activity and attentional processes. Finally, several studies of functional connectivity also suggest a complex spatiotemporal organization [11,27,52–54].

In the following, I introduce a case study from a small-scale pilot experiment that asked subjects to sustain the dissociation between fixation and covert attention ("looking from the corner of the eyes"). During this task, a 10 Hz neural activity was uncovered that is clearly distinct from alpha (Figure 1b), and I used its existence to develop the hypothesis on a multifaceted model of 10 Hz rhythms' contribution to attentional processes. I based this proposed model on a discrete view of neural oscillations that are spatially specific (e.g., [55,56] and Figure 1a), appearing intermittently over time [57]. This view was gained from a large improvement in spectral and spatial resolution of EEG analysis, and I outline the methodological requirements that might allow to further study the interplay of 10 Hz rhythms, alpha, and others, in attentional processes.

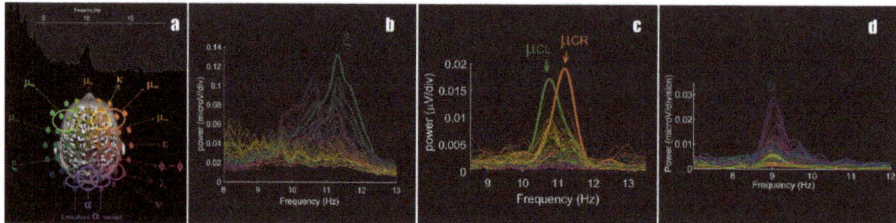

Figure 1. The 10 Hz frequency band carries a number of regionally and functionally specific neuromarkers: (**a**) An overview of their peak scalp locations is provided over a colorimetrically-encoded electrode map (recalling that the inverse problem prevents direct cortical localization); (**b**) xi is found in the upper 10 Hz band, with maxima at left centroparietal scalp locations as shown by the green color of its peak inherited from the colorimetric mapping; (**c**) an exemplar pair of Rolandic mu (here denoted mu central left and right) illustrates the limited spatial overlap that left mu has with xi, though both share the upper 10 Hz band; (**d**) an exemplar of alpha rhythm shows discrepancy both in spatial and spectral organization, with alpha having a slower peak frequency (population mode robustly at 10 Hz [57,58]) and a spatial distance to xi of several centimeters, as manifested with the distinct color (inherited from spatial location and not randomly assigned, see (**a**) for legend). Spectra from (**b**), (**c**), and (**d**) are sampled from different subjects and tasks.

2. Materials and Methods

A subject participated in multiple sessions of an EEG recording (protocol approved by Florida Atlantic University's institutional review board; and written informed consent obtained prior to the experiment). The subject was a right-handed male, healthy young adult (early 20s), with no history of neurological disease, and with normal vision and audition. The sessions were aimed at developing a brain–computer interface [59] and consisted of various ideomotor activities such as executing or imagining movements of the mouth, knees, feet, hands, and fingers by self or other, and lifting of small objects. To control for the potential confound of spatially shifted attention, especially in the case of imagined and executed lower limb movements, a small task was added to the protocol asking the subject to preserve fixation on a crosshair in the center of the computer screen while looking from the corner of the eyes at an unmarked location at the top or bottom of the screen (alternations of 15 s epochs looking from the corner of the eyes and 5 s epochs releasing attention to the central fixation, cumulative duration, 120 s for each direction). This task was created under the rationale that subjects would comply to fixation (validation with EOG) yet might covertly orient their attention to the spatial locus where the targeted body part lay. Since there were no explicit state variables to detect and control for such covert occurrence, we reasoned that sample neuromarkers for this covert activity were important to collect and characterize spatiotemporally. The experiments were conducted in a sound-proof electromagnetically shielded chamber. EEG was recorded using a 60-channel EEG cap with Ag–AgCl electrodes (Falk Minow Services, Herrsching, Germany) arranged according to the 10 percent system [60] (including midline and rows 1 to 8). Electrodes were laid on standard elastic caps whose positioning emphasized the accuracy of vertex electrodes (midway between nasion and inion) and the adequacy of the midline to improve interpretations of lateral symmetries. Electrode impedances were maintained below 10 kΩ, and special attention was paid to the reference electrodes, a pair of digitally linked mastoids (subjected to removal of lipidic film with alcohol swab, double abrasion with hair brush and then gel nuprep, careful adhesive, and compressive securing of the electrodes with tape and elastic cap), leading to their impedance to be low and matched [61]. The ground electrode was located at electrode FPz. The signals were fed to an amplifier (Synamp2, Neuroscan, Texas). The signals were analog-filtered (Butterworth, bandpass from 0.05 Hz (−12 dB/octave) to 100 Hz (−24 dB/octave-)), amplified (gain of 2010), and digitized at 1000 Hz with a 24-bit ADC in the range 0–900 microV (vertical resolution of 0.11 nV). Electro-oculographic (EOG) traces were obtained from two pairs of electrodes placed above and below the right eye (vertical EOG) and on the canthus of each eye (horizontal EOG) to ascertain compliance with instructions not to move the eyes during the tasks.

Three EEG analysis strategies are succinctly presented below, which have been described elsewhere. Multielectrode spectra are obtained via the fast Fourier transform on epochs prepared for enhanced spectral resolution, that is, with the sampling of a longer time interval (e.g., 8.192 or 16.384 s at sampling rate = 1 k Hz) that provides a bin size of 0.06 to 0.12 Hz, much more detailed than a usual 1 Hz resolution and therefore amenable to detecting small discrepancies in frequency of the brain's many 10 Hz activities (Figure 1, see also [55]; strategies to achieve same resolution with smaller epochs can be found in [56]). The spatiotemporal analysis of band-passed filtered EEG uses gently tuned Butterworth filters chosen for their flat passband and applied in both time-positive and time-negative directions to prevent phase distortion [56]. Envelopes are used to scrutinize instantaneous power changes. They were obtained after mean-removed bandpass-filtered signals were rectified and smoothed with a moving average of 100 milliseconds.

3. Results

Figure 2b shows a sample of bandpass-filtered EEG activity collected after on-screen instructions required the subject to covertly move his/her attention to a peripheral location. Xi was observed during covert attention tasks (up and down), execution and imagination of leg movements, imagination of someone else's lifting and releasing a small object, and imagination of self-releasing a grasped object. It was absent in the other ideomotor tasks for this study (i.e., no specific departure from background spectral distribution). Note that xi had not been previously observed in studies of rest with eyes opened or closed, or in a variety of sensorimotor and social coordination tasks (e.g., [56]). The green brainwave that appeared during the covert attention tasks is uncharacteristic of waking EEG in two respects: It has an unusually sustained duration that is infrequently observed during mental activities (compare with, e.g., rest eye opened, with its fast succession of spatiotemporal patterns, see also [56,57,62] for reference dynamics generally lasting one or two cycles). Further, its topography remains several centimeters away from the alpha rhythms. For comparison, Figure 2c provides the dynamics of alpha during an eye opened and eye closed task in a different subject. Note the ample oscillations dominated by blue and magenta color that become sustained and ample at eye closure.

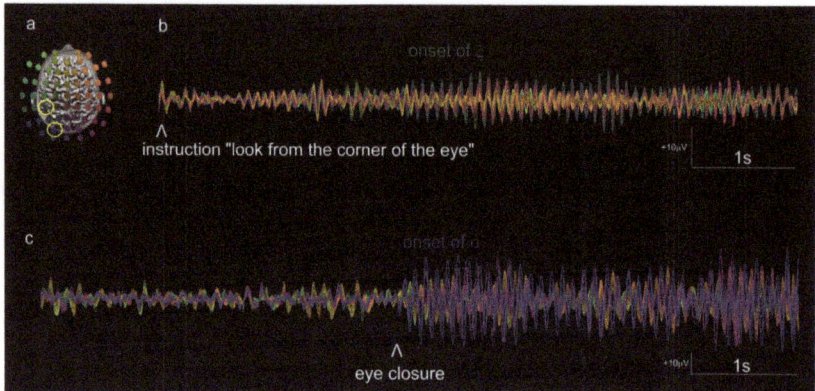

Figure 2. The transition to xi activity during covert shifts of attention is compared to the onset of alpha during closure of the eyes: (**a**) shows a colorimetric map with two electrodes of interest, CP3 (xi, electrode colored green) and PO3 (lateralized variant left alpha, electrode colored blue, see [63]), underlined by yellow circles. (**b**) shows a sample task during which a subject held his attention at the top of the computer screen while fixating the screen's center (i.e., fovea centrally located, and attentional spotlight maintained several degrees away vertically, verified by the absence of saccades or eye movement in EOG traces). Note the onset of ample waves with green color, about 1.5 s after instruction, and sustained for seconds. For comparison, (**c**) shows the 10 Hz band during quiet rest with eye open (left of the marker) and with eye closed (right) in another subject. Note the characteristic low amplitude, moment-to-moment variability in spatiotemporal patterns (color change) prior to eye closure, and the large amplitude activity in posterior locations (colored blue and magenta) afterwards. (**b**) is filtered in the 10–13 Hz band, (**c**) in the 8–12 Hz, in agreement with each target activity's spectral distribution.

The spatial discrepancy between xi and alpha cannot be attributed to irregular electrode positioning or idiosyncratic orientation of the alpha generators shifting the forward projection of alpha generators on the scalp: Analysis within subject confirms that they are two distinct phenomena. They were found to co-occur at the rough timescale of entire tasks, for instance, during covert shift of attention upward (Figure 3a), and they differed in both spatial and spectral distribution as shown by their different color and peak frequencies. They also exhibited distinct temporal organization: Although some alpha patterns were intermittently present in the tasks where xi was discovered, alpha and xi occurred at different times (Figure 3b,c).

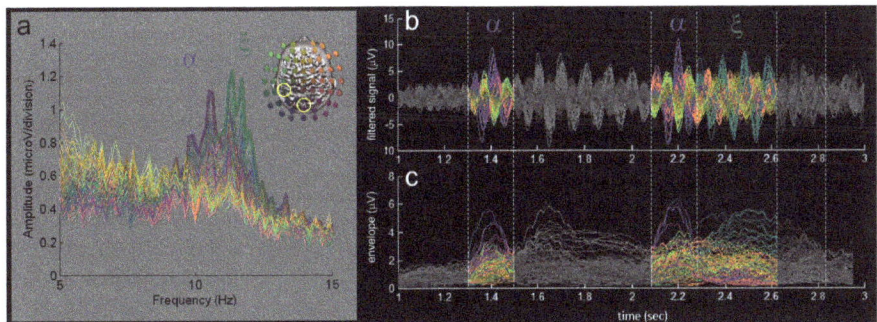

Figure 3. Xi and Alpha differ spectrally and temporally. (**a**) shows a colorimetric spectrum during covert attentional shift upward. Note that in this single subject, the peak of alpha at 10.62 Hz differs from the peak of xi at 11.29 Hz. (**b**) shows a sample bandpass filtered EEG in the 8–13 Hz. Alpha and xi patterns are outlined (other patterns obscured for simplicity). Note that the patterns are not co-occurring in time, as if their functional processes excluded each other. To aid segmentation, signal envelope is plotted in (**c**).

4. Discussion

In a pilot study manipulating the location of the attentional spotlight away from fovea, we found clear evidence of a 10 Hz activity distinct from alpha in a subject [59]. The dissociation was supported by differences in spectral, spatial, and temporal organization (Figures 1–3), and we chose to name the newly characterized neural activity at electrode CP3 'xi'. Naming neuromarkers is instrumental in beginning to confront and document their anatomofunctional specificities [55,56] and to clarify a literature record that oftentimes accretes unrelated oscillatory phenomena (see also the spectacularly detailed insights from [43] along the same lines). In keeping with this logic, like many others, we found alpha to react to subjects' drowsiness (more alpha at the end of experimental sessions than at the beginning), amount of visual stimulation (quantity of movement seen, brightness), and subjective self-report of task engagements (not shown). By contrast, xi reacted to instructions to look from the corner of the eyes, and to tasks where covert attending to distal body parts is implicitly assumed. Alpha was of course increased by inattention; however, inasmuch as it was driven by our instruction to covertly attend to peripheral location, xi was increased, not decreased, by attention. We therefore raise the possibility that alpha and xi are two independent attentional neuromarkers within the 10 Hz band, contributing in unique ways to the functional architecture outlined in the introduction [9,10,64].

In covert tasks such as the above, there are limited tools to cross-validate the subject's mental activity and the temporal footprint of their occurrence. Compliance to fixation was verified from EOG, and a brain–computer interface using xi was successfully developed [59], suggesting that our instructions were coherently understandable in the training and test phases of such research. In hypothesizing on the mental activity associated with xi, I ought to raise three possibilities: (1) xi might represent an idiosyncratic activity that is not shared in the general population and its exposition will be limited to the present report; (2) xi might represent the neural mechanisms that shift the attentional spotlight away from the foveal center; and (3) xi might represent the processes that maintain the dissociation between overt and covert attention, perhaps via oculomotor control areas to repress saccades. In that respect, discussions with a colleague raised the issue of xi's spatial and functional proximity to left Rolandic mu rhythm, a well-known sensorimotor activity, which remains to be more fully studied (although our specimen of xi were more posterior than most left mus on record with the montages used in my laboratory). Rolandic mu rhythms could not be distinguished from background EEG after and during the movement execution tasks, preventing us from making definitive assessments of the similarity between xi and a left mu rhythm.

In the task that was set up, subjects had 15 s to best sustain a covert shift of attention. This prolonged duration (initially designed to gain spectra resolution) likely helped to obtain a robust signal (provided subjects' abilities to sustain the mental effort this long). It is possible that xi activity is also buried in prior cueing tasks, but too brief to rise over the background of a generally dominant alpha activity in human waking EEG. In that respect, I have introduced some sensitive but time-consuming tools to achieve a detailed analysis of spatiotemporal dynamics of the EEG and to uncover crucial activities that are obscured by an unfavorable mixture of small amplitude and short duration: starting with spectra computed with increased spectral resolution, it is possible to distinguish closely-spaced spatiospectral activities (e.g., Figure 3a) and avoid a confound where discretely distinct neuromarkers appear as unitary processes with subtle spatial shift in serial mapping of frequencies with coarse spectral resolution. The study of spatiospectral organization can be followed with the examination of spatiotemporal organization of bandpass-filtered EEG (Figure 2b,c and Figure 3b), its envelope (Figure 3c), and in more details, the phase organization of its oscillations [56,62]. Those painstaking studies allow forming hypotheses on the nature, sources and coordination dynamics of neural oscillations and are aimed to precede robust hypothesis-confirming investigations.

5. Conclusions

In conclusion, this case report of a spatial, spectral, and functional dissociation between alpha and xi supplies the foundation to further experiments, with the potential outcome to break the unitary view of alpha rhythm and attentional processes, which many other electrophysiologists have already suggested [24,31,35,37,54,65].

Funding: Some of this work received a Neuroscience Pilot Award from Florida Atlantic University's Brain Institute. E.T. is supported by the US National Institute of Health, NIBIB EB025819 and NIMH MH080838.

Acknowledgments: Rodrigo Calderon collected some of the data presented in this report, and Rodrigo Calderon, Nurgun Erdol, and Salvatore Morgera contributed some earlier analysis. Intense discussions with Erik Engeberg concerning xi and mu are gratefully acknowledged.

Conflicts of Interest: The author declares no conflict of interest.

References

1. Posner, M.I.; Snyder, C.R.; Davidson, B.J. Attention and the detection of signals. *J. Exp. Psychol. Gen.* **1980**, *109*, 160. [CrossRef]
2. James, W. *The Principles of Psychology*; Henry Holt and Company: New York, NY, USA, 1890; pp. 402–458.
3. Von Helmholtz, H. (1896/1989). Physiological Optics (1896-2nd German Edition, translated by M. Mackeben, from Nakayama and Mackeben. *Vis. Res.* **1989**, *29*, 1631–1647.
4. Hurlbert, A.; Poggio, T. Spotlight on attention. *Trends Neurosci.* **1985**, *8*, 309–311. [CrossRef]
5. Johnston, W.A.; Dark, V.J. Selective attention. *Annu. Rev. Psychol.* **1986**, *37*, 43–75. [CrossRef]
6. Driver, J.; Baylis, G.C. Movement and visual attention: The spotlight metaphor breaks down. *J. Exp. Psychol. Hum. Percept. Perform.* **1989**, *15*, 448. [CrossRef] [PubMed]
7. Cave, K.R.; Bichot, N.P. Visuospatial attention: Beyond a spotlight model. *Psychon. Bull. Rev.* **1999**, *6*, 204–223. [CrossRef] [PubMed]
8. Tong, F. Splitting the spotlight of visual attention. *Neuron* **2004**, *42*, 524–526. [CrossRef]
9. Posner, M.I.; Petersen, S.E. The attention system of the human brain. *Annu. Rev. Neurosci.* **1990**, *13*, 25–42. [CrossRef]
10. Raz, A.; Buhle, J. Typologies of attentional networks. *Nat. Rev. Neurosci.* **2006**, *7*, 367. [CrossRef]
11. Capotosto, P.; Babiloni, C.; Romani, G.L.; Corbetta, M. Frontoparietal cortex controls spatial attention through modulation of anticipatory alpha rhythms. *J. Neurosci.* **2009**, *29*, 5863–5872. [CrossRef]
12. Berger, H. Über das elektrenkephalogramm des menschen. *Eur. Arch. Psychiatry Clin. Neurosci.* **1929**, *87*, 527–570. [CrossRef]
13. Gloor, P. Hans Berger on the electroencephalogram of man. The fourteen original reports on the human electroencephalogram. *Electroencephalogr. Clin. Neurophysiol.* **1969**, *28*, 507.

14. Berger, H. Ueber das Elektrenkephalogramm des Menschen. *J. Psychol. Neurol.* **1930**, *40*, 160–179.
15. Adrian, E.D.; Matthews, B.H. The Berger rhythm: Potential changes from the occipital lobes in man. *Brain* **1934**, *57*, 355–385. [CrossRef]
16. La Vaque, T.J. The history of EEG hans berger: Psychophysiologist. A historical vignette. *J. Neurother.* **1999**, *3*, 1–9. [CrossRef]
17. Millett, D. Hans Berger: From psychic energy to the EEG. *Perspect. Biol. Med.* **2001**, *44*, 522–542. [CrossRef]
18. Cantero, J.L.; Atienza, M.; Gómez, C.M.; Salas, R.M. Spectral structure and brain mapping of human alpha activities in different arousal states. *Neuropsychobiology* **1999**, *39*, 110–116. [CrossRef]
19. Shaw, J.C. *The Brain's Alpha Rhythms and the Mind*; BV Elsevier Science: Amsterdam, The Netherlands, 2003.
20. Jensen, O.; Mazaheri, A. Shaping functional architecture by oscillatory alpha activity: Gating by inhibition. *Front. Hum. Neurosci.* **2010**, *4*, 186. [CrossRef]
21. Foxe, J.J.; Snyder, A.C. The role of alpha-band brain oscillations as a sensory suppression mechanism during selective attention. *Front. Psychol.* **2011**, *2*, 154. [CrossRef]
22. Keitel, C.; Keitel, A.; Benwell, C.S.; Daube, C.; Thut, G.; Gross, J. Stimulus-driven brain rhythms within the alpha band: The attentional-modulation conundrum. *J. Neurosci.* **2019**, *39*, 3119–3129. [CrossRef]
23. Ray, W.J.; Cole, H.W. EEG alpha activity reflects attentional demands, and beta activity reflects emotional and cognitive processes. *Science* **1985**, *228*, 750–752. [CrossRef] [PubMed]
24. Klimesch, W.; Doppelmayr, M.; Russegger, H.; Pachinger, T.; Schwaiger, J. Induced alpha band power changes in the human EEG and attention. *Neurosci. Lett.* **1998**, *244*, 73–76. [CrossRef]
25. Foxe, J.J.; Simpson, G.V.; Ahlfors, S.P. Parieto-occipital ~10 Hz activity reflects anticipatory state of visual attention mechanisms. *Neuroreport* **1998**, *9*, 3929–3933. [CrossRef] [PubMed]
26. Worden, M.S.; Foxe, J.J.; Wang, N.; Simpson, G.V. Anticipatory biasing of visuospatial attention indexed by retinotopically specific-band electroencephalography increases over occipital cortex. *J. Neurosci.* **2000**, *20*, RC63. [CrossRef] [PubMed]
27. Sauseng, P.; Klimesch, W.; Stadler, W.; Schabus, M.; Doppelmayr, M.; Hanslmayr, S.; Gruber, W.R.; Birbaumer, N. A shift of visual spatial attention is selectively associated with human EEG alpha activity. *Eur. J. Neurosci.* **2005**, *22*, 2917–2926. [CrossRef] [PubMed]
28. Thut, G.; Nietzel, A.; Brandt, S.A.; Pascual-Leone, A. α-Band electroencephalographic activity over occipital cortex indexes visuospatial attention bias and predicts visual target detection. *J. Neurosci.* **2006**, *26*, 9494–9502. [CrossRef]
29. Doesburg, S.M.; Roggeveen, A.B.; Kitajo, K.; Ward, L.M. Large-scale gamma-band phase synchronization and selective attention. *Cereb. Cortex* **2008**, *18*, 386–396. [CrossRef]
30. Wyart, V.; Tallon-Baudry, C. Neural dissociation between visual awareness and spatial attention. *J. Neurosci.* **2008**, *28*, 2667–2679. [CrossRef]
31. Pantazis, D.; Simpson, G.V.; Weber, D.L.; Dale, C.L.; Nichols, T.E.; Leahy, R.M. A novel ANCOVA design for analysis of MEG data with application to a visual attention study. *NeuroImage* **2009**, *44*, 164–174. [CrossRef]
32. Banerjee, S.; Snyder, A.C.; Molholm, S.; Foxe, J.J. Oscillatory alpha-band mechanisms and the deployment of spatial attention to anticipated auditory and visual target locations: Supramodal or sensory-specific control mechanisms? *J. Neurosci.* **2011**, *31*, 9923–9932. [CrossRef]
33. Rohenkohl, G.; Nobre, A.C. Alpha oscillations related to anticipatory attention follow temporal expectations. *J. Neurosci.* **2011**, *31*, 14076–14084. [CrossRef] [PubMed]
34. Thorpe, S.; D'Zmura, M.; Srinivasan, R. Lateralization of frequency-specific networks for covert spatial attention to auditory stimuli. *Brain Topogr.* **2012**, *25*, 39–54. [CrossRef] [PubMed]
35. Rana, K.D.; Vaina, L.M. Functional roles of 10 Hz alpha-band power modulating engagement and disengagement of cortical networks in a complex visual motion task. *PLoS ONE* **2014**, *9*, e107715. [CrossRef] [PubMed]
36. Ikkai, A.; Dandekar, S.; Curtis, C.E. Lateralization in alpha-band oscillations predicts the locus and spatial distribution of attention. *PLoS ONE* **2016**, *11*, e0154796. [CrossRef] [PubMed]
37. Samaha, J.; Gosseries, O.; Postle, B.R. Distinct oscillatory frequencies underlie excitability of human occipital and parietal cortex. *J. Neurosci.* **2017**, *37*, 2824–2833. [CrossRef] [PubMed]
38. Kizuk, S.A.; Mathewson, K.E. Power and phase of alpha oscillations reveal an interaction between spatial and temporal visual attention. *J. Cogn. Neurosci.* **2017**, *29*, 480–494. [CrossRef] [PubMed]

39. Cosmelli, D.; López, V.; Lachaux, J.P.; López-Calderón, J.; Renault, B.; Martinerie, J.; Aboitiz, F. Shifting visual attention away from fixation is specifically associated with alpha band activity over ipsilateral parietal regions. *Psychophysiology* **2011**, *48*, 312–322. [CrossRef]
40. Treder, M.S.; Bahramisharif, A.; Schmidt, N.M.; Van Gerven, M.A.; Blankertz, B. Brain-computer interfacing using modulations of alpha activity induced by covert shifts of attention. *J. Neuroeng. Rehabil.* **2011**, *8*, 24. [CrossRef]
41. Martel, A.; Dähne, S.; Blankertz, B. EEG predictors of covert vigilant attention. *J. Neural Eng.* **2014**, *11*, 035009. [CrossRef]
42. Brüers, S.; VanRullen, R. Alpha power modulates perception independently of endogenous factors. *Front. Neurosci.* **2018**, *12*, 279. [CrossRef]
43. Lehmann, D. Multichannel topography of human alpha EEG fields. *Electroencephalogr. Clin. Neurophysiol.* **1971**, *31*, 439–449. [CrossRef]
44. Klimesch, W.; Doppelmayr, M.; Schimke, H.; Pachinger, T. Alpha frequency, reaction time, and the speed of processing information. *J. Clin. Neurophysiol.* **1996**, *13*, 511–518. [CrossRef] [PubMed]
45. Mulholland, T.; Runnals, S. Evaluation of attention and alertness with a stimulus-brain feedback loop. *Electroencephalogr. Clin. Neurophysiol.* **1962**, *14*, 847–852. [CrossRef]
46. Cooper, N.R.; Croft, R.J.; Dominey, S.J.; Burgess, A.P.; Gruzelier, J.H. Paradox lost? Exploring the role of alpha oscillations during externally vs. internally directed attention and the implications for idling and inhibition hypotheses. *Int. J. Psychophysiol.* **2003**, *47*, 65–74. [CrossRef]
47. Rihs, T.A.; Michel, C.M.; Thut, G. A bias for posterior α-band power suppression versus enhancement during shifting versus maintenance of spatial attention. *Neuroimage* **2009**, *44*, 190–199. [CrossRef] [PubMed]
48. Benedek, M.; Schickel, R.J.; Jauk, E.; Fink, A.; Neubauer, A.C. Alpha power increases in right parietal cortex reflects focused internal attention. *Neuropsychologia* **2014**, *56*, 393–400. [CrossRef] [PubMed]
49. Babiloni, C.; Miniussi, C.; Babiloni, F.; Carducci, F.; Cincotti, F.; Del Percio, C.; Sirello, G.; Fracassi, C.; Nobre, A.C.; Rossini, P.M. Sub-second "temporal attention" modulates alpha rhythms. A high-resolution EEG study. *Cogn. Brain Res.* **2004**, *19*, 259–268. [CrossRef]
50. Boncompte, G.; Villena-González, M.; Cosmelli, D.; López, V. Spontaneous alpha power lateralization predicts detection performance in an un-cued signal detection task. *PLoS ONE* **2016**, *11*, e0160347. [CrossRef]
51. Foster, J.J.; Sutterer, D.W.; Serences, J.T.; Vogel, E.K.; Awh, E. Alpha-band oscillations enable spatially and temporally resolved tracking of covert spatial attention. *Psychol. Sci.* **2017**, *28*, 929–941. [CrossRef]
52. Doesburg, S.M.; Bedo, N.; Ward, L.M. Top-down alpha oscillatory network interactions during visuospatial attention orienting. *Neuroimage* **2016**, *132*, 512–519. [CrossRef]
53. van Schouwenburg, M.R.; Zanto, T.P.; Gazzaley, A. Spatial attention and the effects of frontoparietal alpha band stimulation. *Front. Hum. Neurosci.* **2017**, *10*, 658. [CrossRef] [PubMed]
54. Proskovec, A.L.; Heinrichs-Graham, E.; Wiesman, A.I.; McDermott, T.J.; Wilson, T.W. Oscillatory dynamics in the dorsal and ventral attention networks during the reorienting of attention. *Hum. Brain Mapp.* **2018**, *39*, 2177–2190. [CrossRef] [PubMed]
55. Tognoli, E.; Lagarde, J.; DeGuzman, G.C.; Kelso, J.A.S. The phi complex as a neuromarker of human social coordination. *Proc. Natl. Acad. Sci. USA* **2007**, *104*, 8190–8195. [CrossRef] [PubMed]
56. Tognoli, E.; Kelso, J.A.S. The coordination dynamics of social neuromarkers. *Front. Hum. Neurosci.* **2015**, *9*, 563. [CrossRef] [PubMed]
57. Tognoli, E.; Kelso, J.A.S. The metastable brain. *Neuron* **2014**, *81*, 35–48. [CrossRef] [PubMed]
58. Bazanova, O.M.; Vernon, D. Interpreting EEG alpha activity. *Neurosci. Biobehav. Rev.* **2014**, *44*, 94–110. [CrossRef]
59. Calderon, R. Brain computer interface and neuroprosthetics. *ProQuest* **2007**. Available online: http://purl.flvc.org/fau/fd/FA00012509 (accessed on 2 November 2019).
60. Chatrian, G.E.; Lettich, E.; Nelson, P.L. Ten percent electrode system for topographic studies of spontaneous and evoked EEG activities. *Am. J. EEG Technol.* **1985**, *25*, 83–92. [CrossRef]
61. Picton, T.W.; Bentin, S.; Berg, P.; Donchin, E.; Hillyard, S.A.; Johnson, R.; Miller, G.A.; Ritter, W.; Ruchkin, D.S.; Rugg, M.D.; et al. Guidelines for using human event-related potentials to study cognition: Recording standards and publication criteria. *Psychophysiology* **2000**, *37*, 127–152. [CrossRef]
62. Tognoli, E.; Kelso, J.A.S. Brain coordination dynamics: True and false faces of phase synchrony and metastability. *Prog. Neurobiol.* **2009**, *87*, 31–40. [CrossRef]

63. Tognoli, E.; Kelso, J.A.S. Spectral dissociation of lateralized pairs of brain rhythms. *arXiv* **2013**, arXiv:1310.7662.
64. Zani, A.; Proverbio, A.M. How voluntary orienting of attention and alerting modulate costs of conflict processing. *Sci. Rep.* **2017**, *7*, 46701. [CrossRef] [PubMed]
65. Kulke, L.V.; Atkinson, J.; Braddick, O. Neural differences between covert and overt attention studied using EEG with simultaneous remote eye tracking. *Front. Hum. Neurosci.* **2016**, *10*, 592. [CrossRef] [PubMed]

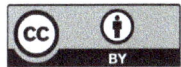

© 2019 by the author. Licensee MDPI, Basel, Switzerland. This article is an open access article distributed under the terms and conditions of the Creative Commons Attribution (CC BY) license (http://creativecommons.org/licenses/by/4.0/).

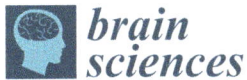

Communication

Cortical Resonance to Visible and Invisible Visual Rhythms

Claudio de'Sperati [1,2]

[1] Laboratory of Action, Perception and Cognition, Vita-Salute San Raffaele University, 20132-Milan, Italy; desperati.claudio@unisr.it
[2] Experimental Psychology Unit, Division of Neuroscience, IRCCS San Raffaele, 20132-Milan, Italy

Received: 19 December 2019; Accepted: 5 January 2020; Published: 9 January 2020

Abstract: Humans are rather poor in judging the right speed of video scenes. For example, a soccer match may be sped up so as to last only 80 min without observers noticing it. However, both adults and children seem to have a systematic, though often biased, notion of what should be the right speed of a given video scene. We therefore explored cortical responsiveness to video speed manipulations in search of possible differences between explicit and implicit speed processing. We applied sinusoidal speed modulations to a video clip depicting a naturalistic scene as well as a traditional laboratory visual stimulus (random dot kinematogram, RDK), and measured both perceptual sensitivity and cortical responses (steady-state visual evoked potentials, SSVEPs) to speed modulations. In five observers, we found a clear perceptual sensitivity increase and a moderate SSVEP amplitude increase with increasing speed modulation strength. Cortical responses were also found with weak, undetected speed modulations. These preliminary findings suggest that the cortex responds globally to periodic video speed modulations, even when observers do not notice them. This entrainment mechanism may be the basis of automatic resonance to the rhythms of the external world.

Keywords: perception; video; visual motion; speed; cortex; rhythm; entrainment

1. Introduction

The capability of judging the correct speed of a dynamic scene in a video clip is surprisingly poor. We have recently shown that (i) speeding up a soccer match video by as much as 12% goes completely undetected [1]; (ii) there are systematic biases in judging the correct video speed, often consisting of speed underestimation [2]; and (iii) 6–7-year-old children judge videos to be slower, as compared to older children and adults [3]. Thus, it appears that there is a mechanism in the brain that implicitly codes a subjective "right" speed of events. This mechanism seems to be specific to event speed, as judgments of video clip speed and video clip duration are not correlated [2].

These findings led us to ask how the speed of a complex video scene is coded in the brain. Taking a somewhat different approach as compared to existing work on visual speed processing [4,5], in this exploratory study we addressed the capability of detecting speed manipulations of complex visual stimuli, both a naturalistic video clip and a laboratory stimulus (random dot kinematogram, RDK). We also had a more specific aim: given that observers appear to be unaware of even large video speed changes, and yet are apparently capable of providing systematic, though often biased, judgments about video speed, there must be a processing stage that automatically and covertly codes the expected speed given the available contextual cues. This processing stage may involve sensory mechanisms, decisional mechanisms, or both. Here, we searched for possible neural correlates of the former, namely, subliminal speed processing. As an initial step towards a more comprehensive understanding of complex visual speed tuning, we recorded perceptual as well as cortical responses to a simple manipulation of the visual stimuli, namely, sinusoidal speed modulation.

2. Materials and Methods

2.1. Participants

Five adult participants aged between 21 and 35 (all females) took part in this experiment on a voluntary basis and gave informed consent prior to the beginning of the experiments. They had normal or corrected-to-normal vision and had no history of neurological diseases. This study was conducted in accordance with the principles of the Declaration of Helsinki and the "Comitato Etico San Raffaele".

2.2. Stimuli and Tasks

Observers were seated 57 cm in front of a laptop screen. Visual stimuli (Figure 1) consisted of (i) a video clip (1280 × 720 @ 30 Hz) depicting sea ripples on a beach that we had previously used [2]; and (ii) a random dot kinematogram (RDK) (3000 black and white dots, 67 ms lifetime, 5 deg/s maximal speed, 0% coherence). In order to modulate video speed, the frame-rate of the visual stimulus was sinusoidally modulated (frequency, 1, 2, or 4 Hz; amplitude, 10%, 30%, or 50% of the original frame-rate) by controlling in real time the video frame flipping on the graphics board (Nvidia GTX 1060, Santa Clara, CA, USA). As a result, videos acquired a pulsatory rhythm. To ensure uniform conditions in extracting cortical oscillations (see below), in each trial there were 50 speed-modulation cycles regardless of the modulation frequency. Therefore, trials lasted 50, 25, or 12.5 s, respectively, for speed modulations of 1, 2, and 4 Hz. Observers kept their gaze in central fixation and watched the videos while wearing an electroencephalographic (EEG) recording headset (18 trials: 3 frequencies × 3 amplitudes for each visual stimulus, randomly interleaved). They were asked to mentally focus on the pulsation of the visual stimulus. Overall, the session lasted about 20 min.

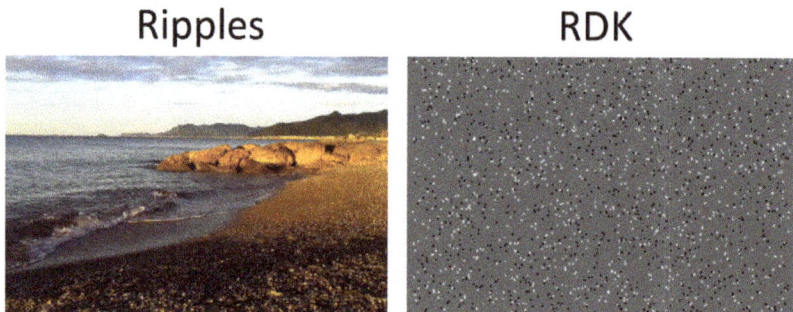

Figure 1. A snapshot of the dynamic visual stimuli used in this study. They were displayed with various sinusoidal speed modulations, which conferred to them a pulsating appearance. In the experiment, there was also a central fixation dot. RDK—random dot kinematogram.

In a second experimental session, administered on a different day, observers rated in a 9-point scale the perceived strength of the pulsation (108 trials: 3 frequencies × 4 amplitudes × 9 repetitions—including catch trials with zero amplitude, i.e., no speed modulation). Observers were specifically instructed to rate the perceived intensity (strength) of sinusoidal speed modulation. Phenomenally, such rhythmic speed modulation appeared as a pulsation, periodically speeding up and slowing down the stimulus at the experimentally imposed frequency (i.e., 1, 2 or 4 Hz). Stimuli and other conditions were the same as in the first session, except that observers could respond whenever they wished. Overall, the session lasted about 30 min.

2.3. EEG Recordings

Scalp electrical activity was recorded through an Enobio device (Neuroelectrics; eight channels, O1, O2, P3, P4, C1, C2, F3, F4; sampling frequency 500 Hz), using the right ear lobe as reference. Electrodes were gel-based passive plates (Ag/AgCl coated; impedance <5 kΩ) and were placed on the scalp by means of an EEG cap. EEG traces were band-pass filtered (0.1–100 Hz).

2.4. Data Analyses

To quantify perceptual responses, we used the subjective estimates of video speed modulation strength (pulsation rating). By separating null (rating = 0) and non-null (rating > 0) responses, we transformed gradual judgments into dichotomous yes/no responses, and we applied a signal detection analysis [6]. Basically, the rating task was treated as a multiple yes/no detection task [7], from which we calculated hit rate (non-null responses in signal trials, i.e., trials in which speed was modulated) and false alarm rate (non-null responses in noise trials, i.e., trials in which speed was not modulated). A correction for extreme values was applied [8]. Given the ten-point rating scale used in this experiment, there were nine possible pairs of hits and false alarms: ratings greater than 0 were first considered to be "yes" responses, while a 0 rating was considered to be a "no" response; next, ratings greater than 1 were considered to be "yes" responses, while ratings less than 2 were considered to be "no" responses, and so on, until encompassing all nine pairs of hits and false alarms. A receiver operating characteristic (ROC) curve was thus fitted and the area under the curve (AUC) computed. For each observer, and for each amplitude and frequency of the two stimuli, the perceptual sensitivity to video speed modulation was obtained by converting the AUC into a corresponding d' index [6].

To quantify cortical responses, we used the Eeglab software ERP averaging tool pop_averager [9] to obtain the averaged traces of each channel over 1-s time windows. Each averaged trace was then fitted to a sinusoidal model (through the Matlab fit function) to compute the cortical response strength, measured as the peak amplitude of the fitted function.

Both the perceptual and the cortical responses were subjected to generalized linear mixed models analysis (GLMM, with diagonal covariance pattern, normal distribution and identity link). The frequency (Freq) and amplitude (Ampl) of video speed modulation were fixed factors, while the video clip (Clip) and participant (Subj) were modeled as random intercept terms to reduce overfitting [10]. Following [11], the recording channel (Chan) for the EEG analysis was also modeled as a random intercept term. The dependent variables were either perceptual sensitivity (PS) or the amplitude of the fitted sinusoidal function (FA). The models were thus "PS ~ 1 + Freq * Ampl + (1 | Clip) + (1 | Subj)" and "FA ~ 1 + Freq * Ampl + (1 | Clip) + (1 | Subj) + (1 | Chan)", respectively, for perceptual and cortical data.

3. Results

Observers' capability of detecting video speed modulation is shown in Figure 2. With weak signals (10% amplitude of video speed modulation), perceptual sensitivity to speed modulation was practically null with both Ripples and RDK video clips (confidence intervals crossed zero in all cases), but increased significantly with speed modulation amplitude. Neither speed modulation frequency nor the interaction frequency × amplitude reached statistical significance (Table 1).

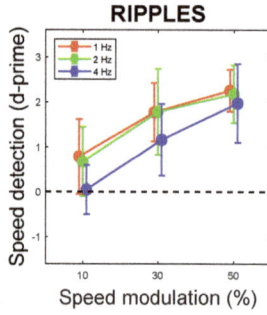 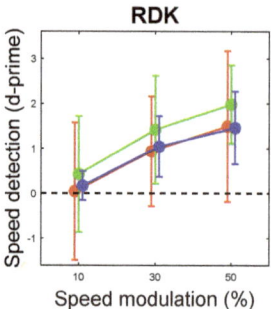

Figure 2. Perceptual sensitivity to video speed modulation as a function of video speed modulation amplitude (10%, 30%, and 50%) and frequency (1, 2, and 4 Hz), shown separately for Ripples and RDK videos. Error bars are 95% confidence intervals.

Table 1. Results of the generalized linear mixed models (GLMM) analysis of perceptual sensitivity.

	e	t	d	p	l	u
Amplitude	0.036	4.437	86	<0.001	0.020	0.051
Frequency	−0.0136	−1.312	86	0.193	−0.341	0.070
Amplitude:Frequency	0.001	0.402	86	0.689	−0.005	0.007

Video speed modulation amplitude, but not frequency, or their interaction, was statistically significant. Abbreviations: e—coefficient estimate, t—t-statistics (Wald t-test), d—degrees of freedom, p—p-value, l—lower confidence bound, u—upper confidence bound.

By contrast, cortical oscillatory responses (steady-state visual evoked potentials, SSVEPs) were found at all video speed modulation amplitudes, with mean adjusted R^2 for the sinusoidal fittings ranging from 13% to 36%, which indicated that a relevant component of cortical activity was pulsating at the stimulus frequency. Although an evident oscillation could not be discerned in all traces (e.g., the 4 Hz, 10% condition of Figure 3), in many cases the cortical potentials followed the rhythm of the video speed (e.g., the 2 Hz, 10% condition of Figure 3). SSVEP amplitude, as computed through sinusoidal fitting, was significantly above zero at all amplitudes and frequencies of speed modulation, as shown by confidence intervals (Figure 4). Also, SSVEP amplitude tended to moderately but significantly increase as speed modulation amplitude increased, though not as steeply as perceptual sensitivity. Speed modulation frequency, but not the interaction frequency × amplitude, also reached statistical significance. The results of these analyses are reported in Table 2. Note also that Figure 3 suggests little SSVEP differentiation across the cortex: indeed, there was a large overlap among the random coefficients of the eight recording channels, with the highest contribution to SSVEP variability coming from F4 (Table 3).

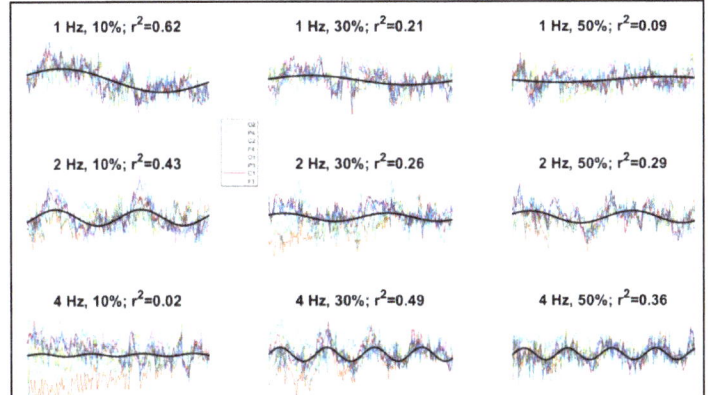

Figure 3. Examples of electroencephalographic (EEG) recordings from one participant showing the traces from all channels (shown in different colors, see legend), averaged across a 1-s time window and superimposed. The sinusoidal best-fitting curves are also shown (black lines; for graphical simplicity, here only a single curve averaged across channels is shown). Also reported are the values of stimulus modulation frequency, stimulus modulation strength, and adjusted R^2 of the fitted functions.

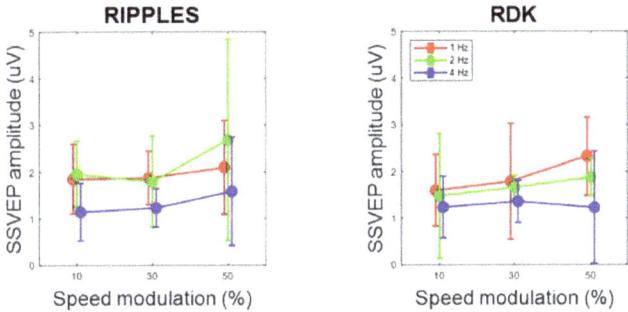

Figure 4. Steady-state visual evoked potential (SSVEP) amplitude as a function of speed modulation amplitude and frequency, shown separately for Ripples and RDK videos. Data have been averaged across participants. Error bars are 95% confidence intervals.

Table 2. Results of the GLMM analysis of SSVEP amplitude.

	e	t	d	p	l	u
Amplitude	16.439	3.030	716	0.003	5.789	27.090
Frequency	−144.841	−2.068	716	0.039	−282.341	−7.341
Amplitude:Frequency	−2.542	−1.240	716	0.215	−6.568	1.484

Video speed modulation amplitude and frequency, but not their interaction, were statistically significant. See Table 1 for abbreviations.

Table 3. Coefficient estimates resulting from the GLMM analysis of SSVEP amplitude for the eight recording channels. See text and Table 1 for abbreviations.

Channel	e	t	d	p	l	u
O1	153.240	1.218	716	0.224	400.210	93.734
O2	85.014	0.676	716	0.499	331.990	161.960
P3	30.566	0.243	716	0.808	277.540	216.410
P4	185.070	1.471	716	0.142	61.900	432.040
C1	141.630	1.126	716	0.261	388.610	105.340
C2	231.030	1.834	716	0.067	478.000	15.944
F3	78.625	0.625	716	0.532	168.350	325.600
F4	377.780	3.003	716	0.003	130.810	624.750

In Table 4, the effect sizes for both perceptual and cortical responses are reported. Perceptual responses tended to be more affected by speed modulation amplitude than speed modulation frequency, whereas the opposite held for cortical responses.

Table 4. Estimates of effect size (partial η^2) of video speed modulation amplitude and frequency on perceptual and cortical responses, shown separately for Ripples and RDK stimuli.

	Perceptual Responses		Cortical Responses	
	Ripples	RDK	Ripples	RDK
Amplitude	0.598	0.649	0.249	0.170
Frequency	0.164	0.172	0.440	0.381

4. Discussion

The present study provided initial evidence for (i) cortical oscillatory responsivity to speed modulation in videos either representing a naturalistic scene (a video clip of ripples on the beach) or RDK (with no directional information), and (ii) dissociation between perceptual and cortical responses, consisting in the presence of cortical responses with the perceptually invisible lowest stimulus strength.

4.1. Shape and Distribution of Cortical Responses

In some cases, SSVEPs presented rather smooth, sinusoidal-like signal variations, while in other cases more abrupt changes were observed. In this preliminary study, we took an agnostic position as to the actual shape of the cortical response and used sinusoidal fitting as a simple method to quantify the periodicity of scalp potentials, at the cost of losing the details of the full cortical response. We remark, however, that the choice of using sinusoidal fitting was by no means meant to imply that in our conditions SSVEPs had sinusoidal-like waveforms, as is the case with traditional SSVEP protocols where higher stimulus frequencies are used [12]. Given the relatively low frequency of our stimuli, an alternative way to analyze the data would be to use the traditional event-related approach (e.g., finding the peaks and latencies of the various components), which would require, however, a more thorough and systematic consideration of the actual appearance of this particular speed-related cortical potential, including identifying the relevant components. Future work will allow full characterization of this cortical response.

A somewhat unexpected finding was an apparent lack of clear regional differentiation in the amplitude of cortical responses. Luminance-evoked VEPs, as well as cortical responses to motion onset [13–17], involve mainly posterior cortical areas. Yet, in our study, the coefficients for the random effect of a channel were largely overlapping, with only a single electrode (F4) showing a contribution larger than the other ones. One possible explanation is that the oscillatory rhythm we impressed on video clips results in global cortical entrainment, with several components at play (e.g., sensory, attentional, motor, imaginative). Indeed, the instruction to mentally focus on visual pulsation may have favored such multi-component entrainment, making these responses quite different from typical motion-evoked cortical responses. Strictly speaking, our RDK stimuli were not even motion stimuli but speed stimuli (no luminance or directional information), and rhythm/pulsation was the main distinguishing phenomenal characteristic of both RDK and naturalistic stimuli used in the present study. For this reason, they are likely to induce high-level resonance that may go beyond sensory stimulation (see, e.g., [18] for a similar consideration in the auditory domain).

Alternatively, our approach might simply not have been fine-grained enough to detect small regional differences. It is possible that with a more in-depth approach (e.g., high-density electroencephalography with event-related component analyses and source reconstruction) and a larger sample size, some differences would emerge.

4.2. Attentive Subliminal Resonance

We found diffuse cortical responses with the weakest video speed modulation (10%), a condition that was associated with null perceptual sensitivity. This phenomenon calls for subliminal speed entrainment, indicative of an automatic resonance process, which may qualify as a form of attentive subliminal processing [19], or at least at the fringe of awareness. By further noting the disparity between the steep increase in perceptual sensitivity at increasing speed modulation amplitudes and the corresponding very moderate increase in cortical responsiveness, it is tempting to speculate that, at least for certain phenomena, global cortical activation to visual stimuli may reflect automatic processing without necessarily being the signature of perceptual awareness.

However, especially when null results are obtained under low statistical power, it should be borne in mind that "absence of evidence" rather than "evidence of absence" is the proper underlying notion. Furthermore, when the goal is to measure perceptual awareness, null results can be problematic on their own, as it is often difficult to clearly tease apart null from fringe perception [20]. Perceptual ratings may help in this regard, as they involve more gradual responses rather than gross dichotomous responses [21]. Exploiting all possible response criteria behind perceptual ratings through the ROC curve afforded a reliable index of perceptual awareness [6]. Thus, pending further investigation with a larger sample size (see below), we believe that most stimuli with 10% speed modulation were closer to a condition of null than fringe speed modulation perception.

4.3. Limitations

The first limitation of this exploratory study is obviously the small sample size. While for some psychophysical designs this numerosity may be reasonable, to provide good statistical power, and also to address possible individual differences, the number of participants should be increased.

Another limitation is the small number of EEG electrodes. With eight electrodes, we did not even attempt to compute a spatial map of cortical activity. This issue should be addressed with more sophisticated EEG recordings and analyses. Our goal here was simply to provide initial evidence of cortical entrainment.

We should also note a limitation of the experimental design. For practical reasons, we administered the cortical recording session before the perceptual session. This could have introduced a carry-over effect, i.e., observers' higher sensitivity in the perceptual session as a result of learning. This could be one reason for the steeper rise of perceptual responses with video speed modulation amplitude, as compared to cortical responses. Note, however, that the direction of such carry-over effect, if any (the cortical session being administered before the perceptual session, and not vice-versa), would reinforce the evidence for a dissociation between cortical and perceptual responses: the perceptual responses in the trials with the lowest speed modulation strength were statistically indistinguishable from the responses in the trials without speed modulation, despite the possible beneficial effect of previous exposure to the stimuli.

Funding: This research was partly funded by *Fondazione Cariplo*, grant #2018-0858.

Acknowledgments: The author thanks Luca Mesin, Tatiana Baroni, and Regina Gregori-Grgič for their help with EEG instrumentation, recordings, and analyses.

Conflicts of Interest: The author declares no conflict of interest.

References

1. De'Sperati, C.; Baud Bovy, G. Low perceptual sensitivity to altered video speed in viewing a soccer match. *Sci. Rep.* **2017**, *7*, 15379. [CrossRef] [PubMed]
2. Rossi, F.; Montanaro, E.; de'Sperati, C. Speed Biases With Real-Life Video Clips. *Front. Integr. Neurosci.* **2018**, *12*, 11. [CrossRef]
3. Zuliani, E.; Caputi, M.; Scaini, S.; de'Sperati, C. Videos look faster as children grow up: Sense of speed and impulsivity throughout primary school. *J. Exp. Child. Psychol.* **2019**, *179*, 190–211. [CrossRef]
4. Burr, D.; Thompson, P. Motion psychophysics: 1985–2010. *Vis. Res.* **2011**, *51*, 1431–1456. [CrossRef] [PubMed]
5. Nishimoto, S.; Vu, A.T.; Naselaris, T.; Benjamini, Y.; Yu, B.; Gallant, J.L. Reconstructing visual experiences from brain activity evoked by natural movies. *Curr. Biol. CB* **2011**, *21*, 1641–1646. [CrossRef] [PubMed]
6. Macmillan, N.A.; Creelman, C.D. *Detection Theory: A User's Guide*, 2nd ed.; Lawrence Erlbaum Associates: Mahwah, NJ, USA, 2005.
7. Gregori Grgic, R.; Crespi, S.A.; de'Sperati, C. Assessing Self-Awareness through Gaze Agency. *PLoS ONE* **2016**, *11*, e0164682. [CrossRef] [PubMed]
8. Brown, G.S.; White, K.G. The optimal correction for estimating extreme discriminability. *Behav. Res. Methods* **2005**, *37*, 436–449. [CrossRef] [PubMed]
9. Delorme, A.; Makeig, S. EEGLAB: An open source toolbox for analysis of single-trial EEG dynamics including independent component analysis. *J. Neurosci. Methods* **2004**, *134*, 9–21. [CrossRef] [PubMed]
10. Bates, D.; Kliegl, R.; Vasishth, S.; Baayen, R. Parsimonious mixed models. *arXiv* **2018**, arXiv:1506.04967.
11. Payne, B.R.; Lee, C.L.; Federmeier, K.D. Revisiting the incremental effects of context on word processing: Evidence from single-word event-related brain potentials. *Psychophysiology* **2015**, *52*, 1456–1469. [CrossRef] [PubMed]
12. Vialatte, F.B.; Maurice, M.; Dauwels, J.; Cichocki, A. Steady-state visually evoked potentials: Focus on essential paradigms and future perspectives. *Prog. Neurobiol.* **2010**, *90*, 418–438. [CrossRef] [PubMed]
13. Snowden, R.J.; Ullrich, D.; Bach, M. Isolation and characteristics of a steady-state visually-evoked potential in humans related to the motion of a stimulus. *Vis. Res.* **1995**, *35*, 1365–1373. [CrossRef]
14. Niedeggen, M.; Wist, E.R. Characteristics of visual evoked potentials generated by motion coherence onset. *Brain Res. Cogn. Brain Res.* **1999**, *8*, 95–105. [CrossRef]
15. Patzwahl, D.R.; Zanker, J.M. Mechanisms of human motion perception: Combining evidence from evoked potentials, behavioural performance and computational modelling. *Eur. J. Neurosci.* **2000**, *12*, 273–282. [CrossRef] [PubMed]
16. Braddick, O.J.; O'Brien, J.M.; Wattam-Bell, J.; Atkinson, J.; Hartley, T.; Turner, R. Brain areas sensitive to coherent visual motion. *Perception* **2001**, *30*, 61–72. [CrossRef] [PubMed]
17. Kuba, M.; Kubova, Z.; Kremlacek, J.; Langrova, J. Motion-onset VEPs: Characteristics, methods, and diagnostic use. *Vis. Res.* **2007**, *47*, 189–202. [CrossRef] [PubMed]
18. Nozaradan, S.; Peretz, I.; Missal, M.; Mouraux, A. Tagging the neuronal entrainment to beat and meter. *J. Neurosci. Off. J. Soc. Neurosci.* **2011**, *31*, 10234–10240. [CrossRef] [PubMed]
19. Dehaene, S.; Changeux, J.P.; Naccache, L.; Sackur, J.; Sergent, C. Conscious, preconscious, and subliminal processing: A testable taxonomy. *Trends Cogn. Sci.* **2006**, *10*, 204–211. [CrossRef] [PubMed]
20. Merikle, P.M.; Smilek, D.; Eastwood, J.D. Perception without awareness: Perspectives from cognitive psychology. *Cognition* **2001**, *79*, 115–134. [CrossRef]
21. Overgaard, M.; Rote, J.; Mouridsen, K.; Ramsoy, T. Is conscious perception gradual or dychotomous? A comparison of report methodologies during a visual task. *Conscious. Cogn.* **2006**, *15*, 700–708. [CrossRef] [PubMed]

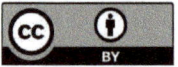

© 2020 by the author. Licensee MDPI, Basel, Switzerland. This article is an open access article distributed under the terms and conditions of the Creative Commons Attribution (CC BY) license (http://creativecommons.org/licenses/by/4.0/).

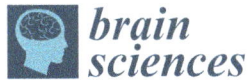

Article

On the Relationship between P3 Latency and Mental Ability as a Function of Increasing Demands in a Selective Attention Task

Tugba Kapanci [1], Sarah Merks [2], Thomas H. Rammsayer [3] and Stefan J. Troche [3,*]

[1] Department of Psychology and Psychotherapy, University of Witten/Herdecke, 58448 Witten, Germany; tugba.kapanci@uni-wh.de (T.K.)
[2] Institute Human in Complex Systems, School for Applied Psychology, University of Applied Sciences and Arts Northwestern Switzerland, 4600 Olten, Switzerland; sarah.merks@fhnw.ch (S.M.)
[3] Institute for Psychology, University of Bern, 3012 Bern, Switzerland; thomas.rammsayer@psy.unibe.ch (T.H.R.)
* Correspondence: stefan.troche@psy.unibe.ch; Tel.: +41-31-631-31-24

Received: 30 December 2018; Accepted: 24 January 2019; Published: 29 January 2019

Abstract: The mental speed approach to individual differences in mental ability (MA) is based on the assumption of higher speed of information processing in individuals with higher than those with lower MA. Empirical support of this assumption has been inconsistent when speed was measured by means of the P3 latency in the event-related potential (ERP). The present study investigated the association between MA and P3 latency as a function of task demands on selective attention. For this purpose, 20 men and 90 women performed on a standard continuous performance test (CPT1 condition) as well as on two further task conditions with lower (CPT0) and higher demands (CPT2) on selective attention. MA and P3 latency negatively correlated in the standard CPT, and this negative relationship even increased systematically from the CPT1 to the CPT2 condition but was absent in the CPT0 condition. The present results indicate that task demands on selective attention are decisive to observe the expected shorter P3 latency in individuals with higher compared to those with lower MA.

Keywords: selective attention; mental ability; P3 latency; continuous performance test; mental speed

1. Introduction

Individuals with higher compared to those with lower mental ability (MA) have been reported to have shorter reaction times (RTs) in a wide range of elementary cognitive tasks (ECTs) [1–3]. ECTs are so easy that individuals with higher and lower MA do not differ in the number of errors or the use of cognitive strategies but only in speed of task completion. The most common explanation of the faster information processing in individuals with higher compared to those with lower MA refers to a more efficient information transmission in the central nervous system [4,5]. It should be noted that MA-related differences in mental speed can be observed in simple RT tasks but usually increase with increasing task demands [6–8]. Only after exceeding a certain level of task demands the relation between MA and RT decreases in favor of an increasing relation between MA and error rates in the experimental task [9,10].

To further elucidate the mechanisms underlying the relation between MA and speed of information processing, psychophysiological studies have probed whether MA-related speed differences can also be identified in the latencies of the event-related potential (ERP) [5,11]. ERP is an electrophysiological response to specific events or stimuli [12], which can be observed in an electroencephalogram (EEG). Different aspects of stimulus processing have been demonstrated to be related to the positive and negative components of ERP [13]. The P3 component, also referred to as P300 and first described by Sutton [14], is a very pronounced positive wave with a maximum peak at about 300 ms after presentation of a stimulus. If the stimulus is presented but not attended to, the P3 component does not (or only rudimentarily) emerge, indicating that the P3 component reflects the allocation of attentional resources [13,15–17]. More specifically, the P3 component is assumed to represent attention-related inhibition of ongoing brain activity to facilitate the consolidation of the target's mental representation in working memory [15,16]. P3 latency, defined as the time interval between stimulus onset and the peak of the P3 wave, has been assumed to be a reliable index of the time needed to evaluate and categorize a presented stimulus [18–22]. As suggested by Verleger's [23] thorough review, however, the view of P3 latency as a pure speed measure of cognitive processes unrelated to response processes might be premature, since P3 latency is also sensitive to delays in response selection when responses are given fast.

As an electrophysiological and reliable measure of speed of information processing [24], P3 latency also received much attention as a possible correlate of MA. In contrast to RT, however, P3 latency was found to be less consistently related to MA, with the majority of studies investigating young adults (but see Reference [25]). In simple and choice RT tasks, for example, a relation between P3 latency and MA could not be obtained [22,26,27]. Houlihan et al. [28] reported a positive relationship between MA and P3 latency in a short-term memory scanning task, whereas McGarry-Roberts et al. [22] reported MA to be negatively related to the P3 latencies derived from a short-term and a long-term memory task. The only task showing consistently the expected negative functional relation between P3 latency and MA was the oddball task with shorter P3 latencies in higher- compared to lower-MA individuals [25,29–33].

From the inconsistent results on the relation between MA and P3 latency, it can be concluded that P3 latency is not in general related to MA. Rather, this relation seems to depend on the respective task used to elicit the P3 component or, in other words, on the specific cognitive processes required by the given task. For example, P3 latency associated with simple or choice reaction time was consistently unrelated to MA [22,27,28], while studies on MA and P3 latency associated with short-term memory scanning produced inconsistent results [22,28]. To date, little empirical support is available for a functional relation between MA and P3 latency associated with long-term memory retrieval [22]. Only the information processing required by the oddball task led to a consistent relation between the associated P3 latency and MA. Thus, the oddball task represents a good starting point for a systematic investigation of the task conditions and, thus, the required cognitive processes necessary to yield faster P3 latencies in individuals with higher than those with lower MA. In the following, we outline why we expect that selective attention is the crucial cognitive process underlying the negative relation between P3 latency and MA.

The oddball task consists of a series of standard stimuli (e.g., the letter "O") infrequently interrupted by the "oddball" (e.g., the letter "X"), to which participants respond. In other words, the task requires to direct attention selectively to an infrequently presented target and to respond with a key press. Given these task characteristics, the oddball task is reminiscent of the continuous performance test (CPT) [34]. With the CPT, the participants' task is to monitor a stream of letters successively presented on a monitor screen and to press a designated key in response to a prespecified target letter (e.g. "X"). According to Riccio et al. [35], the CPT is one of the most popular clinical tasks to assess sustained attention and vigilance by means of RT and error scores. A most obvious difference between the oddball task and the CPT is that the distractors are always the same (frequent) stimulus in the oddball task, whereas different distractor stimuli are used in the CPT. Nevertheless, the attentional demands of both tasks (i.e., identifying a target among distractors for a given period of time) are highly similar.

Given these similarities between the CPT and the oddball task, the first assumption to be investigated in the present study was that the target-related P3 latency in the CPT is negatively associated with MA as suggested by the findings with the oddball task. In addition, we assumed that the selective-attention demands on the identification of a target among distractors are decisive for the relation between P3 latency and MA. To investigate this hypothesis, two further CPT conditions were applied in the present study. In a control condition, the process of selective identification will be eliminated by omitting distractor stimuli from the task and presenting only target stimuli. The absence of distractors should reduce the demands on selective attention. If these demands, in fact, account for the observed relation between MA and P3 latency, the negative association between MA and P3 latency would be expected to vanish in the control condition.

In the case that the process of selectively identifying a target among distractors is the decisive process underlying the relation between P3 latency and MA, this relation should become stronger with increasing task demands on selective attention. To test this hypothesis, in an attention-enhanced CPT condition, the demands on selective attention were experimentally increased. For this purpose, the stream of letters contained a regular as well as an italic 'X' as 'invalid' and 'valid' target letter, respectively. The italic 'X', but not the regular 'X', was defined as the valid target stimulus. Participants were instructed to identify and to respond to the valid target letter (X) but to ignore the invalid target letter (X) as a distractor. Thus, during the process of correctly identifying the valid target stimulus, the letter as well as the font type needed to be attended to. If selective-attention demands for identifying targets among distractors represent the crucial source underlying the functional relationship between P3 latency and MA, the association between MA and the target-related P3 latency should increase in this latter condition compared to the standard CPT condition. With this approach, the present study aims to elucidate the necessary preconditions for a negative relationship between MA and P3 latency to occur. Learning more about these preconditions will contribute to a better understanding and conceptual expansion of the mental-speed approach to MA.

2. Materials and Methods

2.1. Participants

The sample consisted of 116 German-speaking undergraduate students. Due to extremely long RTs in one of the three CPT conditions (four participants) or implausibly low scores in the intelligence test (two participants), six participants were discarded from further analysis. The remaining 90 female and 20 male participants ranged in age from 18 to 36 years (mean = 22.0 years; standard deviation = 3.1 years). They reported normal hearing and normal or corrected-to-normal vision. Only healthy participants were tested and asked to refrain from caffeine and nicotine intake 2 h and from consuming alcohol at least 24 h prior to the EEG recording. As compensation for their participation, participants received course credit. Prior to testing, all participants gave their written informed consent. The study was conducted in accordance with the Declaration of Helsinki and the study protocol was approved by the ethics committee of the Faculty of Human Sciences of the University of Bern (Bern, Switzerland) (date of approval: 26 August 2013; project identification code: No. 2013-8-504570).

2.2. Assessment of Psychometric Intelligence

As a measure of MA, the German version of Cattell's Culture Fair Test-20 R (CFT-20 R) [36] was used. It consisted of three subtests with 27 items (series, classifications, and matrices) and one subtest with 20 items (topologies). Weiss [36] reported test–retest reliabilities ranging from $r_{tt} = 0.80$ to $r_{tt} = 0.90$. Test-taking time was about 60 minutes.

2.3. Continuous Performance Test (CPT)

Apparatus and stimuli. All stimuli were presented on a 17" Dell computer monitor. Stimulus presentation was controlled by E-prime 2.0 experimental software (Psychology Software Tools, Inc., Sharpsburg, PA, USA). Stimuli were the letter X (target stimulus) and the letters G, D, A, W, M, S, K, and R (distractors) presented with a height of 1 cm and a width of 0.5 cm. All stimuli were presented in white font (Courier New, size: 28) against a black background. Participants' responses were recorded by a Cedrus®response pad (RB-830) (Cedrus Corporation, San Pedro, CA, USA) with an accuracy of ± 1 ms.

Procedure. Individual experimental testing and EEG recording took place in a sound-attenuated and electrically shielded room. Participants were seated in front of the computer monitor with a distance of 50 cm ensured by a chin rest.

The experimental task consisted of three conditions (CPT0, CPT1, and CPT2). In all three conditions, a trial started with the presentation of a stimulus for 200 ms, followed by a black screen for 1000 ms. The next trial started after an intertrial interval randomly varying between 0 ms and 1000 ms.

In the 120 trials of the standard CPT condition (henceforth CPT1), the target stimulus ('X') was presented in 24 trials, and each of the eight distractors was presented in 12 trials. Participants were required to respond only to the target by pressing a designated response key as fast as possible (but to avoid errors). The order of trials was randomized. The second condition (CPT0), serving as a control condition, consisted of 32 trials. In each trial, the letter 'X' was presented. Participants were instructed to respond to the onset of the 'X' as fast as possible (but to avoid errors) by pressing the response key. Responses were recorded during the 1200-ms duration of a trial. The attention-enhanced condition (CPT2) was composed of 240 trials. The target stimulus was the letter 'X' (in italic font) presented in 24 trials. In addition to the abovementioned letters, which were presented in 192 trials, the letter 'X' (non-italic font) served as distractor in 24 trials. Participants were requested to respond to the 'X' in italic font as fast as possible but neither to the distractors nor to the 'X' in non-italic font. The duration of the CPT0 condition was about 1'15 min; the durations of the CPT1 and CPT2 conditions were 4'30 and 8'45 min, respectively.

Prior to the task, a general instruction was given and specific instructions; practice trials also preceded each task condition. The order of the three conditions was counter-balanced across participants. The total time to perform the CPT was about 15 to 20 min. As dependent variables, mean RT and error rates in each condition for each participant were determined. Mean RT was based on correct trials with RTs between 100 ms and 1200 ms. Error rates were analyzed separately for errors of omission (failure to respond to a target stimulus) and commission (responding erroneously to a distractor stimulus).

Electrophysiological recording. During the CPT, EEG was recorded using a BrainAmp®amplifier (Brain Products GmbH, Gilching, Germany) and an electrode cap (EasyCap GmbH, Woerthsee-Etterschlag, Germany), with 12 Ag/AgCl electrodes referenced to the ear lobes. To control vertical and horizontal eye movements, electrodes were fixed below and above the right eye (vertical electrooculogram) and at the temples (horizontal electrooculogram). Impedances were kept below 5 kΩ. The sampling rate for the EEG signal was 1000 Hz, and the resolution was 0.1 µV. For further analyses, BrainVision Analyzer 2 (Brain Products GmbH, Gilching, Germany) was used. The EEG data were high-pass (0.1 Hz) and low-pass filtered (30 Hz). Eye movements were corrected by the regression-based method as proposed by Gratton, Coles, and Donchin [37]. The EEG was segmented based on the markers from the CPT sent with every onset of a stimulus. The duration of each segment was 1000 ms, with a 100-ms pre-stimulus and a 900-ms post-stimulus interval. Using a semiautomatic artifact rejection, segments with a voltage change above 500 µV within 1 ms, voltage changes above 200 µV within 200 ms, and values above 100 µV and under −100 µV were marked and rejected semiautomatically. A baseline correction for the pre-stimulus interval was done for each segment. Finally, the segments referring to the targets of each condition were averaged for each participant. A semiautomatic peak detection helped to find out the largest positive deflection for each individual within a time interval ranging from 190 to 550 ms after stimulus onset. If necessary, the peak was manually adjusted. This peak was considered as P3 amplitude. We focused on the PZ electrode site where the P3 component had the largest deflection in all three task conditions. The time between stimulus onset and this peak was defined as P3 latency.

3. Results

3.1. Behavioral Data

The mean CFT-20 R score (± standard deviation) was 77.1 ± 7.8, which is equivalent to a transformed mean intelligence quotient (IQ) of 98.8 (± 11.4). Table 1 provides means and standard deviations of RT in the three conditions of the CPT. A one-way analysis of variance (ANOVA) with CPT conditions as three levels of a repeated-measures factor revealed statistically significant differences in RT, $F(2, 218) = 1978.510$, $p < 0.001$, $\eta_p^2 = 0.948$. As indicated by Bonferroni-adjusted post-hoc t tests, RT increased significantly from the CPT0 to the CPT1 condition, $t(109) = 46.700$, $p < 0.001$, $d = 4.453$, as well as from the CPT1 to the CPT2 condition, $t(109) = 17.869$, $p < 0.001$, $d = 1.704$.

Also given in Table 1 are descriptive statistics of errors of omission in the three CPT conditions and errors of commission in the CPT1 and CPT2 condition. (Due to the lack of distractors in the CPT0 condition, participants could not make errors of commission in this condition.) As indicated by a one-way ANOVA on omissions with the three CPT conditions as levels of a repeated-measures factor, omissions differed significantly between the three task conditions, $F(2, 218) = 11.550$, $p < 0.001$, $\eta_p^2 = 0.096$. There were significantly more errors of omission in the CPT0 than in the CPT1 condition, $t(109) = 4.762$, $p < 0.001$, $d = 0.454$, while omissions in the CPT1 and the CPT2 did not differ significantly after Bonferroni adjustment, $t(109) = 2.152$, $p = 0.034$, $d = 0.205$. Errors of commission, however, were made more frequently in the CPT2 than in the CPT1 condition, $t(109) = 11.317$, $p < 0.001$, $d = 1.079$.

Pearson correlations between RT in the three conditions are reported in Table 2. All three correlation coefficients yielded statistical significance. Unexpectedly, however, the correlations between RTs in the three CPT conditions and CFT-20 R scores were not significant and even positive in the most demanding task condition.

Similarly, CFT-20 R scores did not significantly correlate with errors of omission in the three task conditions (CPT0: $r = -0.006$, $p = 0.949$; CPT1: $r = -0.132$, $p = 0.171$; CPT2: $r = -0.101$, $p = 0.293$) nor with errors of commission in the CPT1, $r = -0.054$, $p = 0.578$, and in the CPT2 condition, $r = -0.116$, $p = 0.229$.

Table 1. Descriptive statistics of reaction times, errors of commission, and errors of omission in the three conditions of the continuous performance test (CPT) in 110 participants. No errors of commission were possible in the CPT0 condition.

Condition	Reaction Times (ms)				Errors of Commission (%)				Errors of Comission (%)			
	M	SD	Min	Max	M	SD	Min	Max	M	SD	Min	Max
CPT0	250	23	211	321	-	-	-	-	0.015	0.028	0	0.120
CPT1	416	41	327	530	0.005	0.007	0	0.031	0.003	0.011	0	0.080
CPT2	482	46	381	613	0.012	0.011	0	0.069	0.006	0.017	0	0.031

M = Means, SD = standard deviation, Min = minimum, Max = maximum.

Table 2. Pearson correlations between reaction times, P3 latencies, and P3 amplitudes in the three conditions of the continuous performance test (CPT0 to CPT2), as well as scores on the CFT-20 R in 110 participants.

Variable	Task/Condition	Reaction Times			P3 Latencies			P3 Amplitudes		
		CPT0	CPT1	CPT2	CPT0	CPT1	CPT2	CPT0	CPT1	CPT2
Reaction times	CFT total	−0.112	−0.002	0.081	−0.073	−0.236 *	−0.336 ***	0.072	0.187 *	0.135
	CPT0		0.437 ***	0.366 ***	0.213 *	0.133	0.041	−0.244 **	−0.272 **	−0.249 **
	CPT1			0.600 ***	0.077	0.293 **	0.215 *	−0.226 **	−0.339 ***	−0.241 **
	CPT2				0.209 *	0.124	0.086	−0.144	−0.218 *	−0.305 **
P3 latencies	CPT0					0.029	−0.046	−0.262 **	−0.170 *	−0.273 **
	CPT1						0.500 ***	−0.010	−0.154	−0.160 *
	CPT2							0.111	−0.103	−0.016
P3 amplitudes	CPT0								0.404 ***	0.339 ***
	CPT1									0.686 ***

* $p < 0.05$; ** $p < 0.01$; *** $p < 0.001$ (one-tailed).

3.2. Electrophysiological Data

Grand averages of the ERPs in the three CPT conditions are presented in Figure 1. The respective descriptive statistics for the P3 amplitudes and latencies are given in Table 3. To examine differences between P3 latencies in the three CPT conditions for significance, a one-way ANOVA was computed, with P3 latencies in the three CPT conditions as three levels of a repeated-measures factor. Due to a violation of sphericity, the Greenhouse–Geisser correction was used with $\varepsilon = 0.740$. The main effect yielded statistical significance, $F(1.480, 161.269) = 122.794$, $p < 0.001$, $\eta_p^2 = 0.530$. Planned comparisons revealed significantly shorter latencies in the CPT0 than in the CPT1 condition, $t(109) = 10.385$, $p < 0.001$, $d = 0.990$, as well as shorter latencies in the CPT1 than in the CPT2 condition, $t(109) = 5.493$, $p < 0.001$, $d = 0.524$.

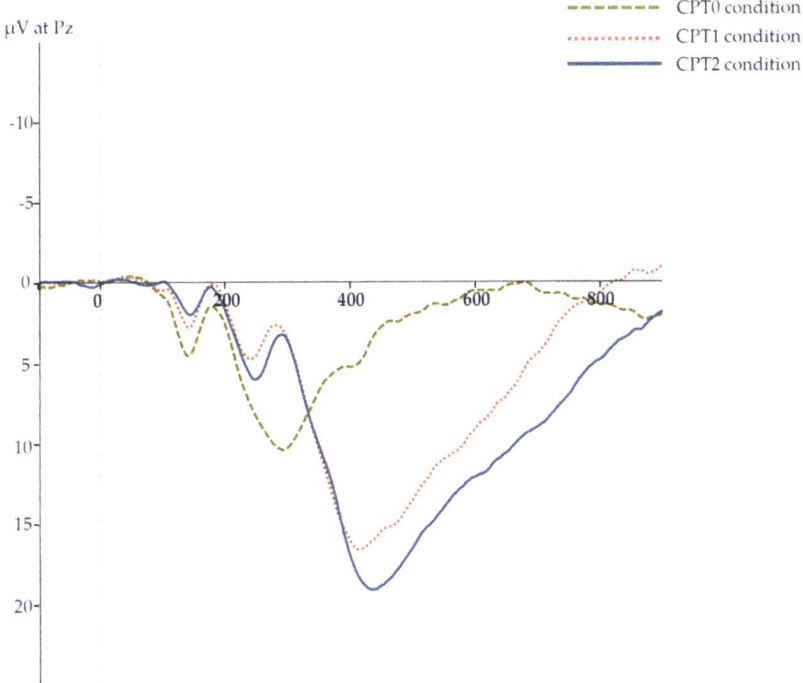

Figure 1. Grand average waves for the event-related potentials (ERPs) in the three CPT task conditions at the PZ electrode site. The zero point of the time scale refers to the onset. Negative is plotted upwards.

Table 3. Descriptive statistics of P3 latencies and P3 amplitudes in the three CPT conditions in 110 participants.

Condition	P3 Latencies (ms)				P3 Amplitudes (µV)			
	M	SD	Min	Max	M	SD	Min	Max
CPT0	371	39	300	543	7.78	3.73	0.69	26.01
CPT1	418	30	360	526	14.50	5.25	3.00	38.80
CPT2	438	29	361	535	16.49	5.87	6.59	42.44

M = Means, SD = standard deviation, Min = minimum, Max = maximum.

The same analysis was computed for the P3 amplitude as a dependent variable to probe differences between P3 amplitude in the three CPT conditions. Again, sphericity was violated, so that the Greenhouse–Geisser adjustment was used with $\varepsilon = 0.927$. The main effect on the P3 amplitude was significant, $F(1.854, 202.091) = 185.224$, $p < 0.001$, $\eta_p^2 = 0.630$. Planned comparisons revealed that P3 amplitude was significantly larger in the CPT1 than in the CPT0 condition, $t(109) = 14.741$, $p < 0.001$, $d = 1.405$, as well as in the CPT2 than in the CPT1 condition, $t(109) = 3.786$, $p < 0.001$, $d = 0.361$. Thus, P3 amplitudes and latencies were sensitive to the experimental manipulation and increased monotonically from the CPT0 to the CPT2 condition.

Correlations between MA, P3 latencies, and P3 amplitudes are presented in Table 2. P3 amplitudes were not associated with MA in the three CPT conditions. The same was true for the P3 latency in the least demanding task condition. In both more demanding task conditions, P3 latency was negatively and significantly related to MA.

In a next step, we submitted the P3 latencies from the three task conditions to stepwise regression analyses to predict MA. In the first model with P3 latency in the CPT0 condition as a predictor of MA, neither the $β$ coefficient, $β = -0.073$, $p = 0.446$, nor the amount of explained variance, adjusted $R^2 = 0.000$, were statistically significant. The second model with P3 latencies from the CPT0 and the CPT1 condition as predictors of MA led to a higher amount of explained variance, adjusted $R^2 = 0.043$, with the R^2 change being significant, $F(1,107) = 6.234$, $p = 0.014$. The $β$ coefficient of P3 latency in the CPT1, $β = -0.234$, $p = 0.014$, but not the $β$ coefficient of P3 latency in the CPT0 condition, $β = -0.067$, $p = 0.479$, yielded statistical significance. Comparing these first two models, P3 latency in the CPT1 condition explained a significantly larger portion of variance in MA compared to P3 latency in the CPT0 condition. Finally, with the third model, a statistically significant additional increase in the amount of explained variance was obtained (adjusted $R^2 = 0.101$) compared to the second model, $F(1,106) = 7.994$, $p = 0.006$. Only the $β$ coefficient of the P3 latency in the CPT2 condition, $β = -0.297$, $p = 0.006$, but not the $β$ coefficients of P3 latency in the CPT1, $β = -0.085$, $p = 0.421$, and in the CPT0 condition, $β = -0.085$, $p = 0.355$, were statistically significant.

Also given in Table 2 are correlations among RT, P3 latency, and P3 amplitude. P3 latencies in the CPT1 and in the CPT2 conditions were significantly correlated with each other but not with P3 latency in the CPT0 condition. This result indicated a functional difference of P3 latency in the CPT0 compared to the CPT1 and CPT2 conditions. P3 latencies in the three CPT conditions were positively correlated with RTs, but only four out of the nine correlation coefficients yielded statistical significance. Correlations between P3 latencies and P3 amplitudes were all negative, but only four out of nine coefficients reached statistical significance. Finally, the P3 amplitudes in the three CPT conditions correlated significantly positively with each other, but negatively with RTs, except for the correlation between the P3 amplitude in the CPT0 condition and RT in the CPT2 condition (see Table 2).

4. Discussion

The present study investigated the functional association between MA and the target-related P3 latency in the standard CPT as well as in two further conditions with variations of task demands. While in the standard condition (CPT1), a target ('X') had to be identified within a sequence of distractor stimuli, the process of selective identification was impeded in the attention-enhanced condition (CPT2) and omitted in the control condition (CPT0). This variation in task demands led to changes in P3 latency: The P3 latency was shorter in the CPT0 condition and longer in the CPT2 condition compared to the standard CPT condition. Concurrently, the correlational relationship between MA and P3 latency observed in the standard CPT condition ceased in the CPT0 condition but was even stronger in the CPT2 than in the CPT1 condition. As indicated by regression analyses, the significant amount of variance in MA explained by P3 latency in the standard CPT condition was also part of the variance explained by P3 latency in the attention-enhanced CPT2 condition. Even more importantly, the P3 latency in the attention-enhanced CPT2 condition explained an additional amount of variance of MA beyond and above the amount explained by the P3 latency in the standard CPT condition. This pattern of results strongly suggests that the functional correlation between MA and P3 latency depended on selective-attention demands.

In the standard CPT condition, attention needed to be directed to each stimulus to decide whether a target or a distractor was presented. In the CPT0 condition, only simple reactions were required so that the demands on selective attention were minimal. Finally, in the CPT2 condition, more selective attention than in the CPT1 condition was required to identify the target not only by its characteristic of being an 'X' but also by the additional feature of being italicized. Increasing RT as well as increasing P3 latencies and amplitudes from the CPT0 to the CPT2 condition indicated increasing selective-attention demands across CPT conditions.

In the standard CPT condition, the expected negative relationship between P3 latency and MA was observed, indicating that individuals with higher MA needed less time to correctly classify, and thus identify, the target stimulus than individuals with lower MA. This result was consistent with previous studies on the relation between MA and P3 latency using the oddball paradigm [25,29–33]. As outlined above, the main difference between the CPT, as used in the present study, and the oddball task was the composition of distractor stimuli. While only one distractor stimulus was used (and frequently presented) in the oddball task, different distractor stimuli were presented in the present standard CPT. In both tasks, however, the target stimulus was infrequently presented to be identified within a series of sequentially presented distractors. The negative relation between MA and P3 latency in the standard CPT condition supports the idea that the speed of identifying targets among distractors accounts for the relation between P3 latency and MA—as it was found for the many applications of the oddball task.

Consistent with the rationale of the present study, the absence of distractors made the identification of the target vs. nontarget stimulus unnecessary. Without this demand on selective attention, however, the latency of the P3 component was no longer related to MA. The absence of an association between MA and P3 latency in the CPT0 condition (i.e., a condition without selective-attention demands) was not unexpected given the results by McGarry-Roberts et al. [22] or Troche et al. [27]. In both studies, similar results were reported for the association between MA and P3 latencies in simple reaction time tasks as in the CPT0 condition of the present study.

P3 amplitude and latency as well as RT and error rates increased from the standard CPT1 to the attention-enhanced CPT2 condition indicating that the CPT2 condition required more selective attention to identify the italic 'X' among distractors (including the regular 'X'). In line with our expectations, the functional relationship between MA and P3 latency became stronger in the CPT2 compared to the CPT1 condition. As indicated by regression analyses, P3 latency in the CPT2 condition not only explained an amount of variance in MA overlapping with P3 latency in the CPT1 condition but also a significant additional portion of variance in MA. This outcome provided further evidence for the notion that the selective-attention demands on target identification are decisive for the relation between MA and P3 latency.

Both RT and P3 latency proved to be similarly sensitive to our experimental manipulation. Nevertheless, the correlation between RT and P3 latency as two distinct speed measures was only weak and not significant in the CPT2 condition. These results provided additional converging evidence for the notion that RT and P3 latency represent functionally different processes [22]. Despite this apparent functional independence of P3 latency and RT, it was the most surprising result of the present study that RT was not (negatively) related to MA in any of the three task conditions. Many previous studies using the CPT analyzed errors of omission and commission regarding their relation to MA or as possible indicators of impaired attentional processes in neurologically ill individuals [38–40]. In the present study with healthy participants, both kinds of errors were extremely rare and no correlations between intelligence and errors of omission or commission could be obtained. Since errors did not differ between individuals with higher and those with lower MA and the use of different cognitive strategies was unlikely, the standard CPT met the preconditions for a systematic relationship between RT and MA [1,2]. It should be noted, however, that a lacking negative relation between MA and RT is not unusual in the field of mental chronometry [41,42]—even though the majority of studies revealed a weak to modest relationship between MA and RT [3].

5. Conclusions

Previous research on the relation between MA and P3 latency has been rather inconclusive reporting negative correlations [25,29,30,33], positive correlations [28] or no significant correlations at all [22,27]. The present study provided first evidence for the notion that task demands on selective attention play a crucial role for the expected negative functional relationship between MA and P3 latency, as proposed within the conceptual framework of the mental speed approach. The negative relation between MA and P3 latency increased systematically with an increase of selective attention required by the task used to elicit the P3 component. As P3 latency and RT were functionally independent from each other, the failure to obtain a relationship between RT and MA did not necessarily hamper the interpretation of the relation between MA and P3 latency.

Supplementary Materials: The following are available online at http://www.mdpi.com/2076-3425/9/2/28/s1, Figure S1: Grand averages (solid lines) and standard deviations (dotted lines) of the event-related potentials in the three CPT conditions; Figure S2: Grand average (solid line) and standard deviation (dotted line) of the event-related potentials in the CPT0 condition; Figure S3: Grand average (solid line) and standard deviation (dotted line) of the event-related potentials in the CPT1 condition; Figure S4: Grand average (solid line) and standard deviation (dotted line) of the event-related potentials in the CPT2 condition.

Author Contributions: S.J.T., S.M., and T.H.R. conceived of and designed the experiment. S.M. set up and performed the experiment. T.K. prepared and analyzed the data. T.K. and S.J.T. wrote the paper. All authors reviewed and edited the paper.

Funding: This research received no external funding.

Acknowledgments: We thank Annkathrin Müller, Christine Krebs and Dominic Freitag for their help in collecting and preparing data.

Conflicts of Interest: The authors declare no conflict of interest.

References

1. Jensen, A.R. *The g Factor*; Praeger: Westport, CT, USA, 1998.
2. Jensen, A.R. *Clocking the Mind: Mental Chronometry and Individual Differences*; Elsevier: Amsterdam, The Netherlands, 2006.
3. Sheppard, L.D.; Vernon, P.A. Intelligence and speed of information-processing: A review of 50 years of research. *Pers. Indiv. Differ.* **2008**, *44*, 535–551. [CrossRef]
4. Garlick, D. Understanding the nature of the general factor of intelligence: The role of individual differences in neural plasticity as an explanatory mechanism. *Psychol. Rev.* **2002**, *109*, 116–136. [CrossRef] [PubMed]
5. Stelmack, R.M.; Houlihan, M.E. Event-related potentials, personality, and intelligence. In *International Handbook of Personality and Intelligence*; Saklofske, D.H., Zeidner, M., Eds.; Springer: New York, NY, USA, 1995; pp. 349–365.
6. Doebler, P.; Scheffler, B. The relationship of choice reaction time variability and intelligence: A meta-analysis. *Learn. Individ. Differ.* **2016**, *52*, 157–166. [CrossRef]
7. Pahud, O.; Rammsayer, T.H.; Troche, S.J. Putting the temporal resolution power (TRP) hypothesis to a critical test: Is the TRP-g relationship still more fundamental than an optimized relationship between speed of information processing and g? *Intelligence* **2018**, *70*, 52–60. [CrossRef]
8. Vernon, P.A.; Weese, S.E. Predicting intelligence with multiple speed of information-processing tests. *Pers. Indiv. Differ.* **1993**, *14*, 413–419. [CrossRef]
9. Borter, N.; Troche, S.J.; Rammsayer, T.H. Speed- and accuracy-related measures of an intelligence test are differentially predicted by the speed and accuracy measures of a cognitive task. *Intelligence* **2018**, *71*, 1–7. [CrossRef]
10. Schweizer, K. The relationship of attention and intelligence. In *Handbook of Individual Differences in Cognition: Attention, Memory, and Executive Control*; Gruszka, A., Matthews, G., Szymura, B., Eds.; Springer: New York, NY, USA, 2010; pp. 247–262.
11. Vernon, P.A.; Wicket, J.C.; Bazana, P.G.; Stelmack, R.M. The neuropsychology and psychophysiology of human intelligence. In *Handbook of Intelligence*; Sternberg, R.J., Ed.; Cambridge University Press: New York, NY, USA, 2000; pp. 245–264.

12. Blackwood, D.H.; Muir, W.J. Cognitive brain potentials and their application. *Brit. J. Psychiat.* **1990**, *9*, 96–101. [CrossRef]
13. Luck, S.J. *An Introduction to the Event-Related Potential Technique*, 2nd ed.; MIT Press: Cambridge, MA, USA, 2014.
14. Sutton, S.; Braren, M.; Zubin, J.; John, E.R. Evoked-potential correlates of stimulus uncertainty. *Science* **1965**, *150*, 1187–1188. [CrossRef]
15. Polich, J. Updating P300: an integrative theory of P3a and P3b. *Clin. Neurophysiol.* **2007**, *118*, 2128–2148. [CrossRef]
16. Polich, J. Neuropsychology of P300. In *The Oxford Handbook of Event-Related Potential Components*; Luck, S.J., Kappenman, E.S., Eds.; Oxford University Press: New York, NY, USA, 2012; pp. 159–188.
17. Polich, J.; Criado, J.R. Neuropsychology and neuropharmacology of P3a and P3b. *Int. J. Psychophysiol.* **2006**, *60*, 172–185. [CrossRef]
18. Duncan, C.C.; Barry, R.J.; Connolly, J.F.; Fischer, C.; Michie, P.T.; Näätänen, R.; Polich, J.; Reinvang, I.; Van Petten, C. Event-related potentials in clinical research: guidelines for eliciting, recording, and quantifying mismatch negativity, P300, and N400. *Int. J. Clin. Neuropsyc.* **2009**, *120*, 1883–1908. [CrossRef] [PubMed]
19. Duncan-Johnson, C.C. P300 latency: a new metric of information processing. *Psychophysiology* **1981**, *18*, 207–215. [CrossRef] [PubMed]
20. Ford, J.M.; Roth, W.T.; Mohs, R.C.; Hopkins, W.F.; Kopell, B.S. Event-related potentials recorded from young and old adults during a memory retrieval task. *Electroen. Clin. Neuro.* **1979**, *47*, 450–459. [CrossRef]
21. Johnson, R. A triarchic model of P300 amplitude. *Psychophysiology* **1986**, *23*, 367–384. [CrossRef] [PubMed]
22. McGarry-Roberts, P.A.; Stelmack, R.M.; Campbell, K.B. Intelligence, reaction time, and event-related potentials. *Intelligence* **1992**, *16*, 289–313. [CrossRef]
23. Verleger, R. On the utility of P3 latency as an index of mental chronometry. *Psychophysiology* **1997**, *34*, 131–156. [CrossRef]
24. Polich, J. P300 clinical utility and control of variability. *J. Clin. Neuriphysiol.* **1998**, *15*, 14–33. [CrossRef]
25. Fjell, A.M.; Walhovd, K.B. Effects of auditory stimulus intensity and hearing threshold on the relationship among P300, age, and cognitive function. *Clin. Neurophysiol.* **2003**, *114*, 799–807. [CrossRef]
26. Euler, M.J.; McKinney, T.L.; Schryver, H.M.; Okabe, H. ERP correlates of the decision time–IQ relationship: The role of complexity in task- and brain-IQ effects. *Intelligence* **2017**, *65*, 1–10. [CrossRef]
27. Troche, S.J.; Merks, S.; Houlihan, M.E.; Rammsayer, T.H. On the relation between mental ability and speed of information processing in the Hick task: An analysis of behavioral and electrophysiological speed measures. *Pers. Indiv. Differ.* **2017**, *118*, 11–16. [CrossRef]
28. Houlihan, M.; Stelmack, R.; Campbell, K. Intelligence and the effects of perceptual processing demands, task difficulty and processing speed on P300, reaction time and movement time. *Intelligence* **1998**, *26*, 9–25. [CrossRef]
29. Bazana, P.G.; Stelmack, R.M. Intelligence and information processing during an auditory discrimination task with backward masking: An event-related potential analysis. *J. Pers. Soc. Psychol.* **2002**, *83*, 998–1008. [CrossRef] [PubMed]
30. Beauchamp, C.M.; Stelmack, R.M. The chronometry of mental ability: An event-related potential analysis of an auditory oddball discrimination task. *Intelligence* **2006**, *34*, 571–586. [CrossRef]
31. De Pascalis, V.; Varriale, V.; Matteoli, A. Intelligence and P3 components of the event-related potential elicited during an auditory discrimination task with masking. *Intelligence* **2008**, *36*, 35–47. [CrossRef]
32. Jaušovec, N.; Jaušovec, K. Correlations between ERP parameters and intelligence: A reconsideration. *Biol. Psychol.* **2000**, *50*, 137–154. [CrossRef]
33. Troche, S.J.; Houlihan, M.E.; Stelmack, R.M.; Rammsayer, T.H. Mental ability, P300, and mismatch negativity: Analysis of frequency and duration discrimination. *Intelligence* **2009**, *37*, 365–373. [CrossRef]
34. Rosvold, H.E.; Mirsky, A.F.; Sarason, I.; Bransome, E.D., Jr.; Beck, L.H. A continuous performance test of brain damage. *J. Consult. Psychol.* **1956**, *20*, 343–350. [CrossRef]
35. Riccio, C.A.; Reynolds, C.R.; Lowe, P.; Moore, J.J. The continuous performance test: a window on the neural substrates for attention? *Arch. Clin. Neuropsych.* **2002**, *17*, 235–272. [CrossRef]
36. Weiss, R. *CFT 20-R. Grundintelligenztest Skala 2*; Hogrefe: Göttingen, Germany, 2006.
37. Gratton, G.; Coles, M.G.; Donchin, E. A new method for off-line removal of ocular artifact. *Electroen. Clin. Neuro.* **1983**, *55*, 468–484. [CrossRef]

38. Klee, S.H.; Garfinkel, B.D. The computerized continuous performance task: A new measure of inattention. *J. Abnorm Child. Psychol.* **1983**, *11*, 487–495. [CrossRef]
39. Naglieri, J.A.; Goldstein, S.; Delauder, B.Y.; Schwebach, A. Relationships between the WISC-III and the Cognitive Assessment System with Conners' rating scales and continuous performance tests. *Arch. Clin Neuropsych* **2005**, *20*, 385–401. [CrossRef] [PubMed]
40. Swanson, H.L.; Cooney, J.B. Relationship between intelligence and vigilance in children. *J. School Psychol.* **1989**, *27*, 141–153. [CrossRef]
41. Barrett, P.T. Electrophysiology, chronometrics, and cross-cultural psychometrics at the Biosignal Lab: Why it began, what we learned, and why it ended. *Pers. Indiv. Differ.* **2016**, *103*, 128–134. [CrossRef]
42. Jensen, A.R. Reaction time and psychometric *g*. In *A Model Intelligence*; Eysenck, H.J., Ed.; Springer: New York, NY, USA, 1982; pp. 93–123.

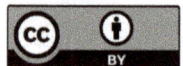

© 2019 by the authors. Licensee MDPI, Basel, Switzerland. This article is an open access article distributed under the terms and conditions of the Creative Commons Attribution (CC BY) license (http://creativecommons.org/licenses/by/4.0/).

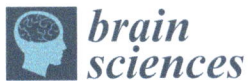

Article

Get Set or Get Distracted? Disentangling Content-Priming and Attention-Catching Effects of Background Lure Stimuli on Identifying Targets in Two Simultaneously Presented Series

Rolf Verleger [1,2,*], Kamila Śmigasiewicz [1,3], Lars Michael [4], Laura Heikaus [1] and Michael Niedeggen [5]

1. Department of Neurology, University of Lübeck, 23538 Lübeck, Germany; k.smigasiewicz@gmail.com (K.Ś.); a.l.heikaus@gmail.com (L.H.)
2. Institute of Psychology II, University of Lübeck, 23538 Lübeck, Germany
3. Laboratoire de Neurosciences Cognitives, Aix-Marseille Université, CNRS, 13331 Marseille, France
4. Department of Psychology, Medical School Berlin, 12247 Berlin, Germany; lars.michael@medicalschool-berlin.de
5. Department of Pedagogy and Psychology, Free University of Berlin, 14195 Berlin, Germany; michael.niedeggen@fu-berlin.de
* Correspondence: rolf.verleger@neuro.uni-luebeck.de

Received: 18 November 2019; Accepted: 9 December 2019; Published: 11 December 2019

Abstract: In order to study the changing relevance of stimulus features in time and space, we used a task with rapid serial presentation of two stimulus streams where two targets ("T1" and "T2") had to be distinguished from background stimuli and where the difficult T2 distinction was impeded by background stimuli presented before T1 that resemble T2 ("lures"). Such lures might actually have dual characteristics: Their capturing attention might interfere with target identification, whereas their similarity to T2 might result in positive priming. To test this idea here, T2 was a blue digit among black letters, and lures resembled T2 either by alphanumeric category (black digits) or by salience (blue letters). Same-category lures were expected to prime T2 identification whereas salient lures would impede T2 identification. Results confirmed these predictions, yet the precise pattern of results did not fit our conceptual framework. To account for this pattern, we speculate that lures serve to confuse participants about the order of events, and the major factor distinguishing color lures and digit lures is their confusability with T2. Mechanisms of effects were additionally explored by measuring event-related EEG potentials. Consistent with the assumption that they attract more attention, color lures evoked larger N2pc than digit lures and affected the ensuing T1-evoked N2pc. T2-evoked N2pc was indistinguishably reduced by all kinds of preceding lures, though. Lure-evoked mesio-frontal negativity increased from first to third lures both with digit and color lures and, thereby, might have reflected expectancy for T1.

Keywords: rsvp; lure stimuli; priming; ERPs; N2pc

1. Introduction

Knowledge about factors limiting visual perception is important to understand how we become aware of the world around us. This issue has often been studied by means of the rapid serial visual presentation task (RSVP) where target stimuli are embedded in background stimuli presented rapidly one after the other. A well-investigated phenomenon is the "attentional blink", which is the difficulty in discerning T2, the second of two target stimuli ("T1" and "T2") when presented at some critical moment after T1 [1,2]. The present study investigates another handicap to identifying T2: Some background stimuli may resemble T2. Such "lure" stimuli, differing from the actual T2 only by occurring before T1 rather than afterwards, have been shown to impair T2 identification [3–9] and may be considered a model case for studying the time-dependent changes of relevance which the many objects in our environment may undergo, because the very same object that is irrelevant when encountered too early may become relevant later on. Several studies have provided evidence that the process launched by perception and associated rejection of lures is inhibition of detecting the targets [4–11].

In the studies by Niedeggen and colleagues [4–9] participants had to detect a color change of the fixation point to red (T1) and then immediately detect or discriminate the direction of coherent motion (T2) of dots surrounding fixation or, in [7], a flip of surrounding bars. Lags from T1 to T2 varied between 0 ms and 700 ms. Performance was nearly perfect for all measured lags (Figure 1 in [6]). Yet T2 identification drastically deteriorated at short T1–T2 lags (most at a lag of 0 ms) when lure stimuli were presented before T1. This negative effect was cumulative, increasing with the number of lures in a trial [5,9], well in line with the notion of a gradual increase of central inhibition [8].

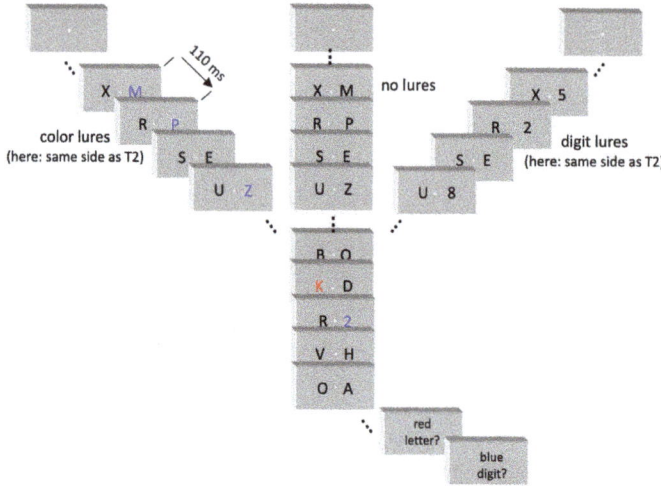

Figure 1. Sequence of events in a trial. Participants had to identify the red letter (T1) and the blue digit (T2) embedded in a stream of background stimuli. At least nine pairs of background stimuli were presented before T1. In 80% of trials, three of these pairs contained stimuli that resembled T2 ("lures"), either by their blue color or by their being a digit. The three lures could be on the same side as the ensuing T2 (as in these examples) or on the other side.

In Zhang et al.'s studies [10,11], T1 was a red letter in a series of white letters at screen center, and T2 was a white digit, either also presented at center [10,11] or left or right [10]. Lures (i.e., white digits presented at center before T1) reduced T2 identification.

In Harris et al.'s study [12] a stream of object drawings was presented at screen center. Participants had to identify the two red objects (T1 and T2) among the other, black objects. The black object that was presented two frames before T1 could be the same object as the red T2. These lures had negative effects on T2 identification when T2 was presented briefly after T1. These negative effects turned to stable positive effects when lures and T2 were rotated or mirrored relative to each other.

In order to embed such time-dependent changes into a spatial dimension, in a previous study, we presented lure stimuli in dual-stream RSVP. In this task, first implemented by Holländer et al. [13] and used in our lab in several studies (from [14] onwards), two streams are presented, left and right from fixation, with T1 and T2 each occurring in either of these streams. In our standard version, background stimuli are black letters, T1 is a red letter, and T2 is a black digit. In our lure study in this set-up [15], lures, presented in half of the trials, were black digits like T2. This is similar to Zhang et al.'s [10,11] stimuli, except that they did not present two streams. In our paradigm with two streams, evidence was found for both positive and negative priming exerted by lures on T2 identification, formally similar to Harris et al.'s [12] results. Specifically, in our task [15] lures had negative effects on T2 identification when the lag between T1 and T2 was 3 frames, This effect was shifted towards positive priming when lures and T2 were in the same stream and when the intervening T1 was "out of the way" in the other stream and when one of three lures was identical to T2. This latter result apparently differs from the above-reported results by Niedeggen et al. and Harris et al. [4–9,12] where identity of lures and T2 impeded rather than facilitated T2 identification.

Because of these conflicting results, here we reasoned that both mechanisms might be effective, either one being triggered by specific relations between lures and T2. To detail, similarity of lures to T2 might result in positive priming of lure contents for discerning T2 [12,15] whereas the property of lures to capture attention due to their similarity to T2 might inhibit and impede T2 identification. In the present study, we aimed at separating these two presumed effects by assigning two different features to T2 and using two types of lures: Unlike in previous studies [10,11,15], the T2 targets stood out not only by being digits but also by their color, being blue rather than black. In different trials, lures were either three same-category lures, i.e., black digits, or three attention-catching, salient lures, i.e., blue letters. We assumed that digit lures will positively prime T2 identification, whereas salient lures, being only superficially similar to T2, will not be able to prime T2 identification but will rather distract attention and, thereby, impede T2 identification. To optimize the presumed distinction of effects, one of the three digit lures in a trial was identical to T2, like in half the lure trials of our previous study [15]. Positive priming from lures on T2 might be considered trivial when one of the lures is T2. But negative identity priming from lures on T2 has been shown as well [12], and moreover, negative priming from identical irrelevant to relevant stimuli when separated by masks or other stimuli has often been demonstrated [16–18].

Sample trials of the three conditions no-lures, digit lures, color lures are depicted in Figure 1.

1.1. Stream Change from Lures to T2

The supposed attention-distracting effect of salient color lures may involve a strong spatial component. I.e., the impeding effect of salient lures on T2 identification may become evident only if lures and T2 are in different streams, because lures will have attracted attention to their stream which then turns out to be the incorrect one. Correspondingly, no negative effect, or even some positive effect on T2 identification, is expected if lures and T2 are in the same stream because, then, the lures will have attracted attention to the correct stream.

In contrast, by being content-dependent, the supposed positive priming effect of digit lures on T2 identification might be less tightly linked to spatial conditions. Thus, this positive effect should not differ much between stream change and stream continuity from lures to T2.

1.2. Role of T1 Stream

The preceding considerations were made without taking the relevant and attention-catching stimulus between lures and T2 into account, which is T1, the red letter. In [15], some evidence was obtained for the assumption that positive priming effects built up by lure presentations are broken and even inverted by T1 presentation (signaling that the preceding digits were too early to be T2). To keep things simple, it may at least be expected here that the spatial position of T1 will have effects on spatially specific effects: The attention-distracting effects of salient lures on other-stream T2 might be enhanced by T1 occurring in the lure stream and attenuated by T1 occurring in the T2 stream.

1.3. Event-Related Potentials

Event-related potentials (ERPs) were recorded in order to provide additional evidence on differential processing of same-category digit lures and salient color lures. This additional evidence was expected to be particularly relevant to evaluate immediate processing of the lures because there were only indirect behavioral measures of lure processing (by their moderating effects on discerning T2 and T1).

1.4. Lure-Evoked ERPs

When a trial included lures, there were always three of them, occurring in the same stream. If lures evoke inhibition then this inhibition should accumulate across the three lures. Lure-evoked ERPs had been measured by Niedeggen et al. [8,9,17], Verleger et al. [13], and Zhang et al. [6]. In all studies, a negative ERP component was evoked by lures at anterior scalp sites around 300 ms. In Niedeggen et al.'s studies [7,8,19], this component became larger across the three lure positions within a trial. (Zhang et al. [10] presented only one lure per trial at a fixed position, immediately before T1). Not occurring in control conditions (where lures did not share features with the target), the increase was interpreted by Niedeggen et al. [7,8,19] as reflecting frontal "gating" against being prematurely activated by these stimuli. However, this increase was not replicated in Verleger et al.'s [15] study. To accommodate this divergence, we assume for the present study that such frontal negativity will not build up with the same-category digit lures but will do so with the distracting salient color lures.

In addition, our use of bilateral streams allowed for measuring the N2pc component. N2pc is a negative deflection around 250 ms after onset of laterally presented relevant stimuli, at contralateral sites above the visual cortex [20,21] reflecting spatially selective processing of these stimuli [22–24]. Measuring N2pc evoked by lures provides a test for the assumption that color lures will attract more attention than digit lures: If this is true, N2pc amplitudes are expected to be larger with color lures than with digit lures, particularly with the first of the three lures because when the first color lure has attracted attention to its side the focus of attention may stay on that side such that the further lures do not require a shift of attention any more.

1.5. T1-Evoked ERPs

Being a relevant and salient lateral event, the red-colored T1 evokes N2pc in this dual-stream task [12,23]. One might speculate that the preceding sequence of three lures is helpful to expecting T1 precisely in time, so T1-evoked N2pc might increase in lure trials. However, no such effect was obtained in our previous study [13]. What is to be expected, though, is that the shifting of attention by preceding color lures will affect T1-evoked N2pc. Without lures, attention will be distributed across the two streams. Color lures will attract attention to their stream. T1 will require less shifting of attention when presented in the same stream as color lures and will require more shifting of attention when color lures had occurred in the other stream. Accordingly, T1-evoked N2pc is expected to be smaller than in trials without lures when color lures and T1 are in the same stream, and to be larger when color lures and T1 are in different streams.

1.6. T2-Evoked ERPs

Likewise, being a relevant event, T2 will evoke N2pc, too [10,14,25,26]. In Zhang et al.'s study [10], N2pc was delayed when lures preceded. In contrast, in Verleger et al.'s study [15], N2pc amplitudes were reduced, but only when lures and T2 were in the same stream. It may be speculated that the possibly inhibition-related effect of [10] might become evident in the present study after color lures while the possibly priming-related effect in [15] might become evident after digit lures.

To summarize, the major purpose of the present study was to obtain divergent effects of the two types of lures on T2 identification, and the ERPs evoked by lures, T1, and T2 were expected to be helpful in describing the mechanisms of these lure effects.

2. Materials and Methods

2.1. Participants

Eighteen students (9 male) of the University of Lübeck participated. This sample size was well in the range of our previous studies using this task where consistent behavioral and ERP effects had been obtained. Informed written consent was obtained and 7 € per hour were paid. All participants reported normal or corrected-to-normal vision, normal color vision, and no history of neurological disorders. Four of those 18 participants turned out to be unable to identify T2 reliably above chance, with mean identification rates markedly below 20%, and were excluded from analysis. The remaining 14 participants (7 males) were aged 20 to 29 years (M = 25, SD = 2.7). One was left-handed (laterality score −100), the others were right-handed, with a mean score of +94 (SD 9) in the Edinburgh Handedness Inventory [27].

2.2. Stimuli and Apparatus

The task is illustrated in Figure 1. Two simultaneous sequences of black capital letters of the Latin alphabet were rapidly (9/s) presented left and right from fixation. The 17" screen had a white background (120 cd/m^2) and was driven with 100 Hz at about 1.2 m from participants' faces. Letters were 8.5 mm wide and 11 mm high (0.5° × 0.6° visual angle) with their inner edges 10 mm from fixation (0.6°). Fixation was marked by a small red cross (0.1° × 0.1°) at screen center. In each trial, two targets had to be identified. The first target (T1) was a red letter (24 cd/m^2; D, F, G, J, K, or L). The second target (T2) was a blue digit (18 cd/m^2; 1, 2, 3, 4, 5, 6, 7, 8, or 9). Background stimuli consisted of all other letters in black (standard), or in blue (color lures) or of the digits 1–9 in black (digit lures). Presentation® software, version 14.5, was used for experimental control (Neurobehavioral Systems Inc., Berkeley, CA, USA).

2.3. Procedure

Participants were seated in a comfortable armchair in a dimly lit room in front of the computer screen. Their task in each trial was to identify the red letter (T1) and the ensuing blue digit (T2).

Each trial started with onset of the fixation cross. The two simultaneous letter streams started 800 ms later. Each stimulus pair was presented for 110 ms, immediately followed by the next frame. Background pairs either consisted of two standard stimuli or, in lure trials, of a standard stimulus and a lure (in three background pairs preceding T1). The three lures were presented in the same stream, which was either on the same side as the subsequent T2 or on the other side. There were five conditions: Same-side (as T2) color lures, other-side color lures, same-side digit lures, other-side digit lures, and no lures; 150 trials of each condition were presented in random order. Standard stimuli were randomly selected with replacement from the letter set (with a restriction against immediate repetition). T1 and T2 were randomly selected from the target sets. One of the three digit lures, randomly selected, was identical to the forthcoming T2 digit (resembling the feature of color lures whose color was always identical to T2) and the other two digit lures were randomly selected from the T2 set. T1 and T2 each were presented on the left or right side together with a standard stimulus on the other side.

In order to avoid fixed temporal expectancies [28] time-points of lures, T1, and T2 were varied across trials. T1 was, on average, at position 12.0 (±1.4 SD; range 10–14). Lures (both color lures and digit lures) occurred between positions 3 and T1 − 2, on average at positions 4.2 (±1.3 SD), 6.5 (±1.7), 8.8 (±1.7), i.e., in temporal intervals of 2.3 frames on average = 250 ms, ending on average 3.2 frames (350 ms) before T1. T2 followed T1 with lags of 110 ms (Lag 1) or 330 ms (Lag 3). Five standard-letter pairs followed T2. Therefore, trial length varied between 16 frames (when T1 came at the 10th position and T1–T2 lag was 1) and 22 frames (when T1 came at 14th position and T1–T2 lag was 3). Out of the four possible side × lag relations of T1 and T2 (same side / other side × lag 1 / lag 3) the same-side lag-1 relation was omitted altogether, in order not to overly lengthen the task, because T2 identification rates are relatively uninformative in this condition, being always close to 100%, due to "lag 1 sparing" [15,29,30]. Thus, of the 150 trials within each of the five lure-T2 relations (same-side color lures, other-side color lures, same-side digit lures, other-side digit lures, no lures) 50 trials each, in random order, applied one of the three T1-T2 relations, half of them with T2 on the left and half with T2 on the right: Same side with lag 3 (in shorthand notation *L3L* and *R3R*, denoting T1 side, lag, T2 side), side change with lag 1 (*R1L* and *L1R*), side change with lag 3 (*R3L* and *L3R*).

A standard keyboard was placed directly in front of participants on an adjustable base. At the end of each trial, 2.5 s after onset of the first stimulus-frame, participants were prompted by a message on the screen to enter their responses on the keyboard, first the T1 letter on the middle row and then the T2 digit on the number pad. When not knowing the answer, they had to guess. The next trial started immediately after the T2 response.

The five (lure conditions) × three (T1-T2 relations) × two (T2 sides) × 25 trials (=750 trials) were presented in random sequence, with a break after 375 trials. Before the task proper, some trials were presented in slow motion for practice, with 500 ms rather than 110 ms presentation rate.

2.4. Analysis of T1 and T2 Identification Rates

Separately for T1 and T2, percentages of trials with correct responses were computed in each of those five × three × two = 30 cells of the design. In order to avoid having an ill-defined three-level factor that would combine variation of lag (1 vs. 3) and of T1-T2 relation (same side vs. other side) we decided to focus analysis on the variation of same vs. other side in lag 3 data. To handle the five levels of the factor Lure Condition, analysis proceeded in two steps. First, no-lure data will be described, with respect to effects of target side (left, right) and of other-target side (same as target, other than target), with "target" and "other target" denoting T1 or T2 depending on analysis. Second, the effects of the lures were tested by subtracting the no-lure data from data of each of the four conditions with the lures, thereby extracting the net effects of lures in each of these conditions, and entering these differences to ANOVAs with the repeated-measurement factors Lure Type (digit, color) and Lure Side (same as target, other than target), additionally to Target Side and Other-Target Side. In additional analyses, the effects of Lag (1 vs. 3) were tested by comparing the other-target-on-other-side data between lag 3 and lag 1. These analyses had the factors Target Side and Lag for no-lure data, and Lure Type, Lure Side, Target Side, and Lag for lure effects. Only effects of the Lag factor will be reported from these analyses.

2.5. EEG Recording and Pre-Processing

EEG was recorded with Ag/AgCl electrodes (Easycap, www.easycap.de) from 60 scalp sites, which were 8 midline positions from AFz to Oz and 26 pairs of symmetric left and right sites. Further electrodes were placed at the nose-tip for off-line reference and at Fpz as connection to ground. On-line reference was Fz. For artifact control, the electrooculogram (EOG) was recorded, vertically (vEOG) from above vs. below the right eye and horizontally (hEOG) from positions next to the outer tails of the eyes. Voltages were amplified from DC to 250 Hz by a BrainAmp MR plus, A–D converted, and stored with 500 samples/s per channel. Off-line processing was done with Brain-Vision Analyzer software (version 2.03). Data were re-referenced to the nose-tip and low-pass filtered at 20 Hz (Butterworth zero phase filters, attenuation of 12 dB / octave). Then 600 ms epochs, starting 100 ms before the respective event, were cut out of the EEG for analyzing the potentials evoked by each of the three lures, by T1, and by T2. These epochs were edited for artifacts, rejecting trials with voltage differences at any recording site that exceeded 150 µV or exceeded 40 µV between successive data points. Mean values of 100 ms pre-stimulus epochs were subtracted, and data were averaged over trials separately by conditions.

For lures, separate averages were formed for left and right 1st, 2nd, and 3rd digit and color lures. Control averages were formed from equivalent positions in no-lure trials and subtracted from the lure epochs. (Lure positions had been assigned by the sequence-generating program also in no-lure trials).

Analysis of T1 and T2 EEG epochs was restricted to trials where T2 followed with a lag of three frames because potentials evoked by T1 and T2 were inextricably mixed when T1 was followed by the other-stream T2 with lag 1. For T1, trials with correct response to T1 were selected, and separate averages were formed over trials for left and right T1 in the five lure conditions (no lures, digit lures in the same stream as T1 and in the other stream than T1, color lures in the same stream as T1 and in the other stream than T1). For T2, trials with correct responses to both T1 and T2 were selected, and separate averages were formed over trials for left and right T2 in the five lure conditions (no lures, digit lures in the same stream as T2 and in the other stream than T2, color lures in the same stream as T2 and in the other stream than T2). Unlike for T1 analysis, this was done separately for trials with T1 and T2 on same sides and T1 and T2 on different sides.

To obtain contralateral–ipsilateral (con–ips) differences of each symmetric left-right pair of recording sites, the left-site average was subtracted from the right-site average when the event (lure, T1, or T2) was left (e.g., PO8 − PO7), vice versa when the event was right (e.g., PO7 − PO8) and the mean of these two con–ips differences was formed. Grand means over participants were calculated for illustrating the results. Con–ips differences were also formed for hEOG and these hEOG difference waveforms were inspected for systematic deviations from baseline within 500 ms after lure onsets, indicating eye movements toward the lures. It was found that only two of the 14 participants had notable deviations after the first color lure. These deviations amounted to about 5 µV only, corresponding to an average eye movement of about 0.3° towards the lure stream, which we considered small enough to keep these participants in the sample. Including those two participants, the grand average waveforms of hEOG deviations toward lures reached a maximum of about 1 µV at 400 ms after onsets of 1st and 2nd lures, and much smaller values after 3rd lures, with 1 µV corresponding to average eye movements of about 0.07° towards the lure stream, which still appeared to be an acceptable level.

As will be detailed in the Results section, parameters were determined in the |PO7 − PO8| con–ips difference waveforms evoked by lures (minus no-lures), by T1, and by T2, as well as in current source densities evoked by lures (minus no-lures) recorded at FCz. Statistical analysis was performed by ANOVA with repeated measurements. *P* values of effects of the three-level factors Lure Position and Epoch (as defined in the Results section) will be reported after Greenhouse–Geisser correction.

3. Results

3.1. Target Identification

Percentages of trials in which the targets were identified are displayed in Figure 2. Additionally, mean values and standard deviations are compiled in the Table S1 (see Supplementary Materials). Each data point was computed from 25 trials per participant.

3.1.1. T1: Trials without Lures

T1 was identified in 84% of no-lure trials on average (black line in the upper left panel of Figure 2). No-lure identification rates were submitted to ANOVA with the factors T1 Side (left, right) and T2 Side (same as T1, other than T1). T1 was identified better when the following T2 was in the same stream and T1 was on the right (R3R in Figure 2, with absence of italics denoting the target under consideration, here T1), as indicated by a main effect of T2 Side, $F_{1,13} = 9.4$, $p = 0.009$, and the interaction of T2 Side × T1 Side $F_{1,13} = 4.5$, $p = 0.05$, resolved to an effect of T2 Side for right T1, $F_{1,13} = 11.8$, $p = 0.004$, and no such effect for left T1, $F_{1,13} = 1.2$, n.s.

Additionally, the other-side-than-T2 data were compared between lag 3 and lag 1 in an ANOVA with the factors T1 Side (left, right) and Lag (1, 3). No effect was significant, all $F_{1,13} \leq 2.1$, $p \geq 0.17$.

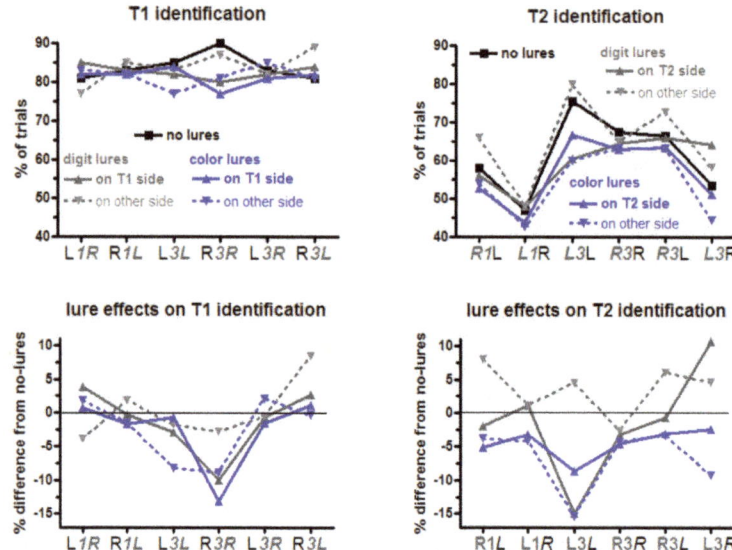

Figure 2. Lure effects on identification rates of T1 and T2. The upper panels display the percentages of trials in which T1 (left) and T2 (right) were identified. The lower panels display the differences between trials with lures from trials without lures. No-lure trials (upper panels only) are denoted by black lines, trials with digit lures by grey lines, and trials with color lures by blue lines. Trials where lures were in the same stream as the target (T1 and T2, respectively) are denoted by solid lines (grey and blue) and trials where lures were in the opposite stream are denoted by dashed lines. Both for T1 and T2, the six values on the x axes denote left-right-left-right-left-right targets. E.g., "L1R" is a trial where T1 was left and T2 was right (separated from each other by 1 frame). Thereby, L1R is the leftmost value for T1 (*L1R*) and the second value for T2 (*L1R*). The main ANOVAs were conducted on the lag 3 data (four rightmost values in each panel) and additional ANOVAs compared lag 1 and lag 3 other-target-on-other-side data (two leftmost and two rightmost values in each panel).

3.1.2. Lure Effects on T1 Identification

Lure effects were tested by subtracting the no-lure data from data of each of the four conditions with lures and entering these differences to ANOVAs. The main ANOVA was conducted on lag 3 trials with the repeated-measurement factors Lure Type (digit, color) and Lure Side (same as T1, other than T1), additionally to T1 Side and T2 Side. ANOVA results are compiled in Table 1.

Table 1. ANOVA on effects of lures (deviations of lure conditions from the no-lure condition) on T1 identification rates.

Effect	F (p)	Effect	F (p)
T1 Side (left, right)	0.4	T2 Side × Lure Side	0.2
T2 Side (same as T1, other than T1)	**9.1 (0.01)**	Lure Type × Lure Side	4.0 (0.07)
Lure Type (digit, color)	**5.1 (0.04)**	T1 Side × T2 Side × Lure Type	0.9
Lure Side (same as T1, other than T1)	2.3	T1 Side × T2 Side × Lure Side	**7.5 (0.02)**
T1 Side × T2 Side	3.9 (0.07)	T1 Side × Lure Type × Lure Side	0.6
T1 Side × Lure Type	3.1 (0.10)	T2 Side × Lure Type × Lure Side	2.9
T1 Side × Lure Side	3.8 (0.07)	T1 Side × T2 Side × Lure Type × Lure Side	**6.9 (0.02)**
T2 Side × Lure Type	0.2		

Degrees of freedom are 1,13 throughout. F and p values are printed in bold when $p \leq 0.050$. p-values were entered when $p \leq 0.10$.

Color lures had larger negative effects on T1 identification than digit lures (blue vs. grey in Figure 2), Lure Type $F_{1,13} = 5.1$, $p = 0.04$, and lure effects were more negative when the following T2 was on the same side as T1 (L3L and R3R) than when sides changed (L3R and R3L), T2 Side $F_{1,13} = 9.1$, $p = 0.01$.

When lures, T1, and T2 all were in one stream (solid blue and grey lines in Figure 2), right-side T1 was more affected by lures than left-side T1 (rR3R > lL3L): Lure Side × T1 Side × T2 Side $F_{1,13} = 7.5$, $p = 0.02$, resolved to an effect of T1 Side × T2 Side of $F_{1,13} = 6.7$, $p = 0.02$, for lures on the same side as T1 (in contrast to $F_{1,13} = 1.0$, n.s., for lures on other side than T1) and further, for these same-side lures, to an effect of T1 Side of $F_{1,13} = 10.1$, $p = 0.007$, when T2 was on same side as T1 (in contrast to $F_{1,13} = 0.7$, n.s., for T2 on the other side than T1).

Finally, the significant four-fold interaction (T1 Side × Lure Side × Lure Type × T2 Side $F_{1,13} = 6.9$, $p = 0.02$) reflected two separate effects, namely, first, the outlying positive value of the dashed grey line in Figure 2 at R3L and, second, the outlying negative value of the dashed blue line at L3L. To detail: The outlying positive value of the dashed grey line at R3L was reflected by resolving the fourfold interaction to threefold interactions of Lure Type × T1 Side × T2 Side separately for same-side and other-side lures, which yielded a significant result for other-side lures (dashed lines in Figure 2), $F_{1,13} = 14.2$, $p = 0.002$, in contrast to $F_{1,13} = 0.9$, n.s., for same-side lures. Then resolving that threefold interaction for other-side lures to effects of T1 Side for each of the four combinations of Lure Type × T2 Side yielded a significant effect of T1 Side for digit lures and other-side T2 (dashed grey line: R3L more positive than L3R), $F_{1,13} = 9.1$, $p = 0.01$, in contrast to $F_{1,13} \leq 0.7$, n.s., for each of the other three combinations. Second, the outlying negative value of the dashed blue line at L3L was reflected by resolving the overall fourfold interaction to threefold interactions of Lure Side × T1 Side × T2 Side separately for color lures and digit lures which yielded a significant result for color lures, $F_{1,13} = 12.5$, $p = 0.004$, in contrast to digit lures, $F_{1,13} = 0.0$, n.s. Resolving that threefold interaction for color lures to effects of Lure Side for each of the four combinations of T1 Side × T2 Side yielded a significant effect of Lure Side for L3L—other side (dashed blued line in Figure 2) more negative than same-side (solid blue line)—, $F_{1,13} = 8.9$, $p = 0.01$, in contrast to the other three combinations of T1 Side × T2 Side (R3R, L3R, R3L), $F_{1,13} \leq 2.5$, $p \geq 0.15$, n.s.

A second ANOVA was run to compare other-side-than-T2 data between lag 3 (L3R, R3L) and lag 1 (L1R, R1L), replacing the previous factor T2 Side by Lag (lag 1, lag 3) to have the factors Lure Type, Lure Side, T1 Side, and Lag. No effect of Lag reached significance, all $F_{1,13} \leq 2.8$, $p \geq 0.12$.

3.1.3. T2: Trials without Lures

T2 was identified in 61% of no-lure trials on average. Similar to T1 analysis, ANOVA on no-lure rates of T2 identification in lag 3 trials had the factors T2 Side (left, right) and T1 Side (same as T2, other than T2). Left T2 was identified better than right T2, $F_{1,13} = 7.5$, $p = 0.02$. T2 on the same side as T1 was better identified than T2 on the other side, $F_{1,13} = 10.3$, $p = 0.007$. These two factors did not interact, $F_{1,13} = 0.3$, n.s.).

Additionally, the lag 1 data were compared to the other-side-than-T1 data of lag 3 in an ANOVA with the factors T2 Side (left, right) and Lag (1, 3). T2 tended to be better identified after Lag 3 than after Lag 1, $F_{1,13} = 4.3$, $p = 0.06$. The advantage of left T2 over right T2 was again significant, $F_{1,13} = 5.4$, $p = 0.04$, and did not interact with Lag, $F_{1,13} = 0.3$, n.s.

3.1.4. Lure Effects on T2 Identification

Like with T1, the main ANOVA on differences between lure and no-lure trials was conducted on lag 3 trials, with the factors Lure Type (digit, color) and Lure Side (same as T2, other than T2), additionally to T1 Side (same as T2, other than T2) and T2 Side (left, right). ANOVA results are compiled in the top half of Table 2.

As predicted, color lures were much more detrimental than digit lures, $F_{1,13} = 27.5$, $p < 0.001$. Besides, the pattern of effects differed much between color lures and digit lures (Figure 2), as reflected by five out of seven possible interactions of Lure Type being significant (top half of Table 2). Therefore, separate ANOVAs were computed for the two lure types, with the factors Lure Side, T1 Side, and T2 Side (bottom half of Table 2).

Table 2. ANOVA effects on lure effects (deviations of lure conditions from the no-lure condition) on T2 identification rates: main analysis followed by separate ANOVAs for the two lure types.

Effect	F (p)	Effect	F (p)
T1 Side (same as T2, other than T2)	5.7 (0.03)	T2 Side × Lure Side	8.3 (0.01)
T2 Side (left, right)	1.4	Lure Type × Lure Side	10.4 (0.007)
Lure Type (digit, color)	27.5 (<0.001)	T1 Side × T2 Side × Lure Type	5.5 (0.04)
Lure Side (same as T1, other than T1)	1.2	T1 Side × T2 Side × Lure Side	0.6
T1 Side × T2 Side	0.9	T1 Side × Lure Type × Lure Side	3.5 (0.08)
T1 Side × Lure Type	13.9 (0.003)	T2 Side × Lure Type × Lure Side	8.6 (0.01)
T1 Side × Lure Side	4.7 (0.050)	T1 Side × T2 Side × Lure Type × Lure Side	5.0 (0.04)
T2 Side × Lure Type	0.2		
Color Lures		**Digit Lures**	
T1 Side (same as T2, other than T2)	1.3	T1 Side	15.9 (0.002)
T2 Side (left, right)	0.6	T2 Side	2.0
Lure Side (same as T1, other than T1)	5.9 (0.03)	Lure Side	9.3 (0.009)
T1 Side × T2 Side	5.4 (0.04)	T1 Side × T2 Side	0.2
T1 Side × Lure Side	0.0	T1 Side × Lure Side	8.1 (0.01)
T2 Side × Lure Side	0.0	T2 Side × Lure Side	25.4 (<0.001)
T1 Side × T2 Side × Lure Side	3.9 (0.07)	T1 Side × T2 Side × Lure Side	0.9

Degrees of freedom are 1,13 throughout. F and p values are printed in bold when $p \leq 0.050$. p-values were entered when $p \leq 0.10$.

Color lures had an overall negative effect (constant term of ANOVA differing from zero: $F_{1,13} = 22.0$, $p < 0.001$). As predicted, this effect was larger when lures were in the other stream than when they were in the same stream (Lure Side: $F_{1,13} = 5.9$, $p = 0.03$). Furthermore, the negative effect was largest on L3L, i.e., left T2 preceded by left T1 (T1 Side × T2 Side $F_{1,13} = 5.4$, $p = 0.04$; simple effect of T1 Side on left T2 $F_{1,13} = 5.3$, $p = 0.04$; on right T2 $F_{1,13} = 0.1$, n.s.).

Digit lures had an overall zero effect (constant term of ANOVA $F_{1,13} = 0.2$, n.s.). But effects differed between lure sides, $F_{1,13} = 9.3$, $p = 0.009$, and between T1 sides, $F_{1,13} = 15.9$, $p = 0.002$, in both cases being negative when sides (of lures or of T1) were the same as T2 and positive when sides differed from T2. Important were the strong interactions of Lure Side × T2 Side, $F_{1,13} = 25.4$, $p < 0.001$, and of Lure Side × T1 Side, $F_{1,13} = 8.1$, $p = 0.01$. Both interactions reflected that there were large moderating effects (of T2 Side and of T1 Side) on lure effects on T2 identification when lures and T2 were in the same stream (solid grey line in Figure 2; effect of T2 Side $F_{1,13} = 16.2$, $p = 0.001$; of T1 Side $F_{1,13} = 29.7$, $p < 0.001$) in contrast to absence of effects when lures and T2 were in different streams (dashed grey line; effect of T2 Side $F_{1,13} = 2.0$, $p = 0.19$; of T1 Side $F_{1,13} = 2.0$, $p = 0.18$). Thus, when lures and T2 were in the same stream (solid grey line), lure effects were negative both for left T2 (L3L and R3L) and when T1 was on the same side (L3L and R3R), and were more positive both for right T2 and when T1 was on the other side. Thereby, when looking at these interactions from the viewpoint of differential effects of lure side, these effects of lure side—negative with same-side lures, positive with other-side lures—were focused on left T2 (effect of Lure Side on left T2 $F_{1,13} = 43.6$, $p < 0.001$; on right T2 $F_{1,13} = 1.1$, n.s.) and on same-side T1 (effect of Lure Side with same-side T1 $F_{1,13} = 26.5$, $p < 0.001$; with other-side T1 $F_{1,13} = 0.0$, n.s.). Whether these effects were indeed significantly different from zero was tested by evaluating the deviations from zero of the constant terms of ANOVAs conducted on single levels of those two two-way interactions Lure Side × T2 Side and Lure Side × T1 Side. Effects were reliably negative when T2 was in the same stream as lures (solid grey line) and either was left (L3L and R3L), $F_{1,13} = 16.8$, $p < 0.001$, or when T1 was in the T2 stream (L3L and R3R), $F_{1,13} = 23.9$, $p < 0.001$. Effects were reliably positive when T2 was in the other stream than lures (dashed grey line) and was left (L3L and R3L), $F_{1,13} = 5.7$, $p = 0.03$, and when lures were in the same stream as T2 (solid grey line) but T1 was in the other stream (R3L and L3R), $F_{1,13} = 7.5$, $p = 0.02$.

Additionally, the lag 1 data were compared to the other-side-than-T1 data of lag 3, replacing the previous factor T1 Side by Lag (lag 1, lag 3) to have the factors Lure Type, Lure Side, Lag, and T2 Side. No effect of Lag came below the $p = 0.05$ threshold (all $F_{1,13} \leq 4.5$, $p \geq 0.054$).

3.2. ERP Reflections of Lure Processing

Lure-evoked ERPs were computed from 150 trials per participant (minus artifact-affected epochs).

3.2.1. Lure-evoked N2pc

Lure-evoked contralateral–ipsilateral differences from posterior–lateral sites |PO7–PO8| are displayed in Figure 3. There is obviously a negative component (N2pc) peaking around 250 ms with the 1st lure. N2pc was measured by computing mean amplitudes at 200–300 ms and submitting these values to ANOVA with the factors Lure Type (color, digit) and Serial Position (1st, 2nd, 3rd lure).

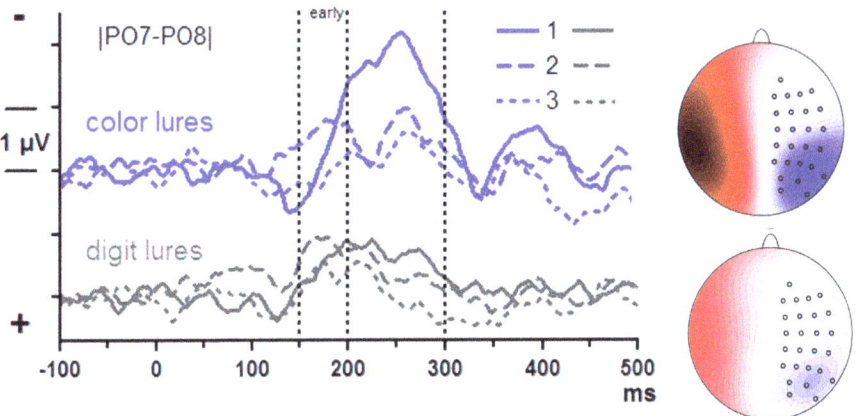

Figure 3. Contralateral–ipsilateral event-related potential (ERP) differences evoked by the lures. Data are grand means across participants, recorded from left and right posterior sites PO7 and PO8. Depicted are differences between lure-trials and corresponding epochs of no-lure trials. Unit on x-axis is milliseconds, time-point zero is lure onset. Unit on y-axis is microvolts, negative voltage is plotted upwards. Waveforms evoked by the 1st lure are shown as solid lines, by the 2nd lure as dashed lines, and by the 3rd lure as dotted lines. ERPs evoked by color lures and digit lures are plotted with blue and grey lines, respectively. The scalp maps show the view on the head (120°) from above. Recording sites (small circles) are depicted on one hemisphere only because the contralateral–ipsilateral differences were pooled across left and right sides. Blue is contralateral negativity, red is positivity. Scale is ±4 µV. Displayed are topographic distributions of N2pc evoked by the first lure at its peak latency: 256 ms with the first color lure, 224 ms with the first digit lure.

Overall, N2pc was largest with the 1st lure (Serial Position: $F_{2,26} = 12.4$, $p = 0.001$) and larger with color than digit lures, $F_{1,13} = 4.8$, $p = 0.048$. Both factors tended to interact, $F_{2,26} = 3.4$, $p = 0.07$. Indeed, in separate analyses for each serial position, Lure Type was significant at the first position only. $F_{1,13} = 5.5$, $p = 0.04$ ($F_{1,13} \leq 2.0$, n.s., for 2nd and 3rd positions). In separate analyses of the two lure types, the Position effect was significant in either analysis, though being somewhat larger with color lures ($F_{2,26} = 9.2$, $p = 0.004$) than with digit lures ($F_{2,26} = 6.1$, $p = 0.009$).

It may be suggested that the early negative deflections in the 2nd position waveforms, peaking at about 170 ms, are accelerated N2pc peaks. But a second peak is visible at about 250 ms in these waveforms as well. Given that attention was already shifted towards the lure stream because of the first lure, we agree with one reviewer of this paper that the negativity may reflect increased N1 components evoked by this attended lure stream (e.g., [31]) rather than an early N2pc. When quantifying this early activity as mean amplitudes 150–200 ms, there was no effect of Lure Type, $F \leq 2.1$, n.s., but a distinct effect of Position, $F_{1,13} = 11.7$, $p < 0.001$, with largest values for the 2nd position.

3.2.2. Frontal Activity

The upper panel of Figure 4 shows lure-evoked ERPs at FCz. A large negative peak seems to be evoked by the first color lure at about 300 ms. However, the scalp map of these data suggests that this peak may stem from volume-conducted posterior negativity. In contrast, negative peaks with fronto-central focus are visible with 2nd and 3rd lures, though at later latencies. In order to enhance the weights of location-specific activity and get rid of volume conducted posterior negativity, current source densities (CSDs) [32] were computed (lower panel of Figure 4). Indeed, as the maps in Figure 4 show, current-sinks had a focus at or near FCz, with their amplitudes appearing to vary between serial positions: negligible activity with the first lure, distinct but relatively late activity with the second lure (400–500 ms after lure onset), somewhat earlier activity (300–400 ms) with the third lure.

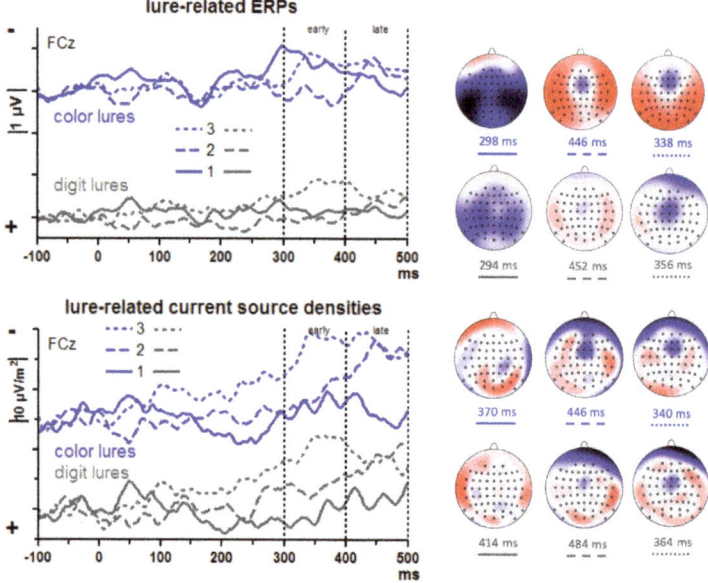

Figure 4. ERPs and current source densities evoked by the lures. Data are grand means across participants, recorded from the fronto-central midline site FCz. The upper panel displays the ERPs, and the lower panel displays current source densities, i.e., ERP data from which ERP data from surrounding sites were subtracted. Depicted are differences between lure-trials and corresponding epochs of no-lure trials. Unit on x-axis is milliseconds, time-point zero is lure onset. Unit on y-axis is microvolts in the upper panel and microvolts per square meter in the lower panel, negative values are plotted upwards. Waveforms evoked by the 1st lure are shown as solid lines, by the 2nd lure as dashed lines, and by the 3rd lure as dotted lines. Data evoked by color lures and digit lures are plotted with blue and grey lines, respectively. The scalp maps show the view on the head (120°) from above. Recording sites are denoted by the small circles. Displayed are topographic distributions at the indicated latencies for each of the six conditions. In the upper panel, blue denotes negative polarity, red positive polarity, and scale is ±2 µV. In the lower panel, blue denotes negative sinks, red denotes positive sources, and scale is ±15 µV/m².

To quantify these impressions, an ANOVA was computed on mean CSD amplitudes of the 300–400 ms and 400–500 ms epochs, with the factors Epoch (early, late), Serial Position (1st, 2nd, 3rd lure), Lure Type (digit, color), and Lure Stream (left, right). The main effect of Serial Position ($F_{2,26} = 3.8$, $p = 0.047$) and the interaction of Epoch × Serial Position ($F_{2,26} = 3.9$, $p = 0.043$) were further explored by computing pairwise ANOVAs on lure #1 vs. #2 and on #2 vs. #3 separately for the two epochs. Negativity increased from lure #1 to #2 in the late epoch ($F_{1,13} = 6.6$, $p = 0.02$; early epoch: $F_{1,13} = 0.6$, n.s.) and from lure #2 to #3 in the early epoch ($F_{1,13} = 7.3$, $p = 0.02$; late epoch: $F_{1,13} = 0.1$, n.s.). Different from what we had expected, there was hardly any difference between digit and color lures. The only effect of Lure Type was a moderation of the just-mentioned Epoch × Serial Position interaction, Epoch × Serial Position × Lure Type $F_{2,26} = 4.6$, $p = 0.02$, which appeared to reflect a tendency with 3rd lures where negativity tended to decrease from early to late epoch with digit lures, $F_{1,13} = 4.3$, $p = 0.06$, not so with color lures, $F_{1,13} = 0.0$, n.s. There were no reliable differences between left and right streams (all effects of Lure Stream $F_{1,13} \leq 3.6$, $p \geq 0.08$).

3.3. ERP Reflections of Lure Effects on T1 Processing

T1-evoked ERPs were computed from about 120 trials per participant (150 trials per cell minus about 20% trials with incorrect responses) minus artifact-affected trials.

T1-evoked contralateral–ipsilateral differences from posterior–lateral sites |PO7–PO8| are displayed in Figure 5. There is a large N2pc, peaking at about 220 ms. Lure effects were measured by computing the differences between lure trials and no-lure trials in the mean amplitudes at 175–275 ms for each of the four lure conditions and submitting these difference values to an ANOVA with the factors Lure Type (color, digit) and Lure-T1 Relation (same side, other side).

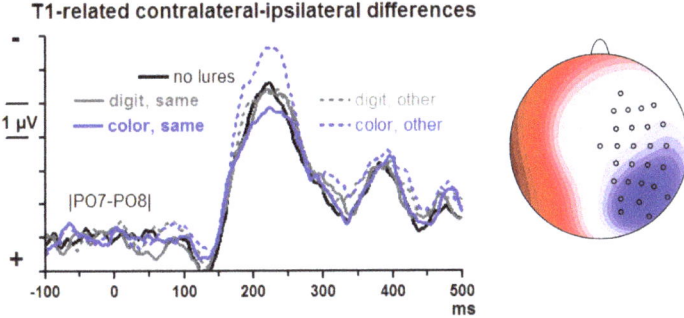

Figure 5. Contralateral–ipsilateral ERP differences evoked by T1. Data are grand means across participants, recorded from left and right posterior sites PO7 and PO8. Unit on x-axis is milliseconds, time-point zero is lure onset. Unit on y-axis is microvolts, negative voltage is plotted upwards. Waveforms evoked in no-lure trials are black, from color-lure trials blue, and from digit-lure trials grey. Trials where lures were in the same stream as T1 are denoted by solid lines (grey and blue) and trials where lures were in the opposite stream are denoted by dashed lines. The scalp map shows the view on the head (120°) from above. Recording sites (small circles) are depicted on one hemisphere only because the contralateral–ipsilateral differences were pooled across left and right sides. Blue is contralateral negativity, red is positivity. Scale is ±7 µV. Displayed is the topographic distribution of N2pc evoked in no-lure trials at the peak latency of N2pc (222 ms).

T1-evoked N2pc reliably increased when color lures had preceded on the other side. (Main effect of Lure-T1 Relation $F_{1,13} = 19.8$, $p = 0.001$, modified by the interaction of Lure-T1 Relation × Lure Type $F_{1,13} = 5.9$, $p = 0.03$, resolved to a simple effect of Lure-T1 Relation with color lures, $F_{1,13} = 55.8$, $p < 0.001$, and absence of such effect with digit lures, $F_{1,13} = 0.3$, n.s.). The main effect of Lure Type was not significant ($F_{1,13} = 1.0$, n.s.).

Confirming the ANOVA results, t tests of the four lure conditions against no lures yielded a significant increase of negativity for color lures in the other stream, $t = -4.6$, $p < 0.001$, and no significant differences for any of the three other conditions, $t \leq |1.2|$, $p \geq 0.24$.

3.4. ERP Reflections of Lure Effects on T2 Processing

T2-evoked ERPs were computed from 28 trials per participant (50 trials per cell minus about 33% trials with incorrect responses minus artifact-affected trials).

T2-evoked contralateral–ipsilateral differences from posterior–lateral sites |PO7–PO8| are displayed in Figure 6, separately for T2 on the same side as T1 and T2 on the other side from T1. Since T2 followed on T1 with a lag of 3, = 330 ms, the leftmost time-point of Figure 6 (−100 ms) is time-point 230 ms of Figure 5 (except that Figure 5 also includes trials where T2 followed T1 at lag 1 whereas Figure 6 includes trials with lag 3 only). At that time, T1-evoked N2pc just reaches its peak in Figure 5. Thus, Figure 6 starts with the decreasing slope of T1-evoked N2pc. This decrease is plotted with same polarity (descending towards positivity) when T2 and T1 are on the same side (left panel of Figure 6) and with opposite polarity in the other case (ascending towards negativity; right panel).

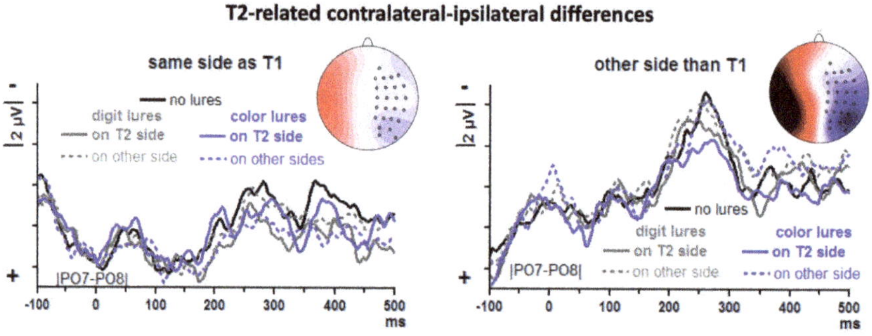

Figure 6. Contralateral–ipsilateral ERP differences evoked by T2. Data are grand means across participants, recorded from left and right posterior sites PO7 and PO8. Unit on x-axis is milliseconds, time-point zero is lure onset. Unit on y-axis is microvolts, negative voltage is plotted upwards. Waveforms evoked in no-lure trials are black, from color-lure trials blue, and from digit-lure trials grey. Trials where lures were in the same stream as T2 are denoted by solid lines (grey and blue) and trials where lures were in the opposite stream are denoted by dashed lines. The left panel displays data where T1 was in the same stream as T2, and the right panel displays data where T1 was in the other stream. Time-point −100 ms is approximately the peak of that preceding T1. The scalp maps show the view on the head (120°) from above. Recording sites (small circles) are depicted on one hemisphere only because the contralateral–ipsilateral differences were pooled across left and right sides. Blue is contralateral negativity, red is positivity. Scale is ±8 µV. Displayed is the topographic distribution of N2pc evoked in no-lure trials at the peak latencies of N2pc (282 ms in same-stream-as-T1 trials, 260 ms in opposite-stream trials).

There is a distinct N2pc when T2 was preceded by T1 in the other stream (right panel of Figure 6), peaking at about 250 ms, and a similar though apparently smaller component is visible when T2 was preceded by T1 in the same stream (left panel of Figure 6). To quantify these impressions, N2pc was measured by computing mean amplitudes 200–300 ms.

First, T2-evoked N2pcs were compared between same-side T1 and other-side T1 in an ANOVA on no-lure trials with the one factor T1-T2 Relation (same side, other side). Indeed, N2pc was larger after other-side T1 than after same-side T1, $F_{1,13} = 13.8$, $p = 0.003$. Then, lure effects were measured by computing the differences between lure trials and no-lure trials, separately for each of the four lure conditions and for T1-T2 same-side and other-side trials, and submitting these difference values to an ANOVA with the factors Lure Type (color, digit), Lure-T2 Relation (same side, other side) and T1-T2 Relation (same side, other side). In this ANOVA on difference values, the constant term was different from zero, $F_{1,13} = 7.2$, $p = 0.02$, indicating that there was an overall N2pc difference between lure and no-lure trials which, as Figure 6 shows, was an overall reduction of N2pc by the presence of lures. None of the factors had significant influence on this lure effect, though, all $F_{1,13} \leq 2.8$, $p \geq 0.12$.

When nevertheless testing each of the eight lure conditions separately against the no-lure condition, reductions were significant when digit lures preceded on the same side and also T1 was on that side ($t = 2.3$, $p = 0.04$; solid grey line in left panel of Figure 6) and when color lures preceded on the same side and T1 was on the other side ($t = 2.7$, $p = 0.02$; solid blue line in right panel of Figure 6).

4. Discussion

In a demanding task with spatially varying rapid presentation, we tested the impact of early occurrence of features that were typical of the second target. The original variation of the present study from several earlier studies [3–12,15] was that lures resembled T2 in two different, alternative ways. Our major expectation about these two types of lures was confirmed: Their effects on T2 identification grossly diverged (main effect of Lure Type $p < 0.001$). T2 identification was impeded by color lures and was mainly improved by digit lures.

We had assumed as a mechanism underlying this divergence of effects that color lures falsely attract attention to their stream while digit lures positively prime the identification of digits. From this viewpoint, the obtained results will be discussed in detail. It will be concluded that these mechanisms were indeed at work but cannot account for the whole pattern of results.

4.1. T2 Identification

We focused analysis on the lag 3 trials. This was an a posteriori decision (suggested by one reviewer of this paper) because the three-level factor T1-T2 Relation in the ANOVA on all data was hard to interpret, being composed of the distinction between same-side and different-side T1 at lag 3 and the distinction between lags 3 and 1 for different-side T1. By dropping the lag 1 data, analysis could focus on the effects of same-side vs. different-side targets.

This mixed three-level factor had been a consequence of our decision to omit lag 1 same-side T1-T2 from the experiment altogether because T2 identification uses to be near perfect in this condition and otherwise the experiment would have been too long. In the light of this a posteriori decision to drop the remaining lag 1 condition from the main analysis, in planning the experiment it might have been wiser to achieve the necessary reduction of trials not by complete omission of lag 1 same-side trials but rather by balanced reduction of lag 1 trials both for same-side and different-side targets.

In any case, corresponding to the analysis in the Results section, also the following discussion will focus on the lag 3 trials.

4.1.1. No-Lure Trials

The mean identification rate of 66% in no-lure trials at lag 3 was lower than we had expected based on preceding studies where T2 identification was frequently close to 80% for lags > 1 [33]. A problem in designing this study had been that T2 stood out from its background not only by being a digit among letters, as usual, but additionally by its color, being blue among black stimuli. From pilot data, we worried that identification rates would be too much improved by this additional feature, reaching ceiling, therefore we increased the presentation rate from our usual 7.7/s (130 ms per frame) to 9/s (110 ms per frame). This might have been too fast.

Alternatively, identification rates might have suffered even in no-lure trials from the presence of lures. This appears plausible because T2 identification rates were low not only in the present study but also in our previous lure study [15] where mean rates in no-lure trials at lag 3 barely reached 60% although T2 appearance and presentation rates conformed to our usual standard that has usually resulted in rates of 80%. Perhaps the presence of potentially distracting lure stimuli causes participants to invest more attention in the task than usual. Such increased investment of attention might actually be detrimental to performance [34,35]. Or the concepts may be applied that have been suggested by episodic distinction approaches to the attentional blink [2,18]: Having expected the irrelevant lures first which were not to be included in the "evaluation window" [18], participants might have still waited for those events in the no-lure trials and might have opened their "evaluation window" too late for processing the actually relevant events.

Left-side T2 was better identified than right-side T2, as has been found again and again in dual-stream RSVP tasks [11,12,33]. Until recently, we had ascribed this to dominance of the right hemisphere in shifting attention. But recent studies made a clear case for learned strategies of left-to-right reading as the underlying cause [36–38].

4.1.2. Lure Effects

As predicted, color lures were much more detrimental than digit lures. Different from our predictions, though, were the spatial specificities of those effects.

For color lures, we had predicted that their negative effect would be most evident when lures and T2 are in different streams and that there might be even a positive effect on same-stream T2. Indeed, color lures' negative effects on T2 identification were smaller when T2 was in the same stream than when T2 was in the other stream. Yet same-stream lures still had negative effects rather than positive ones. Thus, while it might still be true that color lures attracted attention (cf. below, 4.3), as expected, this shift of attention did not appear to be the only mechanism responsible for their negative effects on T2 identification. Nor were these effects moderated by T1 position in the predicted way: We had assumed that the attention-distracting effects of color lures on other-stream T2 (dashed blue line in Figure 2) might be enhanced by T1 occurring in the lure stream and attenuated by T1 occurring in the T2 stream. This hypothesis was more incorrect than correct. In line with the hypothesis was the relatively large negative effect of other-stream (left-side) lures on *L3R*. But against expectation, the maximum negative effect of lures on other-stream T2 occurred when T1 and T2 were in the same stream (*L3L*).

For digit lures, we had predicted that spatial effects would be largely absent because the relevant mechanism of their presumed positive effects on T2 identification was assumed to be priming of digits as a category. Based on the actual results we cannot firmly exclude category priming as a mechanism. But the spatial specificity of the obtained effects came as a surprise. The expected positive effects on T2 identification were considerably more distinct when lures and T2 were in different streams than when they were in the same stream, and were restricted to effects of right-side lures (improving identification of left-side T2 in the sequences rR1L, rL3L, rR3L, and of right-side T2 in the sequence rL3R). The effect in the first three cases is remarkable because left-side T2s have already an advantage over right-side T2s in the no-lure control condition, so the positive lure effect did not serve for restoring the balance but rather exacerbated the differences.

Further below, we will offer a hypothesis about the mechanisms underlying these effects of color lures and digit lures. Since our original hypothesis failed, this proposed mechanism will remain speculative.

4.2. T1 Identification

4.2.1. No-Lure Trials

T1 was identified best when presented in the right stream, followed by T2 in the same, right stream. The right-side advantage for T1 has been found in several of our studies using this task where T1 data for right and left sides were separately reported. Either as a main effect or interacting with T2 side or lag, the effect was obtained in Exp.1 of [14], in Taiwanese and Israelis in [38], and in [39–41], with a total of 163 participants. The effect was not obtained in some other studies of ours using this task ([25,42–45]) with a total of 123 participants. Similarly, an advantage for identification of T1 followed by T2 on the same side has been found several times, either as a main effect or interacting with T1 side or lag [12,15,40,46], with a total of 73 participants. Yet one study on 50 participants yielded the opposite effect [47] and several studies, with a total of 206 participants, yielded no effect [25,38,39,41–43]. Thus, the present good identification of right T1 followed by right T2 seems to be a both replicable and variable phenomenon.

The advantage of right T1 might be related to left-hemisphere specialization for language [48], and its variability across experiments may confirm Hellige's [49] conclusion that laterality of letter identification depends on the detailed circumstances. Accounting for the effect of side of the following T2 on identification of the previous T1 seems more challenging. Worse T1 identification when T2 is on the same side [47] might be due to backward masking. The opposite better T1 identification when T2 is on the same side [14,15,40,46] may be taken to suggest that, like a post-cue [50,51], T2 is able to draw attention not only to its ongoing stimulus stream but, given beneficial circumstances, also to the short-term memory representation of previous stimuli in this stream.

4.2.2. Lure Effects

We had not stated any hypothesis about effects of lures on T1 identification.

Based on our initial attention-attraction hypothesis of color lures, it makes sense to assume that T1 identification was impaired when color lures had preceded in the other stream, withdrawing attention from the stream in which T1 was presented. As Figure 2 showed (blue dashed line), this did indeed apply to those two of the four *lag 3* instances where T1 and T2 were in the same stream (L3L and R3R) but did not apply when T2 was in the other stream (L3R and R3L). Moreover, this hypothesis does not account for the large negative effect on T1 identification both for color and digit lures when, lures, T1 and L2 were all in the same, right-side stream. Nor is there any clue why the was positive priming on T1 when digit lures were left, T1 was right, and T2 was left again (grey dashed line in Figure 2 at R3L).

4.3. Lure-Evoked ERPs: N2pc

The N2pc component is a marker of shifts of spatial attention [20–24], possibly in order to individuate the attention-attracting stimuli [52]. Based on the notion of attentional shifts, it was assumed that color lures will evoke larger N2pc than digit lures and, more trivially, that the first lure in a row will evoke larger N2pc than the second and third ones because the three lures are all on the same side (as in [15]). Both assumptions were confirmed. These results confirm that color lures attracted more attention than digit lures.

In recent studies, a contralateral positive potential, following the N2pc or even instead of N2pc, has been described to be the major ERP signature of distracting stimuli in visual search arrays [23]. It has been suggested that this "P_D" indicates an inhibitory mechanism to prevent stimuli from catching attention [53]. The question may, therefore, be asked why lures evoked contralateral negativity (N2pc) rather than positivity (P_D). As pointed out by one reviewer of this manuscript, one reason might be that lures were, by definition, similar to targets. Such similarity has resulted in N2pc rather than P_D being evoked by distractors in previous studies (e.g., [54,55]). A P_D is typically observed with targets that are easy to find and clearly distinct from the distractor [23,56,57] whereas an N2pc will result, like in the present study (as well as in [10,15]), when targets are difficult to find [58].

4.4. Lure-Evoked ERPs: Frontal Negativity

In previous studies, lures evoked a negative component at 300 ms [7,8,10,15,19]. This negativity became larger across the three lure events within a trial in [15] and was accordingly interpreted by those authors as reflecting frontal gating for inhibition. That increase was not replicated in [15] (and could not be replicated in [10], because one lure only was presented in each trial). To accommodate these divergent results, we assumed that frontal gating is only necessary when lures are potentially harmful to T2 identification. Therefore, it was predicted that such frontal negativity will increase over lure repetitions mainly with color lures.

Genuinely fronto-central negative activation (excluding the peak evoked by first color lures at 300 ms which was volume-conducted from posterior sites) did occur in the present data, as corroborated by computing CSDs. But this activation occurred later than in most of those previous studies (except [8]), from 340 ms onwards, and took the form of slow shifts.

As expected, frontal negativity increased across lure repetitions. But unexpectedly, this increase occurred with digit lures as well as with color lures whereas we had expected that the effect would be larger with color lures because only color lures had negative effects on T2 identification. Interpreting frontal negativity as indicator of gating for inhibitory purposes [8,10] we would have to conclude that the positively priming digit lures underwent inhibition to the same degree as the distracting color lures. This does not seem probable.

As an alternative, it may be suspected that these late potentials evoked by the later lures actually are not evoked by lures but rather by the ensuing T1. (The minimum interval between 3rd lure and T1 was 220 ms only, and 330 ms from 2nd lure to T1. Thus, although mean intervals were much longer, 350 ms and 600 ms, there might have remained some vestige of T1 in the analyzed epochs). However, any such effects had been prevented by having subtracted data of no-lure control trials from the lure trials. Thereby, any T1-evoked potentials were subtracted out. This leaves us to assume that these components were evoked by the later lures specifically in expectancy of T1, i.e., that these FCz-focused relatively slow potentials are CNVs (Contingent Negative Variations, [59–61]) in expectancy of T1 because the third and second lures provided some temporal structure to the otherwise undifferentiated stream of background stimuli, thereby enabling participants to build some short-term expectations. To conclude, these slow frontal negative shifts might rather be CNV-type expectancy potentials for better localizing T1 in time than reflect inhibitory activity.

4.5. T1-Evoked N2pc

T1-evoked N2pc was expected to increase to the extent that an attention shift is required (e.g., [46]). Without lures, attention will be randomly distributed across the two streams whereas color lures will attract attention to their stream. T1, presented on average 350 ms after the final lure, will, therefore, require either less or more shifting of attention depending on its being presented either in the same stream as color lures or in the other stream. Accordingly, T1-evoked N2pc was expected to be either smaller or larger than in trials without lures depending on color lures and T1 being either in the same stream or in different streams.

Results were in reasonably good agreement with these predictions: T1-evoked N2pc was not at all affected by digit lures, was increased when color lures preceded in the other stream and showed a weak tendency to be reduced (far from significance, though) when color lures preceded in the same stream.

Additionally, we had speculated that T1-evoked N2pc might increase after any lures because the sequence of three lures is helpful to expecting T1 precisely in time. Evidence for this supportive function of lures was provided by the CNV-type negativity evoked by the final lures as discussed in the previous section. However, amplitude of T1-evoked N2pc was not generally increased by preceding lures. (Nor was it in our previous lure study, [15]). In fact, we do not know of evidence showing that N2pc is larger when evoked by events whose timing can be better predicted. Thus, this hypothesis might have been unfounded.

4.6. T2-Evoked N2pc

We had expected that, by using the two types of lures, our data might reconcile conflicting results of previous studies. Specifically, color lures might lead to a delay in N2pc, reflecting ongoing inhibition, like in Zhang et al. [10], and digit lures might lead to a decrease of N2pc amplitude when lures and T2 are in the same stream, like in Verleger et al. [15].

However, this is not what we obtained. Rather, the ANOVA yielded a general reducing effect of preceding lures on N2pc amplitude. Close inspection of Figure 6 suggests that this may be particularly true, like in [15], when lures were presented on the same side as T2, and indeed this is where significant deviations from no-lure trials were found in *t* tests on single conditions. But this was as well true for digit lures (as predicted) as for color lures (not predicted). In any case, differences of lure effects between lure types and lure sides were not significant in the ANOVA, casting doubt on any differential interpretation other than that lures generally reduced T2-evoked N2pc.

Such general reduction of T2-evoked N2pc amplitudes after preceding lures needs some interpretation. Above, with N2pc evoked by lures and by T1, we have interpreted N2pc reductions as consequence of the fact that attention had already been shifted before to the respective location, which is compatible with a facilitating effect of lures. On the other hand, N2pc may be reduced because participants are less capable of shifting their attention (e.g., [26]) which is compatible with an interfering effect of lures. For these reasons, with the different lure effects on N2pc not reliably differing from each other, the interpretation of this general reduction remains unclear.

This lack of specificity in lure effects might well be a Type-2 error caused by noisy signals. By design, each of the 10 analyzed conditions (no lures, digit and color lures on same and on other side × T2 on same vs. other side as T1 at lag 3) consisted of 50 trials, namely 25 left-T2 and 25 right-T2 trials. This is certainly at the lower limit of what is required for N2pc. Moreover, this number of 50 trials was reduced by the fact that only correctly responded T2 trials entered analysis which were, e.g., for the no-lure condition, about 66% of the lag 3 trials (cf. Table 1). Together with rejection of trials for artifacts in the EEG, this led to a mean number of 28 trials per condition.

4.7. Speculation on Underlying Mechanisms

It appears that the ERP results may serve for defining some boundary conditions: Indeed, color lures attracted more attention than digit lures (lure-evoked N2pc), both types of lures might have been equally helpful in localizing T1 in time (lure-following frontal negativity), color lures indeed made a shift of attention necessary when T1 was in the other stream (T1-evoked N2pc), and lures somehow affected attention shifts to T2 although the nature of that affection remained unclear (T2-evoked N2pc). However, it seems that the unexpected result pattern of lure effects on target identification cannot be brought into a coherent picture by means of these ERP results. Thus, we are left to speculate, based on the pattern of the above-discussed identification effects and on previous literature.

Building on perceptual-episode accounts of the attentional blink [2,18] it appears to us that the major function of lures might be to make participants uncertain about the order of events. Unlike in the tasks with multiple targets explored by Wyble et al. [2] and Dell'Acqua et al. [62], T1 can hardly be mistaken to be T2 in our task (one being a letter, the other a digit). But, if sufficiently similar to T2, lures may fool participants into thinking that one of the lures might have already been T2 and that, therefore, T1 had been missed. When then T1 is nonetheless encountered, it might get processed (after the lure which would act as first target) as a second target in time, thereby suffering from the asymmetry of T2 identification, being much worse identified when presented on the right than when presented on the left. This agrees with the cumulation of negative effects of lures on T1 identification in the R3R sequence. In order to account for the fact that this is particularly true with R3R, and not equally with R3L and R1L, we have to additionally assume that the presentation of T2 in the same stream as T1 (R3R) is apt to increase participants' confusion about the roles assigned to the successive targets.

The crucial factor in the difference between color and digit lures might have been which one is more similar to T2, thereby confusing participants more about the order of events. We may assume that, in our task, participants searched for T2 by its color above all, perhaps in order to use the same strategy as in searching for T1 which was exclusively defined by its color (red letter among black letters). This might be the major reason why color lures had a negative impact on T2 identification: Blue letters, more than black digits, might have led participants to believe that the blue digit had already been presented, thereby terminating their search for the true T2. This reasoning may account for the minor role of spatial specificity of color-lure effects. In fact, similar conclusions have emerged from a research tradition where lures were not similar to T2 but rather to the only target that had to be detected in a central RSVP stream, and lure-type distractors were placed in the periphery of this central stream: Also here, color lures in the periphery had spatially non-specific negative effects, by interfering with detection of the centrally presented target [63–68].

In contrast to color lures, the black digit lures could hardly be mistaken for T2 and, thereby, could serve as positive primes for T2 identification. Perhaps a certain extent of confounding the lures and T2 was still possible when digit lures and T2 were in the same stream. This might explain why positive priming was regularly obtained when digit lures and T2 were in different stream and not when they were in the same stream. Finally, the reason for the asymmetry of the positive digit-lure effect (exclusively by right-side lures and mainly on left-side T2) is not really clear. It may be due to better processing of the alphanumeric character of lures in the left hemisphere or, alternatively due to the preferred processing of left-side T2 in this dual-RSVP paradigm.

5. Conclusions

In conclusion, the spatial variation enabled by the dual-stream task and the use of two types of lures provided rich opportunity for observing a variety of lure effects which require more solid theoretical interpretation than could here be achieved post hoc.

Supplementary Materials: The following are available online at http://www.mdpi.com/2076-3425/9/12/365/s1, Table S1: Percentages of trials with correctly identified targets.

Author Contributions: Conceptualization, R.V. and L.M.; software, L.M.; formal analysis, R.V.; investigation, K.Ś. and L.H.; writing—original draft preparation, R.V.; writing—review and editing, K.Ś., M.N., L.M.; visualization, R.V.; funding acquisition, R.V. and M.N.

Funding: This work was supported by grants Ve110/15-2 and Ni513/8-2 awarded from the Deutsche Forschungsgemeinschaft to R.V. and M.N. as parts of the network PAK270 "Neuro-cognitive mechanisms of conscious and unconscious visual perception".

Acknowledgments: Critical comments provided by three reviewers (Dirk Kerzel and two anonymous ones) on an earlier version of this manuscript considerably helped in improving the paper.

Conflicts of Interest: The authors declare no conflict of interest. The funders had no role in the design of the study; in the collection, analyses, or interpretation of data; in the writing of the manuscript, or in the decision to publish the results.

References

1. Chun, M.M.; Potter, M.C. A two-stage model for multiple target detection in rapid serial visual presentation. *J. Exp. Psychol. Hum. Percept. Perform.* **1995**, *21*, 109–127. [CrossRef] [PubMed]
2. Wyble, B.; Bowman, H.; Nieuwenstein, M. The attentional blink provides episodic distinctiveness: Sparing at a cost. *J. Exp. Psychol. Hum. Percept. Perform.* **2009**, *35*, 787–807. [CrossRef] [PubMed]
3. Maki, W.S.; Padmanabhan, G. Transient suppression of processing during rapid serial visual presentation: Acquired distinctiveness of probes modulates the attentional blink. *Psychon. Bull. Rev.* **1994**, *1*, 499–504. [CrossRef] [PubMed]
4. Hay, J.L.; Milders, M.M.; Sahraie, A.; Niedeggen, M. The effect of perceptual load on attention-induced motion blindness: The efficiency of selective inhibition. *J. Exp. Psychol. Hum. Percept. Perform.* **2006**, *32*, 885–907. [CrossRef] [PubMed]
5. Hesselmann, G.; Niedeggen, M.; Sahraie, A.; Milders, M. Specifying the distractor inhibition account of attention-induced motion blindness. *Vis. Res.* **2006**, *46*, 1048–1056. [CrossRef] [PubMed]
6. Hesselmann, G.; Allan, J.L.; Sahraie, A.; Milders, M.; Niedeggen, M. Inhibition related impairments of coherent motion perception in the attention-induced motion blindness paradigm. *Spat. Vis.* **2009**, *22*, 493–509. [CrossRef]
7. Niedeggen, M.; Michael, L.; Hesselmann, G. Closing the gates to consciousness: Distractors activate a central inhibition process. *J. Cogn. Neurosci.* **2012**, *24*, 1294–1304. [CrossRef]
8. Niedeggen, M.; Busch, N.A.; Winther, G.N. The state of a central inhibition system predicts access to visual targets: An ERP study on distractor-induced blindness (DIB). *Conscious. Cogn.* **2015**, *35*, 308–318. [CrossRef]
9. Winther, G.N.; Niedeggen, M. Distractor-induced blindness: A special case of contingent attentional capture? *Adv. Cogn. Psychol.* **2017**, *13*, 52–63. [CrossRef]
10. Zhang, D.; Zhou, X.; Martens, S. The impact of negative attentional set upon target processing in RSVP: An ERP study. *Neuropsychologia* **2009**, *47*, 2604–2614. [CrossRef]

11. Zhang, D.; Zhou, X.; Martens, S. Negative attentional set in the attentional blink: Control is not lost. *Atten. Percept. Psychophys.* **2011**, *73*, 2489–2501. [CrossRef] [PubMed]
12. Harris, I.M.; Benito, C.T.; Dux, P.E. Priming from distractors in rapid serial visual presentation is modulated by image properties and attention. *J. Exp. Psychol. Hum. Percept. Perform.* **2010**, *36*, 1595–1608. [CrossRef] [PubMed]
13. Holländer, A.; Corballis, M.C.; Hamm, J.P. Visual-field asymmetry in dual-stream RSVP. *Neuropsychologia* **2005**, *43*, 35–40. [CrossRef] [PubMed]
14. Verleger, R.; Sprenger, A.; Gebauer, S.; Fritzmannova, M.; Friedrich, M.; Kraft, S.; Jaśkowski, P. On why left events are the right ones: Neural mechanisms underlying the left-hemifield advantage in rapid serial visual presentation. *J. Cogn. Neurosci.* **2009**, *21*, 474–488. [CrossRef] [PubMed]
15. Verleger, R.; Śmigasiewicz, K.; Michael, L.; Niedeggen, M. Effects of premature lure stimuli on 2nd-target identification in rapid serial visual presentation: Inhibition induced by lures or by 1st target? *Psychophysiology* **2012**, *49*, 1254–1265. [CrossRef]
16. Eimer, M.; Schlaghecken, F. Effects of masked stimuli on motor activation: Behavioral and electrophysiological evidence. *J. Exp. Psychol. Human. Percept. Perform.* **1998**, *24*, 1737–1747. [CrossRef]
17. Jaśkowski, P.; Białuńska, A.; Tomanek, M.; Verleger, R. Mask- and distractor-triggered inhibitory processes in the priming of motor responses: An EEG study. *Psychophysiology* **2008**, *45*, 70–85. [CrossRef]
18. Klauer, K.C.; Dittrich, K. From sunshine to double arrows: An evaluation window account of negative compatibility effects. *J. Exp. Psychol. Gen.* **2010**, *36*, 892–905. [CrossRef]
19. Niedeggen, M.; Hesselmann, G.; Sahraie, A.; Milders, M.; Blakemore, C. Probing the prerequisites for motion blindness. *J. Cogn. Neurosci.* **2004**, *16*, 584–597. [CrossRef]
20. Luck, S.J.; Fan, S.; Hillyard, S.A. Attention-related modulation of sensory-evoked brain activity in a visual search task. *J. Cogn. Neurosci.* **1993**, *5*, 188–195. [CrossRef]
21. Wascher, E.; Wauschkuhn, B. The interaction of stimulus- and response-related processes measured by event-related lateralisations of the EEG. *Electroencephalogr. Clin. Neurophysiol.* **1996**, *99*, 149–162. [CrossRef]
22. Eimer, M. The N2pc component as an indicator of attentional selectivity. *Electroencephalogr. Clin. Neurophysiol.* **1996**, *99*, 225–234. [CrossRef]
23. Hickey, C.; Di Lollo, V.; McDonald, J.J. Electrophysiological indices of target and distractor processing in visual search. *J. Cogn. Neurosci.* **2009**, *21*, 760–775. [CrossRef] [PubMed]
24. Tay, D.; Harms, V.; Hillyard, S.A.; McDonald, J.J. Electrophysiological correlates of visual singleton detection. *Psychophysiology* **2019**, *56*, e13375. [CrossRef] [PubMed]
25. Verleger, R.; Śmigasiewicz, K.; Möller, F. Mechanisms underlying the left visual-field advantage in the dual stream RSVP task: Evidence from N2pc, P3, and distractor-evoked VEPs. *Psychophysiology* **2011**, *48*, 1096–1106. [CrossRef]
26. Dell'Acqua, R.; Sessa, P.; Jolicœur, P.; Robitaille, N. Spatial attention freezes during the attentional blink. *Psychophysiology* **2006**, *43*, 394–400. [CrossRef]
27. Oldfield, R.C. The assessment and analysis of handedness: The Edinburgh inventory. *Neuropsychologia* **1971**, *9*, 97–113. [CrossRef]
28. Kiefer, M.; Brendel, D. Attentional modulation of unconscious "automatic" processes: Evidence from event-related potentials in a masked priming paradigm. *J. Cogn. Neurosci.* **2006**, *18*, 184–198. [CrossRef]
29. Visser, T.A.W.; Zuvic, S.M.; Bischof, W.F.; Di Lollo, V. The attentional blink with targets in different spatial locations. *Psychon. Bull. Rev.* **1999**, *6*, 432–436. [CrossRef]
30. Wyble, B.; Bowman, H.; Potter, M. Categorically defined targets trigger spatiotemporal visual attention. *J. Exp. Psychol. Hum. Percept. Perform.* **2009**, *35*, 324–337. [CrossRef]
31. Müller, M.M.; Picton, T.W.; Valdes-Sosa, P.; Riera, J.; Teder-Sälejärvi, W.A.; Hillyard, S.A. Effects of spatial selective attention on the steady-state visual evoked potential in the 20–28 Hz range. *Cogn. Brain Res.* **1998**, *6*, 249–261. [CrossRef]
32. Kayser, J.; Tenke, C. Issues and considerations for using the scalp surface Laplacian in EEG/ERP research: A tutorial review. *Int. J. Psychophysiol.* **2015**, *97*, 189–209. [CrossRef] [PubMed]
33. Verleger, R.; Śmigasiewicz, K. Consciousness wanted, attention found: Reasons for the advantage of the left visual field in identifying T2 among rapidly presented series. *Conscious. Cogn.* **2015**, *35*, 260–273. [CrossRef] [PubMed]

34. Olivers, C.N.L.; Nieuwenhuis, S. The beneficial effects of additional task load, positive affect, and instruction on the attentional blink. *J. Exp. Psychol. Hum. Percept. Perform.* **2006**, *32*, 364–379. [CrossRef] [PubMed]
35. Taatgen, N.A.; Juvina, I.; Schipper, M.; Borst, J.P.; Martens, S. Too much control can hurt: A threaded cognition model of the attentional blink. *Cogn. Psychol.* **2009**, *59*, 1–29. [CrossRef] [PubMed]
36. Holcombe, A.O.; Nguyen, E.H.L.; Goodbourn, P.T. Implied reading direction and prioritization of letter encoding. *J. Exp. Psychol. Gen.* **2017**, *146*, 1420–1437. [CrossRef] [PubMed]
37. Ransley, K.; Goodbourn, P.T.; Nguyen, E.H.L.; Moustafa, A.A.; Holcombe, A.O. Reading direction influences lateral biases in letter processing. *J. Exp. Psychol. Learn. Mem. Cogn.* **2018**, *44*, 1678–1686. [CrossRef]
38. Śmigasiewicz, K.; Shalgi, S.; Hsieh, S.; Möller, F.; Jaffe, S.; Chang, C.C.; Verleger, R. Left visual-field advantage in the dual-stream RSVP task and reading direction: A study in three nations. *Neuropsychologia* **2010**, *48*, 2852–2860. [CrossRef]
39. Verleger, R.; Möller, F.; Kuniecki, M.; Śmigasiewicz, K.; Groppa, S.; Siebner, H.R. The left visual-field advantage in rapid visual presentation is amplified rather than reduced by posterior-parietal rTMS. *Exp. Brain Res.* **2010**, *203*, 355–365. [CrossRef]
40. Asanowicz, D.; Śmigasiewicz, K.; Verleger, R. Differences between visual hemifields in identifying rapidly presented target stimuli: Letters and digits, faces, and shapes. *Front. Psychol.* **2013**, *4*, 452. [CrossRef]
41. Asanowicz, D.; Kruse, L.; Śmigasiewicz, K.; Verleger, R. Lateralization of spatial rather than temporal attention underlies the left hemifield advantage in rapid serial visual presentation. *Brain Cogn.* **2017**, *118*, 54–62. [CrossRef] [PubMed]
42. Verleger, R.; Dittmer, M.; Śmigasiewicz, K. Cooperation or competition of the two hemispheres in processing characters presented at vertical midline. *PLoS ONE* **2013**, *8*, e57421. [CrossRef] [PubMed]
43. Śmigasiewicz, K.; Asanowicz, D.; Westphal, N.; Verleger, R. Bias for the left visual field in rapid serial visual presentation: Effects of additional salient cues suggest a critical role of attention. *J. Cogn. Neurosci.* **2015**, *27*, 266–279. [CrossRef] [PubMed]
44. Śmigasiewicz, K.; Liebrand, M.; Landmesser, J.; Verleger, R. How handedness influences perceptual and attentional processes during rapid serial visual presentation. *Neuropsychologia* **2017**, *100*, 155–163. [CrossRef]
45. Śmigasiewicz, K.; Wondany, K.; Verleger, R. Left-hemisphere delay of EEG potentials evoked by standard letter stimuli during rapid serial visual presentation: Indicating right-hemisphere advantage or left-hemisphere load? *Front. Psychol.* **2019**, *10*, 171. [CrossRef]
46. Śmigasiewicz, K.; Hasan, G.S.; Verleger, R. Rebalancing spatial attention: Endogenous orienting may partially overcome the left visual field bias in rapid serial visual presentation. *J. Cogn. Neurosci.* **2017**, *29*, 1–13. [CrossRef]
47. Śmigasiewicz, K.; Weinrich, J.; Reinhardt, B.; Verleger, R. Deployment and release of interhemispheric inhibition in dual-stream rapid serial visual presentation. *Biol. Psychol.* **2014**, *99*, 47–59. [CrossRef]
48. Gannon, P.J. Evolutionary depth of human brain language areas. In *The Two Halves of the Brain: Information Processing in the Cerebral Hemispheres*; Hugdahl, K., Westerhausen, R., Eds.; The MIT Press: Cambridge, MA, USA, 2010; pp. 37–63. [CrossRef]
49. Hellige, J.B. Feature similarity and laterality effects in visual masking. *Neuropsychologia* **1983**, *21*, 633–639. [CrossRef]
50. Kuo, B.-C.; Rao, A.; Lepsien, J.; Nobre, A.C. Searching for targets within the spatial layout of visual short-term memory. *J. Neurosci.* **2009**, *29*, 8032–8038. [CrossRef]
51. Dell'Acqua, R.; Sessa, P.; Toffanin, P.; Luria, R.; Jolicœur, P. Orienting attention to objects in visual short-term memory. *Neuropsychologia* **2010**, *48*, 419–428. [CrossRef]
52. Mazza, V.; Pagano, S.; Caramazza, A. Multiple object individuation and exact enumeration. *J. Cogn. Neurosci.* **2013**, *25*, 697–705. [CrossRef] [PubMed]
53. Gaspelin, N.; Luck, S.J. The role of inhibition in avoiding distraction by salient stimuli. *Trends Cogn. Sci.* **2018**, *22*, 79–92. [CrossRef] [PubMed]
54. Hilimire, M.R.; Mounts, J.R.; Parks, N.A.; Corballis, P.M. Dynamics of target and distractor processing in visual search: Evidence from event-related brain potentials. *Neurosci. Lett.* **2011**, *495*, 196–200. [CrossRef] [PubMed]
55. Liesefeld, H.R.; Liesefeld, A.M.; Töllner, T.; Müller, H.J. Attentional capture in visual search: Capture and post-capture dynamics revealed by EEG. *Neuroimage* **2017**, *156* (Suppl. C), 166–173. [CrossRef]

56. Burra, N.; Kerzel, D. The distractor positivity (Pd) signals lowering of attentional priority: Evidence from event-related potentials and individual differences. *Psychophysiology* **2014**, *51*, 685–696. [CrossRef]
57. Gaspar, J.M.; McDonald, J.J. Suppression of salient objects prevents distraction in visual search. *J. Neurosci.* **2014**, *34*, 5658–5666. [CrossRef]
58. Barras, C.; Kerzel, D. Salient-but-irrelevant stimuli cause attentional capture in difficult, but attentional suppression in easy visual search. *Psychophysiology* **2017**, *54*, 1826–1838. [CrossRef]
59. Walter, W.G.; Cooper, R.; Aldridge, V.J.; McCallum, W.C.; Winter, A.L. Contingent negative variation: An electric sign of sensorimotor association and expectancy in the human brain. *Nature* **1964**, *203*, 380–384. [CrossRef]
60. Brunia, C.H.M. Waiting in readiness: Gating in attention and motor preparation. *Psychophysiology* **1993**, *30*, 327–339. [CrossRef]
61. Trillenberg, P.; Verleger, R.; Wascher, E.; Wauschkuhn, B.; Wessel, K. CNV and temporal uncertainty with "ageing" and "non-ageing" S1-S2 intervals. *Clin. Neurophysiol.* **2000**, *111*, 1216–1226. [CrossRef]
62. Dell'Acqua, R.; Dux, P.E.; Wyble, B.; Jolicœur, P. Sparing from the attentional blink is not spared from structural limitations. *Psychon. Bull. Rev.* **2012**, *19*, 232–238. [CrossRef]
63. Folk, C.L.; Leber, A.B.; Egeth, H.E. Made you blink! Contingent attentional capture produces a spatial blink. *Percept. Psychophys.* **2002**, *64*, 741–753. [CrossRef] [PubMed]
64. Folk, C.L.; Leber, A.B.; Egeth, H.E. Top-down control settings and the attentional blink: Evidence for nonspatial contingent capture. *Vis. Cogn.* **2008**, *16*, 16–616. [CrossRef]
65. Moore, K.S.; Weissman, D.H. Involuntary transfer of a top-down attentional set into the focus of attention: Evidence from a contingent attentional capture paradigm. *Atten. Percept. Psychophys.* **2010**, *72*, 1495–1509. [CrossRef] [PubMed]
66. Moore, K.S.; Weissman, D.H. Set-specific capture can be reduced by pre-emptively occupying a limited-capacity focus of attention. *Vis. Cogn.* **2011**, *19*, 417–444. [CrossRef] [PubMed]
67. Zivony, A.; Lamy, D. Attentional engagement is not sufficient to prevent spatial capture. *Atten. Percept. Psychophys.* **2014**, *76*, 19–31. [CrossRef]
68. Zivony, A.; Lamy, D. Attentional capture and engagement during the attentional blink: A "camera" metaphor of attention. *J. Exp. Psychol. Hum. Percept. Perform.* **2016**, *42*, 1886–1902. [CrossRef]

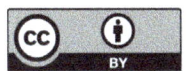

© 2019 by the authors. Licensee MDPI, Basel, Switzerland. This article is an open access article distributed under the terms and conditions of the Creative Commons Attribution (CC BY) license (http://creativecommons.org/licenses/by/4.0/).

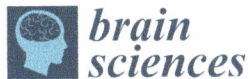

Article

Early Attentional Modulation by Working Memory Training in Young Adult ADHD Patients during a Risky Decision-Making Task

Manon E. Jaquerod [1], Sarah K. Mesrobian [1], Alessandro E. P. Villa [1], Michel Bader [2] and Alessandra Lintas [1,3,*]

[1] NeuroHeuristic Research Group, HEC-Lausanne, University of Lausanne, Quartier UNIL-Chamberonne, 1015 Lausanne, Switzerland; manon.jaquerod@unil.ch (M.E.J.); smesrobian@neuristic.org (S.K.M.); Alessandro.Villa@unil.ch (A.E.P.V.)
[2] University Service of Child and Adolescent Psychiatry, University Hospital of Lausanne, 1014 Lausanne, Switzerland; bader_m@bluewin.ch
[3] Faculty of Law, Criminal Justice and Public Administration, University of Lausanne, Quartier UNIL-Chamberonne, 1015 Lausanne, Switzerland
* Correspondence: alessandra.lintas@unil.ch or alessandro.villa@unil.ch

Received: 11 November 2019; Accepted: 3 January 2020; Published: 9 January 2020

Abstract: Background: Working memory (WM) deficits and impaired decision making are among the characteristic symptoms of patients affected by attention deficit/hyperactivity disorder (ADHD). The inattention associated with the disorder is likely to be due to functional deficits of the neural networks inhibiting irrelevant sensory input. In the presence of unnecessary information, a good decisional process is impaired and ADHD patients tend to take risky decisions. This study is aimed to test the hypothesis that the level of difficulty of a WM training (WMT) is affecting the top-down modulation of the attentional processes in a probabilistic gambling task. **Methods**: Event-related potentials (ERP) triggered by the choice of the amount wagered in the gambling task were recorded, before and after WMT with a the dual n-back task, in young ADHD adults and matched controls. For each group of participants, randomly assigned individuals were requested to perform WMT with a fixed baseline level of difficulty. The remaining participants were trained with a performance-dependent adaptive n-level of difficulty. **Results**: We compared the ERP recordings before and after 20 days of WMT in each subgroup. The analysis was focused on the time windows with at least three recording sites showing differences before and after training, after Bonferroni correction ($p < 0.05$). In ADHD, the P1 wave component was selectively affected at frontal sites and its shape was recovered close to controls' only after adaptive training. In controls, the strongest contrast was observed at parietal level with a left hemispheric dominance at latencies near 900 ms, more after baseline than after adaptive training. **Conclusion**: Partial restoration of early selective attentional processes in ADHD patients might occur after WMT with a high cognitive load. Modified frontal sites' activities might constitute a neural marker of this effect in a gambling task. In controls, conversely, an increase in late parietal negativity might rather be a marker of an increase in transfer effects to fluid intelligence.

Keywords: working-memory training; selective attention; cognitive remediation; EEG; ERP; P1; P3b; N500; late posterior negative slow wave; late parietal negativity

1. Introduction

The information necessary for complex cognitive tasks, which require the expectation that a relevant stimulus is remembered, must be encoded and maintained in working memory (WM) with a prior selective attention that is necessary to ignore irrelevant information for further processing. Patients diagnosed with attention deficit/hyperactive disorder (ADHD) are characterized by poor WM, poor concentration, high impulsivity, tendency to excessive talking, impairement in maintaining focused attention and a multiple range of associated disorders [1–4]. Limited or untidy attentional resources in ADHD patients would reduce the anticipation of ensuing stimuli to be remembered and the amount of information that can be encoded [5,6]. Impaired selective attention processes during encoding information in WM and the resulting WM deficits have been observed in ADHD patients in association with altered functional connectivity of cortical and subcortical networks involving, in particular, the prefrontal cortex (PFC) [7–10]. Besides, neurophysiological evidence show that improvement in WM performance is achieved by invariant and distributed neuronal dynamics in the PFC [11].

A growing body of evidence shows that a few weeks of WM training for children and adults suffering from ADHD has positive behavioral and cognitive effects [12–15], Transfer effects reported after WM training [16,17] suggest that such training could be an alternative therapeutic approach to drugs for ADHD patients [18–20]. However, some comprehensive reviews and meta-analyses draw a more skeptical conclusion [21–24]: the training has a limited efficacy, the generalization and the duration of the effects are questionable, and the underlying neurophysiological processes remain unclear.

It is known that WM deficits are associated with impaired decision making in individuals with substance addictions and alcohol-dependency [25,26]. Risky decision making in an experimental task, the Iowa gambling task, is poorly performed by ADHD patients [27,28] and WM impairments characterizing ADHD were suggested to moderate the expression of risky decision-making in patients affected by this disorder [29–31]. Indeed, ADHD patients often choose riskier options with unfavorable outcomes in economic and financial settings [32,33]. More generally, substance use disorders, pathological gambling, and ADHD [26,34–36], as well as healthy participants charged with a high WM load [37], shared deficits in tasks associated with ventral prefrontal cortical dysfunction. On the one hand, the structural abnormalities observed in young adults with ADHD suggest complex audio-visual, motivational, and emotional dysfunctions [38]. The dual n-back task, on the other hand, is a WM training task in which the participants have to remember two independent sequences of audio-visual stimuli and must identify when an auditory or visual stimulus matches the one that appeared n trials back [39,40].

In the current work, we extend our previous study with EEG recordings, which showed differences in brain dynamics between controls and young adult patients with ADHD during the performance of a probabilistic gambling task [41]. Our working hypothesis is that WM training with the Dual n-back task is acting on a top-down modulation of the attentional processes with participation of prefrontal and parietal areas as sources of the efferent control signals. In the current study, we present new evidence that WM training affects selectively the activity of prefrontal cortex of young adult ADHD during a probabilistic gambling task. The P1-like waveform, elicited by the choice of the amount wagered, was restored in ADHD patients after WM training with the *adaptive level* variant of the Dual n-back task. We interpret this finding as an improvement of early higher-level mechanisms of attentional control in ADHD after adaptive training. In controls, the level of difficulty of WM training tended to affect late components of the event-related potentials (ERPs) mainly located at parietal areas.

2. Materials and Methods

2.1. Participants

This study was carried out in accordance with the latest version of the Declaration of Helsinki [42] and approved by the mandatory Ethics Committees requested by Swiss Federal Authorities, following the constitutional article (art. 118b Cst) of 8 March 2010 and the Federal Act involving Human Beings on 30 September 2011 (revised 1 January 2014). The ADHD patients were recruited either in the Psychiatric Department of the University Hospital of Lausanne or at a psychiatrist's practice in collaboration with the Lausanne University Hospital after an initial screening appointment to ensure that they were fulfilling the criteria defined by the DSM-IV-TR for inattentive, hyperactive/impulsive or mixed subtypes [43]. Subjects with comorbid disorders and subjects taking medications were excluded from this study. We selected 65 young adults between 18 and 30 years old in the two groups of study, controls ($N_{CTRL} = 37$) and ADHD patients ($N_{ADHD} = 28$). Notice that control participants were recruited in the same age-range of the patients and with a similar social and educational background. Controls were screened prior to the experimental session to ensure that they would not report any disorder or exclusion criteria mentioned in the authorization released by the Ethics Committees. All participants were requested to fill French versions of the adult ADHD self-report scale (ASRS) and the Conners' adult ADHD rating scales-self seport: screening version (CAARS-S:SV) [44–46] two weeks prior the begin of the protocol. All participants received a monetary compensation following the scale approved by the mandatory Ethics Committees (Commission cantonale d'ethique de la recherche sur l'être humain, code 101/12) requested by Swiss Federal Authorities.

2.2. Working Memory Task

In this study the WM task consisted in two variants of the dual n-back task aimed at testing the divided attention [47,48]. Briefly, the task is the following. At each trial, an auditory and a visual cue were presented simultaneously during 500 ms, with an interstimulus interval (ISI) set to 3000 ms. The level of difficulty of the task is referred as n-back. The participants were asked to memorize the dual modality cues in order to compare the current auditory and visual stimuli with those presented n-trials back in time with the value n always the same for auditory and visual stimuli. In the conditions under which the current stimulus is not the same as the cue presented n-trials earlier, no response was requested by the participants. The participants had to press the "A" key for any visual stimulus matching the same stimulus presented n-trials back in time and/or the "L" key for any auditory stimulus matching the same stimulus presented n-trials back in time. If the participants did not respond within the fixed ISI, the trial was accounted as no response. Immediately after the response, a green light was switched on for correct response, otherwise a red light indicated a mistake. If "no response" was the correct choice, the green light switched on at the end of the ISI. In the case of baseline level, the difficulty of the task was set to $n = 1$. Figure 1 illustrates the dual n-back task at level $n = 2$ of difficulty.

In the case of adaptive level, the difficulty n of the task was adjusted as a function of the performance. The whole task consisted of 20 blocks of $20 + n$ trials with the same level of difficulty. An increase by 1 in the level of difficulty in the next block was triggered by a performance of less than three mistakes in each modality. With levels of difficulty higher than 1, a decrease by 1 in the level was triggered by five or more errors cumulated in any modality. The total duration of the working memory task was approximately half an hour.

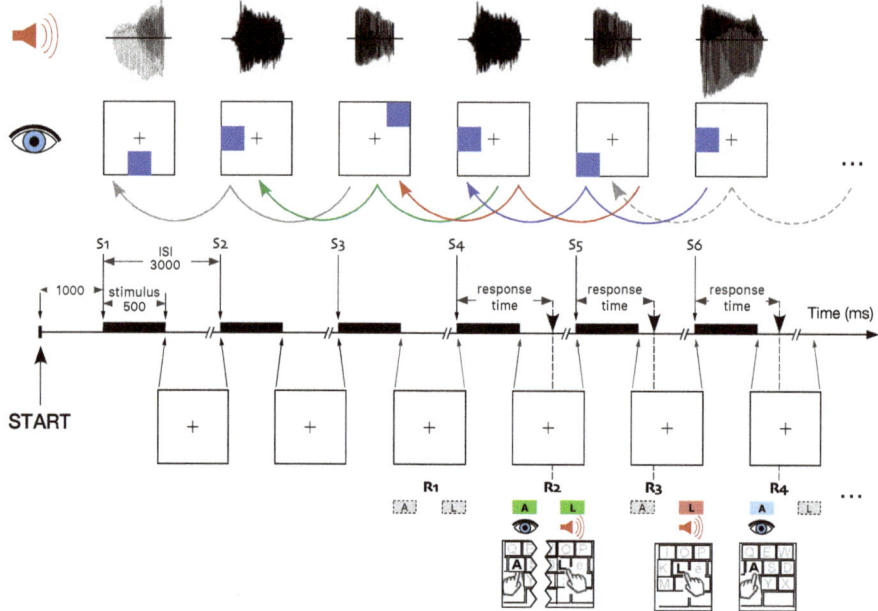

Figure 1. Level $n = 2$ of the dual n-back task. Each stimulus was composed by an auditory and a visual cue presented during 500 ms. This means the participants had to compare the third stimulus (S3) with the first one (S1), S4 with S2, S5 with S3, and so on. For the first correct response (R1), no stimuli matched those presented two trials back in time and no key press was requested. For R2, both auditory and visual stimuli matched the target (S4 identical to S2, green arrow)), such that both "A" and "L" key were pressed. For R3, only the auditory stimulus matched the target (red arrow) and only the "L" key was pressed. For R4, only the visual stimulus matched the target (blue arrow) and only the "A" key was pressed. Notice that in this example only correct responses are illustrated.

2.3. Working Memory Training Protocol

In a pre-training session, at the laboratory, all participants played the adaptive version of the dual n-back task. At this session, the participants performed the WAIS-IV (Wechsler Adult Intellicence Scale-Fourth Edition) digit span subtest from the Wechsler adult intelligence scale, which requires participants to sequentially order the numbers (i.e., backward and forward digit span sequencing) presented by the examiner [49], the forward span of the Corsi block-tapping task, which is a visuospatial short-term memory task [50] and the attentional network test (ANT) [51]. The analysis of ANT will be presented in another paper. The WM training started the day after the pre-training session. At home, the participants played the dual n-back task by mean of an Internet remote connection to a server with protected access. The strict requirement was to complete at least 18 training sessions within a month. Randomly assigned participants in both controls and ADHD group were requested to perform a WM training either with a fixed baseline level of difficulty, i.e., dual 1-Back, or with a performance-dependent adaptive n-level of difficulty. A post-training session similar to the pre-training session was scheduled at the end of WM training [48]. All participants played the adaptive version of the dual n-back task at the post-training session. Please notice that all the analyses in this paper refer to the data acquired during the pre-training and the post-training sessions.

2.4. Probability Gambling Task

The probability gambling task (PGT) used in this study was derived from a modified Gneezy–Potters' task [48,52]. In summary, at the beginning of each trial an amount of 20 points was endowed to each participant. At each trial, the participant had to choose the amount wagered (as illustrated by Figure 2). The probability to win was set to 1/3, which meant a gain equal to 4× the gamble. In the event of a loss, at the end of the trial, the participant loses the entire amount wagered for that trial and keeps the rest of the initial endowment (which was always equal to 20). If the bet was equal to 16, then at the end of the trial the participant would receive 4 points in the event of a loss (i.e., $4 = (20 - 16)$) and 68 points in case of a win (i.e., $= (20 - 16) + (4 \times 16)$). Notice that in this study the participant was just informed that the outcome of the bet was determined without any feedback on the amount earned, on the contrary of another study published elsewhere [41]. The click on the selected value of the bet with a mouse button is used as the triggering event for the electrophysiological analysis.

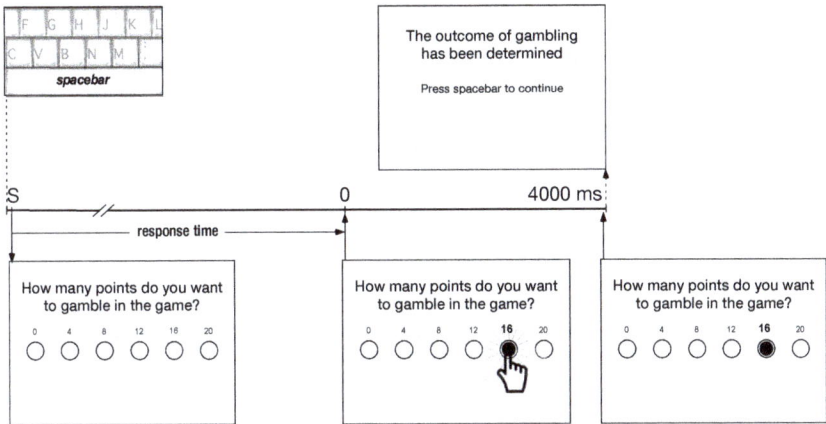

Figure 2. Probabilistic gambling task. A trial started when the participant pressed the spacebar (event S in the timeline), followed (20 milliseconds later) by a screen with a message request to select the gamble. This screen stayed on until a response was made by clicking on the selected value of gamble (event 0). The response time was determined by the interval between that message and the selection of gamble. This button click (event 0) was used as triggering event for the electrophysiological analysis. A fixed interval of 4000 ms followed until the end of the trial with the same screen and with the highlighted selected gamble.

2.5. EEG Recording and Analyses

EEG was recorded using using 64 scalp Ag/AgCl active electrodes with impedances kept below 5 kΩ and referenced to the linked earlobes (ActiveTwo MARK II Biosemi EEG System, BioSemi B.V., Amsterdam, The Netherlands) mounted on a headcap (10/20 layout, NeuroSpec Quick Cap). Two pairs of bipolar electrodes were used to record ocular movements. EEG signals were recorded at 1024 Hz sampling frequency (24 bit resolution) and band-pass filtered between 0.05 Hz and 200 Hz. The selection of the amount to gamble (Figure 2, event 0) detected by a button-click was used to trigger the event-related potentials (ERPs). BrainVision Analyzer 2.0.4 (Brain Products, Gilching, Germany) was used for ERP preprocessing and removal of ocular artefacts by Infomax Independent Component Analysis (ICA) [53]. The ERP trials were cut into epochs starting 500 ms before and ending 1000 ms after the trigger. The interval of 500 ms prior to trigger onset was used for baseline correction. After removal of the trials characterized by easily identifiable artefacts, the epochs were visually inspected for contamination by residual minor artefacts. Artefact-free trials were filtered with lower cutoff at 0.1 Hz and upper cut-off at 30 Hz (−12dB/octave). Participants with less than 15 segments in any of the two recordings were excluded from this study. Analyses on the individual average whole-scalp ERP signals were performed with the software Cartool [54]. Those tests were applied with Bonferroni correction for the number of electrodes with a p value threshold at 0.05 [55].

3. Results

3.1. Participants' Clinical Assessment

We used the R language and standard packages for the statistical analyses [56] and for each variable we report the values m, $(M \pm SEM)$, corresponding to the median (m) and mean (M) $\pm$ standard error of the mean (SEM). Participant's age for controls and ADHD was 22 years old (22.3 ± 0.51) and 21 years old (22.1 ± 0.71), respectively. The female-to-male gender ratio was 17:20 and 7:21 in controls and ADHD, respectively. The 2×2 contingency table showed no difference of gender ratio between the groups, $\chi^2(1, 65) = 2.17, p > 0.05$.

A two-way analysis of variance, (*group*: controls, ADHD) × (*gender*: female, male), was run to assess ADHD symptoms. This analysis showed that normalized T-score values for CAARS-S:SV were always significantly higher for ADHD patients, such that it yielded a significant main effect for *group*, $F(1, 61) = 35.98, p < 0.001$ for DSM-IV Inattentive Symptoms and $F(1, 61) = 21.65, p < 0.001$ for the ADHD index. ADHD reported also higher values for ASRS than controls with a significant *group* effect, $F(1, 61) = 11.19, p = 0.001$. The main effect of *gender* was always non-significant, $F(1, 61) = 0.26, p > 0.05$, $F(1, 61) = 2.18, p > 0.05$ and $F(1, 61) = 0.004, p > 0.05$, for DSM-IV inattentive symptoms, ADHD index, and ASRS, respectively. The interaction effect was also non-significant $F(1, 61) = 0.59, p > 0.05$, $F(1, 61) = 1.94, p > 0.05$ and $F(1, 61) = 1.12, p > 0.05$, for DSM-IV inattentive symptoms, ADHD index, and ASRS, respectively. In our previous paper [41] we have extensively analyzed and discussed the fact that there is a general agreement in the literature that there is no clear gender effect in young adult ADHD behavioral expression. For this reason we will not analyze further gender effects in this study, whose focus is the effect of the level of difficulty of the WM training protocol on the evoked brain activity.

3.2. Working Memory Performance

The effect of WM training was assessed by comparing the performance between the post- and pre-training sessions for the level n of difficulty achieved during the Dual n-Back task, the normalized score for the WAIS-IV digit span and the percentiles for the total score of the Corsi Block-Tapping Task (Table 1). A three-way analysis of variance, (group: controls, ADHD) × (WMT: pre-training, post-training) × (training level: baseline, adaptive) was carried out with a $F(1, 122)$ F-statistics for all main and interaction effects because all factors had two levels.

The ANOVA for the dual n-back task yielded a significant interaction between factors WMT and training level. A one-way analysis of variance for the pre-training and post-training sessions separately yielded a significant effect of the kind of training protocol ($F(1, 63) = 7.70, p < 0.01$, and $F(1, 63) = 19.35, p < 0.001$, respectively) on the average n-back level achieved by the participants. Another one-way analysis of variance for the baseline or the adaptive training protocol separately yielded a significant effect of the WM training ($F(1, 62) = 15.20, p < 0.001$, and $F(1, 64) = 94.25, p < 0.001$, respectively). This can be interpreted as some bias effect due to the initial random assignment of the participants to either the baseline or the adaptive training protocol. Table 1 shows that before WM training, the participants assigned to the baseline training protocol performed better than those assigned to the adaptive protocol (on average 2.20 ± 0.12 vs. 1.90 ± 0.06 and 2.10 ± 0.13 vs. 1.84 ± 0.11 for controls and ADHD, respectively). Despite this bias, the outcome of WM training was such that after being trained with the adaptive protocol both groups showed a better performance than being trained with the baseline protocol (on average 3.80 ± 0.23 vs. 2.91 ± 0.17 and 3.55 ± 0.29 vs. 2.52 ± 0.16 for controls and ADHD, respectively). This means that a one-month training of working memory had an effect on the outcome of the dual n-back task and that a training by the adaptive protocol produced a larger effect than baseline. Hence, the simple main effects on training level and WMT were truly significant by themselves, irrespective of the group of participants.

The WAIS-IV digit span showed no interaction between factors (Table 1), such that all significant simple main effects for factors *group*, *WMT* and *training level* can be considered as independent. This means that ADHD's performance to this digit span sequencing test was poorer than in controls, and that Dual n-Back adapative training improved performance to WAIS-IV Digit Span irrespective of the group of participants. On the opposite, no significant effect was found for the visuospatial short-term memory assessed by the Corsi block-tapping task.

Table 1. Pre and post-training performance (median, mean, and SEM) to the memory tasks and results of the three-way analysis of variance (ANOVA).

	Group:	Controls		ADHD			ANOVA	
	Level:	Baseline	Adaptive	Baseline	Adaptive	Effect	$F(1, 122)$	$Pr(> F)$
Sample size (N)		18	19	14	14			
Dual n-Back level						group:	2.76	> 0.05
						level:	7.67	0.006 **
	pre-training	2.12	1.95	1.97	1.80	WMT:	101.2	< 0.001 ***
		2.20 (0.12)	1.90 (0.06)	2.10 (0.13)	1.84 (0.11)	group × level:	0.13	> 0.05
WMT:						group × WMT:	1.06	> 0.05
	post-training	2.77	3.95	2.45	3.33	level × WMT:	26.4	< 0.001 ***
		2.91 (0.17)	3.80 (0.23)	2.52 (0.16)	3.55 (0.29)	group × level × WMT:	0.04	> 0.05
WAIS-IV digit span (*normalized score*)						group:	11.28	0.001 **
						level:	14.99	< 0.001 ***
	pre-training	13.50	11.00	10.50	10.00	WMT:	6.95	0.009 **
		13.67 (0.68)	11.11 (0.31)	11.14 (0.94)	9.86 (0.72)	group × level:	2.22	> 0.05
WMT:						group × WMT:	0.11	> 0.05
	post-training	15.50	13.00	13.00	11.50	level × WMT:	0.03	> 0.05
		14.83 (0.62)	12.26 (0.55)	12.43 (1.04)	11.57 (0.84)	group × level × WMT:	0.05	> 0.05
Corsi block-tapping task (*percentiles*)						group:	0.06	> 0.05
						level:	0.00	> 0.05
	pre-training	90.0	80.0	70.0	80.0	WMT:	0.80	> 0.05
		78.3 (5.1)	72.9 (4.9)	60.7 (7.4)	67.1 (6.8)	group × level:	0.00	> 0.05
WMT:						group × WMT:	3.56	> 0.05
	post-training	80.0	80.0	85.0	80.0	level × WMT:	0.00	> 0.05
		78.9 (4.6)	69.0 (4.9)	70.4 (8.0)	75.4 (4.7)	group × level × WMT:	0.00	> 0.05

**: $p < 0.01$; ***: $p < 0.001$.

3.3. Probabilistic Gambling Task

The response time during the PGT, measured as indicated in Figure 2, decreased in all groups from the pre- to the post-training session, $F(1, 122) = 18.65$ ($p < 0.001$), thus showing a significant main effect for factor *WMT*, irrespective of the training condition. In addition, Table 2 shows that the response time in controls was shorter than in ADHD, as revealed by the significant main effect of factor *group*. The WT training did not affect the total gains earned by all participants at the Probabilistic Gambling Task, irrespective of the group and the training condition. A Risk index $RI = (HIR - -LIR)/(HIR + LIR)$ is calculated as a function of LIR, corresponding to low valued gambles (i.e., small amounts equal to 0, 4, or 8 points were gambled by the participant), and HIR, corresponding to high value gambles (i.e., the participant gambled 12, 16, or 20 points). The index RI is centralized such that a risk averse strategy is characteristic by $RI \approx -1$, a risk neutral attitude by $RI \approx 0$ and a risky decision-making by $RI \approx 1$. It is interesting to notice that ANOVA shows the only significant main factor for Risk index is training level (Table 2). A two-way analysis of variance, (*group*: controls, ADHD) × *training level*: baseline, adaptive), was run for the pre- and post-training sessions separately. Before training, the two-way analysis of variance shows that the factor ttraining level was not significant ($F(1, 61) = 3.37$, $p > 0.05$). On the contrary, after training the factor *training level* affected the Risk index ($F(1, 61) = 5.40$, $p = 0.023$). In the baseline training condition, the RI increased on average by 0.07 and by 0.04 for controls and ADHD, respectively, from the pre- to the post-training session. This means that a WMT in the baseline condition tended to increase a risk taking attitude in both groups. Conversely, the adaptive training tended to increase a risky decision making in controls but in ADHD it tended to increase risk aversive attitude. However, *t*-test were not significant for each of these comparisons taken separately.

Table 2. Pre and post-training performance (median, mean and SEM) during the probabilistic gambling task and results of the three-way analysis of variance (ANOVA).

Group:		Controls		ADHD			ANOVA	
	Level:	Baseline	Adaptive	Baseline	Adaptive	Effect	$F(1, 122)$	$\Pr(> F)$
Sample size (N)		18	19	14	14			
Response time (ms)						group :	5.26	0.024 *
						level :	1.4	> 0.05
	pre-training	914	1289	1305	1332	WMT :	18.65	< 0.001 ***
		1199 (155)	1396 (203)	1542 (192)	1573 (233)	group × level :	0.01	> 0.05
WMT :						group × WMT :	1.40	> 0.05
	post-training	738	812	926	996	level × WMT :	0.01	> 0.05
		764 (73)	826 (79)	942 (107)	1201 (217)	group × level × WMT :	0.61	> 0.05
Total Gains (points)						group :	2.24	> 0.05
						level :	1.17	> 0.05
	pre-training	1886	1868	1812	1878	WMT :	0.05	> 0.05
		1947 (48)	1875 (39)	1853 (46)	1902 (45)	group × level :	3.79	> 0.05
WMT :						group × WMT :	0.55	> 0.05
	post-training	1890	1868	1848	1806	level × WMT :	0.36	> 0.05
		2010 (92)	1850 (58)	1809 (52)	1857 (65)	group × level × WMT :	0.27	> 0.05
Risk index						group :	1.14	> 0.05
						level :	8.68	0.004 **
	pre-training	0.18	−0.22	0.15	−0.08	WMT :	0.29	> 0.05
		0.18 (0.12)	−0.15 (0.09)	−0.02 (0.14)	−0.09 (0.12)	group × level :	1.20	> 0.05
WMT :						group × WMT :	0.10	> 0.05
	post-training	0.18	−0.18	0.16	−0.04	level × WMT :	0.12	> 0.05
		0.25 (0.14)	−0.09 (0.09)	0.06 (0.15)	−0.14 (0.10)	group × level × WMT :	0.04	> 0.05

*: $p < 0.05$; **: $p < 0.01$; ***: $p < 0.001$.

3.4. Event Related Potentials Triggered by Gambling Choice

In controls ($N = 37$), the median number of epochs per participant was equal to 69 (63.8 ± 2.6) and 71 (65.4 ± 2.7) during the pre- and post-training sessions, respectively. In ADHD ($N = 28$), we analyzed 48 (52.6 ± 2.9) and 60 (58.3 ± 2.6) epochs per participant during the pre- and post-training sessions, respectively. A three-way analysis of variance, (group: controls, ADHD) × (WMT: pre-training, post-training) × (training level: baseline, adaptive) yielded a significant main *group* effect, $F(1, 122) = 11.17 (p < 0.01)$ for the number of epochs. This is due to the fact that EEG recordings of ADHD are always contaminated by more muscular artefacts than controls. It is important to notice that neither a main effect for the training level, $F(1, 122) = 0.24 (p > 0.05)$, nor for the WMT, $F(1, 122) = 1.52 (p > 0.05)$, was observed, thus validating the ERP analysis as a function of the WM training protocol in both groups of participants. Several positive and negative peaks were identified in the ERP grand averages waveforms in both control and ADHD participants before the training (Figure 3).

A negative readiness potential maximal at frontocentral electrodes, or decision preceding negativity (DPN), peaked at 40 ms before the trigger in both groups (Figure 3). After the trigger, we observed a positive wave component peaking at 90 ms in control participants (a P1-like component) corresponding to an early positive frontocentral deflection (Figure 3). Notice that in electrodes Fz and Cz, this P1-like component component was much less visible in ADHD participants, as confirmed by the topographic maps for the interval 70–120 ms, at the top of Figure 3. These topographic maps show also that this early positive component reaches its maximum at central electrodes, slightly lateralized on the left, and that ADHD patients are characterized by a stronger lateralization and a negative amplitude in frontal sites.

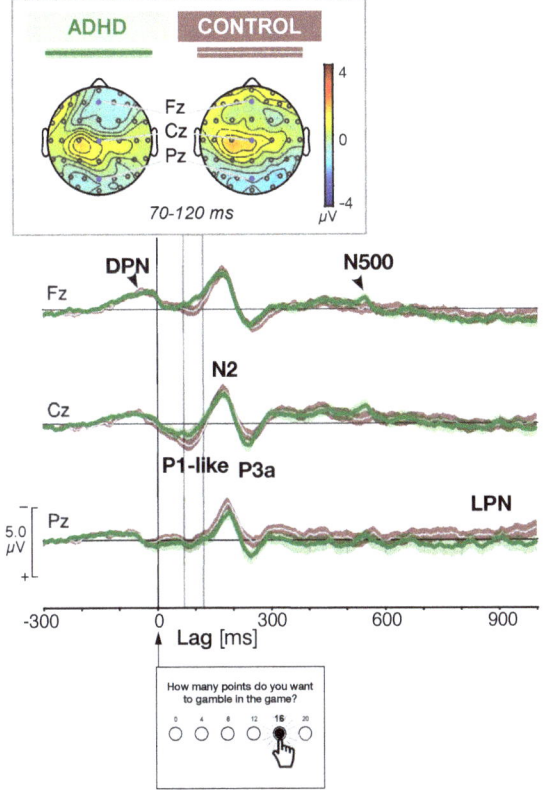

Figure 3. Grand average event-related potentials (ERPs) recorded before the working memory (WM) training at Fz, Cz and Pz sites triggered at lag 0, corresponding to button-click of the selected gamble, in attention deficit/hyperactivity disorder (ADHD) ($N = 28$, green curves over light green shaded areas) and control participants ($N = 37$, white curves over brown shaded areas) on a millisecond scale. The confidence interval (mean curve ± SEM) is shown by the shaded areas. We identified the decision preceding negativity (DPN), P1-like, N2, P3a, N500, and a late parietal negativity (LPN). Signal amplitude is scaled in microvolts (µV). The topographic maps on the top represent the distribution of the mean amplitude of the signal between 70 and 120 ms (estimated P1-like component) using a color-coded scale in µV.

At all electrode sites, we observed a clear N2/P3 complex with N2 peaking at 180 ms and P3a peaking at about 250 ms. ADHD were characterized by a larger posterior P3 component than controls. The peak-to-peak amplitude between the N2 and P3a ERPs was measured for Pz, Cz and Fz. We ran a three-way ANOVA for factors (*group*: controls, ADHD), (WMT: pre-training, post-training) and (training level: baseline, adaptive) to determine any affect on the peak-to-peak amplitudes. We found no effect ($p > 0.05$) of *group* with statistics $F(1, 122) = 0.01$, $F(1, 122) = 1.03$, and $F(1, 122) = 0.37$ for Pz, Cz and Fz, respectively. We found neither any effect ($p > 0.05$) of WMT with statistics $F(1, 122) = 0.03$, $F(1, 122) = 0.00$, and $F(1, 122) = 0.05$ nor of *training level* with statistics $F(1, 122) = 3.60$, $F(1,122) = 0.00$, and $F(1, 122) = 0.23$, for Pz, Cz and Fz, respectively. In Figure 3 we have also marked the N550 and the late parietal negativity (LPN). This latter component (LPN) is barely visible before training, in particular only in controls at site Pz in Figure 3. After training, LPN is very much affected and for this reason we have marked it already in this figure.

3.5. Effect of WM Training Condition on Differential Topographic Maps

At first, we compute the topographic head map distribution of the grand-average ERP amplitude (in µV) at post- and pre-training sessions for both subgroups of ADHD and controls, those who were trained in the baseline protocol (i.e., with the fixed level $n = 1$ of the dual n-back task), and those with the adaptive protocol. After the ERP onset, corresponding to the choice of the selected gamble with the button-click, we determined five intervals of interest corresponding to the time course of the most relevant components observed in the ERPS. These wave components and their respective intervals were P1-like (70–120 ms), N2 (150–200 ms), P3a (240–290 ms), P3b (350–400 ms), and LPN (800–950 ms). All but LPN corresponded to time windows of 50 ms. The differential head maps were obtained with the topographic map for a specific time interval of the ERP at the post-training session minus the topographic map at the pre-training session for the same interval (Figure 4).

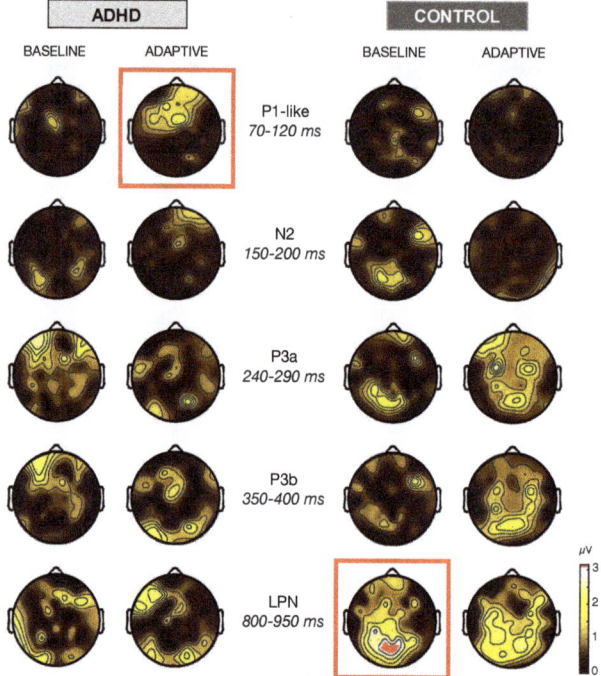

Figure 4. Differential head maps of the topographical distribution of the Grand-Average ERP amplitude (in µV) at post- minus pre-training sessions for ADHD and controls trained either by the baseline or adaptive protocol of the dual n-back task. ERPs were triggered by the choice of the selected gamble with the button-click. Differential head maps using a color-coded scale in µV are plotted for the five major ERP time windows. The red squares correspond to those head maps with significant Bonferroni-corrected p-values in the given time window, computed from paired t-tests on the individual average signals (see Figure 5).

Before the training, no difference was observed between averaged ERPs of either group assigned to adaptive and baseline training protocol. The most significant differential head maps were selected by applying a paired t-test with Bonferroni correction for the number of electrodes. We set a criterion of at least three electrode sites with a significant difference ($p < 0.05$) during the very same time window within the interval of the selected wave component to define such significant differential head maps. The P1-like component was particularly affected in ADHD after the adaptative training protocol (Figure 4, red square at first raw). Figure 5a shows that this component was increased in a significant way at frontocentral electrodes (F3, $p < 0.05$; Fz, $p < 0.05$; FCz, $p < 0.01$). In this panel, notice that at site F4 the P1-like amplitude after training was also more positive than in the pre-training session, but the criterion of significance for the Bonferroni t-test correction was not reached. The grand average ERPS at site Cz is reported (Figure 5a) as a benchmark for a non-significant neighboring channel.

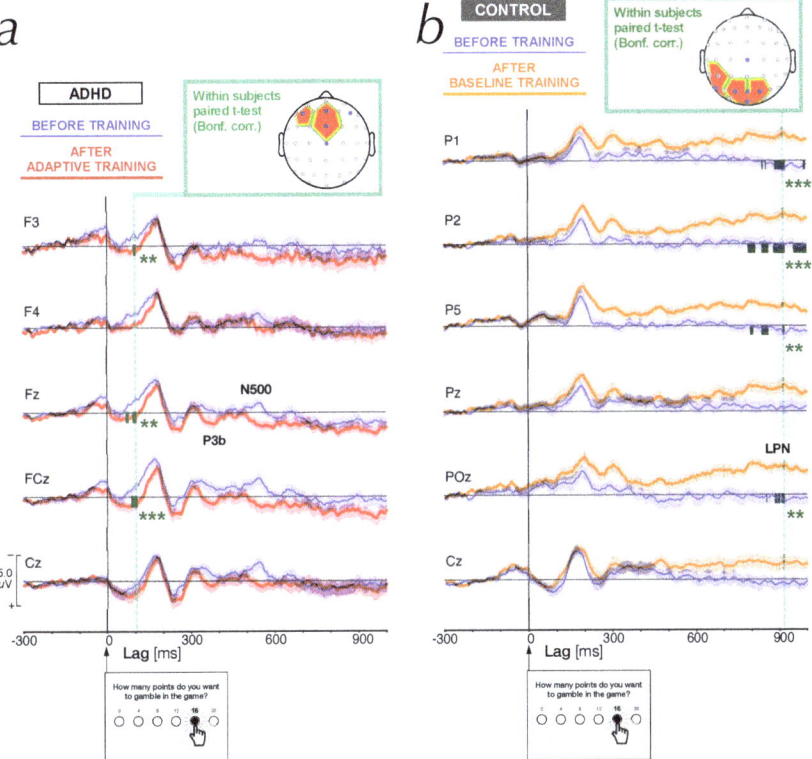

Figure 5. Grand average ERPs, triggered (at lag 0 ms) by the button-click at the time of the selection of the amount to gamble, recorded *before working memory training* (blue curves and shaded areas). The confidence interval (mean curve ± SEM) is shown by the shaded areas. The vertical scale represents the amplitude of the signal in µV and the lag is scaled in milliseconds. (**a**). Grand average ERPs at sites F3, F4, Fz, FCz and Cz sites (blue marks in the head map) for ADHD participants recorded after training with the adaptive level protocol (red curves and shaded areas) for the dual n-back task. Green ticks show the significant Bonferroni-corrected $1 - p$ values computed from paired t-test on individual average ERP signal with significance $p < 0.05$ (**) and $p < 0.01$ (***). The panel at the top, shows a head map with the significant sites after Bonferroni correction (red areas around F3, Fz and FCz), at a latency of 100 ms (dashed green vertical line), corresponding to the P1-like component discussed in the text. (**b**). Grand average ERPs at sites P1, P2, P5, Pz, POz, and Cz sites (blue marks in the head map) for controls recorded after training with the baseline level protocol (orange curves and shaded areas), i.e., after the dual 1-back task. In this figure, the head map on the top shows the significant sites (in red areas around P1, P2, P5, CP3 and POz) at a latency of 912 ms (dashed green vertical line), corresponding to the slow negative wave component associated with the expectation of the gambling outcome.

In the interval 150–200 ms, no training protocol produced any major effect on N2 head maps, neither for controls nor for ADHD. Notice that the differential head maps at P3a and P3b were very similar to each other in any of the subgroups. In controls, the maps showed increases in amplitudes at posterior sites, in particular, after adaptive training. Although these differences were significant for one or another channel, the criterion of three channels simultaneously significant for the paired *t*-test with Bonferroni correction was not reached. The late parietal negativity (LPN) was little affected in ADHD, but the differences in controls were large and mainly distributed over the parietal areas. In controls, Figure 5b shows that baseline training affected the ERPs already appear at wave components P3a and P3b, then disappeared at about 400 ms after the trigger onset. The maximal level of significance was observed at a lag near 900 ms, corresponding to LPN, where we observed significant Bonferroni-corrected *p* values at five posterior electrode sites (CP3, $p < 0.05$; P1, $p < 0.01$; P2, $p < 0.01$; P5, $p < 0.05$; POz, $p < 0.05$) (Figure 4, red square at last raw). A similar but less significant effect was observed in controls after training with the adaptive dual *n*-back task.

4. Discussion

Working memory problems and impaired sustained attention are characteristic symptoms of ADHD [2,57]. Improvement of symptomatology by cognitive training and psychological interventions aimed to increase the correlation between sustained attention and arousal has been evalued several times in the recent past [58–61]. However, benefits for behavioral transfer effects to measures of fluid intelligence after several weeks of a computerized working memory treatment requiring high cognitive load could not be confirmed satisfactorily and raised questions about the controversial usefulness of such training [22,24,62]. The demand on cognitive processes is increased by the dual *n*-back task, which is a particular task aimed at challenging the divided attention by running visual and auditory modalities concurrently with the potential of WMT to compensate for a decline in executive functions [47,63]. In the current study, we have tested controls and ADHD patients who were trained during three weeks with the Dual *n*-Back Task. We included two subgroups, from controls and ADHD, who were trained with a non adaptive version of the task-with a fixed level of difficulty set to 1, that is a dual 1-back task (the *baseline* protocol).

We found evidence that WMT, irrespective of *baseline* or adaptive protocol, improved the score of the dual *n*-back task played by the participants at the post-training in comparison with the pre-training session, in agreement with past studies using fewer sessions of WMT [39]. Our training protocol lasted 20 days, a duration comparable with other studies reported in the literature using Dual *n*-Back Task [64]. In addition to increase in dual *n*-back scores in controls, we observed that WMT improved performance in the WAIS-IV Digit Span in agreement with previous studies [39,65,66]. It is important to notice that ADHD patients and controls are reliably differentiated by the WAIS-IV [67]. The novelty in our study is that for the first time, to our best knowledge, we report that ADHD patients improved their performance in the WAIS-IV Digit Span after a WM training protocol. After training, ADHD could perform at the same level of controls before training. However, measurement of the visuospatial working memory by the Corsi block-tapping task did not show any significant difference between controls and ADHD neither before nor after training. This finding is in agreement with the observation that visuospatial working memory is not specifically impaired in ADHD [68–70] and that dual *n*-back task is a working memory task affecting circuits other than those involved in visuospatial processing [66,71–74].

Before training, the results of the probability gambling task did not show any difference between ADHD and controls with respect to the total gain and risk index, in line with our previous study [41]. The analysis of the response time confirmed that ADHD responded at a significant slower pace than controls already before WMT, as previously reported [41]. However, training in both baseline and adaptive conditions provoked a faster reaction in both groups with similar magnitude, thus suggesting a similar process for an increase in the capacity to handle divided attentional stimuli in both ADHD and controls. The WM training failed to affect the total gains, but in the baseline condition it revealed a tendency to increase a risk taking attitude in both groups, matching our previous observation along the same line [75]. Controls tended to increase a risky decision making also after the adaptive training, somehow like after baseline training. On the contrary, after adaptive training, ADHD tended to decrease risk-taking attitude. This result suggests that improved divided attentional processes in both groups and opposite risk-taking behavior are elicited by a high cognitive load generated by the adaptive dual *n*-back task. An interpretation of this result is that these processes are controlled by different pathways, in agreement with literature on the behavioral deficits of ADHD patients [76–80].

Before the onset of the ERP trigger, we observed a negative readiness potential maximal at frontocentral electrodes, or decision preceding negativity (DPN), consistent with the literature and unaffected by WMT [81]. The ERPs following the gamble selection in the Probability Gambling Task [52] are characterized by several wave components [82–85]. Few studies analyzed the ERPs in adult ADHD and showed that N2, P3a, P3b, feed-back related negativity and N400-like components distinguish ADHD and controls in association with the evaluation of the reward outcome [28,86] and with the emotional feelings generated by risk-taking attitude [41]. In our current paper, we did not observe group effects (i.e., differences between controls and ADHD) on the measurements of PGT due to the working memory training, other than on the response times (Table 2). Our finding is in agreement with the observation that working memory training in general improves processing speed and attention performance [87] independently of the transfer to fluid intelligence [24,62,79] and that inattentive symptoms in ADHD are not associated with fluid intelligence [78,79,88] Hence, we do not discuss further the gambling task-related ERP components but P1 and LPN, the wave components which appeared to be the most affected by dual *n*-back task working memory training.

We observed a very significant effect of adaptive training on the P1-like wave component in the ADHD group. It is known that P1/N1 early sensory ERP components tend to be attenuated in ADHD patients [89–92] and our observations before training confirm those studies. Attentional modulation progress along the build-up of the ensuing P1-like [93,94]. The attenuation observed in ADHD can be interpreted following the perceptual load theory in selective attention [95,96]. In the current study, the P1-like wave is triggered by the button-click on the selected gamble. ADHD participants might have a degree of perceptual overload when facing the decision to invest, thus impairing their attentional resources as revealed by the attenuated P1-like. A WMT during three weeks with the adaptive training protocol of the dual *n*-back task generates a sustained high cognitive load on divided attention. The particular characteristic of this task is that the working memory capacity is solicited by the number of objects to be memorized and by the cross-modal features associated with the stimuli. P1 was found to likely reflect spatially based information shared by the auditory attention and visual memory systems that do not have to be mutually recruited in situations involving cross-modal tasks [97,98] and sensitive to the number of objects rather to the number of features to be memorized [99]. This is also in agreement with our finding, mentioned before, of an improvement in the score of the WAIS-IV digit span after WMT. The puzzling finding of an increase in P1-like wave amplitude in ADHD after the adaptive training, with restoration of a waveform similar to controls, is in favor of the hypothesis of an improvement of early higher-level mechanisms of attentional control in ADHD after adaptive training. The topological maps have clearly located this change of activity at the level of the prefrontal cortical areas. The P1 wave has been associated with an inhibitory feedback wave from "higher" cortical areas acting as an inhibitory filter to control feedforward sensory processes [100]. A change in P1 might be related to a change in the early modulation of attention, such to improve the sensory-perceptual level of processing that is necessary to improve the decisional process. There is evidence that modulation of neural activity by selective attention may occur at the subcortical level [101], where inhibitory gating mechanisms take place [102–104]. Then, an increase of the P1-like wave, in our paradigm, could be associated with a more effective processing of the decision due to a greater inhibition of potentially competing and task irrelevant networks.

The last ERP component strongly affected by WMT is the late parietal negative slow wave, whose amplitude was selectively increased in controls after both training level conditions. This wave started approximately 700 ms after the onset and extended for several hundreds of milliseconds. The topographic distribution of this wave is clearly parietal-posterior and with a left hemispheric dominance at latencies near 900 ms. In the literature, it is interesting to note that LPN has been observed as a neural marker related to the transfer of cross-modal associated information in working memory, [105,106] with memory tasks that required continued evaluation of contextual information [107–109] and with memory tasks that required high demands on action monitoring in presence of conflictual response options [110]. Before training, ERPs recorded in both groups did not show a relevant presence of LPN in the PGT. This suggests that WMT is a necessary condition to let appear LPN. Moreover, ADHD patients did not show any effect of WMT on LPN. If we consider all these observations together we may raise the hypothesis that WMT with the dual n-back task is able to generate a transfer effect in the PGT [111,112], as revealed by the LPN associated with a continued evaluation of contextual information in our PGT. This effect is strong in controls, but it is absent in our ADHD group, thus suggesting that the kind of WMT performed by our group of patients only confers benefits for those tasks that were trained [15,62,113]. We could speculate that a deficit in transfer effects associated with WM training could be associated with the abnormal parietal brain function observed in ADHD [114].

5. Conclusions

In conclusion, we have confirmed that working memory training produces cognitive effects for the task that was trained in both controls and ADHD patients. In particular, improvement in early attentional processes in ADHD is likely to be the most beneficial effect of WMT with the dual n-back task if the training required a high cognitive effort for divided attention, such as in the case of the adaptive condition. Transfer effects to fluid intelligence occurring only in controls might be associated with the development of a late parietal negativity elicited by a risky decision-making task.

Author Contributions: Author Contributions: methodology, M.E.J., S.K.M., A.E.P.V., M.B., and A.L.; validation, A.L.; formal analysis, M.E.J., S.K.M., and A.L.; writing—original draft, M.E.J., A.L.; investigation, S.K.M., A.E.P.V., M.B., and A.L.; supervision, A.E.P.V., M.B.; conceptualization, A.E.P.V., M.B., and A.L.; funding acquisition, A.E.P.V., M.B.; writing—review and editing, A.E.P.V. All authors have read and agreed to the published version of the manuscript.

Funding: This research was funded by the Swiss National Science Foundation grant number CR13I1-138032.

Acknowledgments: The Authors are grateful to the ADHD patients and their families who kindly agreed to be part of the project. They also wish to thank Maria Soares Duarte for the psychological screening, and Damiano Cereghetti for the technical assistance in the development of the dual n-back task.

Conflicts of Interest: The authors declare no conflict of interest.

References

1. Barkley, R.A. Major life activity and health outcomes associated with Attention-Deficit/Hyperactivity Disorder. *J. Clin. Psychiatry* **2002**, *63* (Suppl. 12), 10–15. [PubMed]
2. Kessler, R.C.; Adler, L.A.; Barkley, R.; Biederman, J.; Conners, C.K.; Faraone, S.V.; Greenhill, L.L.; Jaeger, S.; Secnik, K.; Spencer, T.; et al. Patterns and predictors of Attention-Deficit/Hyperactivity Disorder persistence into adulthood: Results from the national comorbidity survey replication. *Biol. Psychiatry* **2005**, *57*, 1442–1451. [CrossRef] [PubMed]
3. Northover, C.; Thapar, A.; Langley, K.; van Goozen, S. Emotion Regulation in Adolescent Males with Attention-Deficit Hyperactivity Disorder: Testing the Effects of Comorbid Conduct Disorder. *Brain Sci.* **2015**, *5*, 369–386. [CrossRef] [PubMed]
4. Engelhardt, P.E.; Nobes, G.; Pischedda, S. The Relationship between Adult Symptoms of Attention-Deficit/Hyperactivity Disorder and Criminogenic Cognitions. *Brain Sci.* **2019**, *9*. [CrossRef]
5. Gazzaley, A.; Nobre, A.C. Top-down modulation: bridging selective attention and working memory. *Trends Cogn. Sci.* **2012**, *16*, 129–135. [CrossRef]
6. Mueller, A.; Hong, D.S.; Shepard, S.; Moore, T. Linking ADHD to the Neural Circuitry of Attention. *Trends Cogn. Sci.* **2017**, *21*, 474–488. [CrossRef]
7. Arnsten, A.F.T. Fundamentals of attention-deficit/hyperactivity disorder: Circuits and pathways. *J. Clin. Psychiatry* **2006**, *67* (Suppl. 8), 7–12.
8. De La Fuente, A.; Xia, S.; Branch, C.; Li, X. A review of Attention-Deficit/Hyperactivity Disorder from the perspective of brain networks. *Front. Hum. Neurosci.* **2013**, *7*, e00192. [CrossRef]

9. Lenartowicz, A.; Delorme, A.; Walshaw, P.D.; Cho, A.L.; Bilder, R.M.; McGough, J.J.; McCracken, J.T.; Makeig, S.; Loo, S.K. Electroencephalography correlates of spatial working memory deficits in attention-deficit/hyperactivity disorder: Vigilance, encoding, and maintenance. *J. Neurosci.* **2014**, *34*, 1171–1182. [CrossRef]
10. Duffy, F.H.; Shankardass, A.; McAnulty, G.B.; Als, H. A unique pattern of cortical connectivity characterizes patients with attention deficit disorders: A large electroencephalographic coherence study. *BMC Med.* **2017**, *15*, 51. [CrossRef]
11. Tang, H.; Qi, X.L.; Riley, M.R.; Constantinidis, C. Working memory capacity is enhanced by distributed prefrontal activation and invariant temporal dynamics. *Proc. Natl. Acad. Sci. USA* **2019**, *116*, 7095–7100. [CrossRef] [PubMed]
12. Klingberg, T.; Forssberg, H.; Westerberg, H. Training of working memory in children with ADHD. *J. Clin. Exp. Neuropsychol.* **2002**, *24*, 781–791. [CrossRef] [PubMed]
13. Green, C.T.; Long, D.L.; Green, D.; Iosif, A.M.; Dixon, J.F.; Miller, M.R.; Fassbender, C.; Schweitzer, J.B. Will working memory training generalize to improve off-task behavior in children with attention-deficit/hyperactivity disorder? *Neurotherapeutics* **2012**, *9*, 639–648. [CrossRef] [PubMed]
14. Liu, Z.X.; Lishak, V.; Tannock, R.; Woltering, S. Effects of working memory training on neural correlates of Go/Nogo response control in adults with ADHD: A randomized controlled trial. *Neuropsychologia* **2017**, *95*, 54–72. [CrossRef] [PubMed]
15. Jones, M.R.; Katz, B.; Buschkuehl, M.; Jaeggi, S.M.; Shah, P. Exploring N-Back Cognitive Training for Children With ADHD. *J. Atten. Disord.* **2018**, 1087054718779230. [CrossRef] [PubMed]
16. Buschkuehl, M.; Jaeggi, S.M.; Jonides, J. Neuronal effects following working memory training. *Dev. Cogn. Neurosci.* **2012**, *2* (Suppl. 1), S167–S179. [CrossRef] [PubMed]
17. Schwaighofer, M.; Fischer, F.; Bühner, M. Does Working Memory Training Transfer? A Meta-Analysis Including Training Conditions as Moderators. *Educ. Psychol.* **2015**, *50*, 138–166. [CrossRef]
18. Muris, P.; Roodenrijs, D.; Kelgtermans, L.; Sliwinski, S.; Berlage, U.; Baillieux, H.; Deckers, A.; Gunther, M.; Paanakker, B.; Holterman, I. No Medication for My Child! A Naturalistic Study on the Treatment Preferences for and Effects of Cogmed Working Memory Training Versus Psychostimulant Medication in Clinically Referred Youth with ADHD. *Child Psychiatry Hum. Dev.* **2018**, *49*, 974–992. [CrossRef]
19. Ackermann, S.; Halfon, O.; Fornari, E.; Urben, S.; Bader, M. Cognitive Working Memory Training (CWMT) in adolescents suffering from Attention-Deficit/Hyperactivity Disorder (ADHD): A controlled trial taking into account concomitant medication effects. *Psychiatry Res.* **2018**, *269*, 79–85. [CrossRef]
20. Capodieci, A.; Re, A.M.; Fracca, A.; Borella, E.; Carretti, B. The efficacy of a training that combines activities on working memory and metacognition: Transfer and maintenance effects in children with ADHD and typical development. *J. Clin. Exp. Neuropsychol.* **2019**, *41*, 1074–1087. [CrossRef]
21. Rapport, M.D.; Orban, S.A.; Kofler, M.J.; Friedman, L.M. Do programs designed to train working memory, other executive functions, and attention benefit children with ADHD? A meta-analytic review of cognitive, academic, and behavioral outcomes. *Clin. Psychol. Rev.* **2013**, *33*, 1237–1252. [CrossRef] [PubMed]
22. Sonuga-Barke, E.; Brandeis, D.; Holtmann, M.; Cortese, S. Computer-based cognitive training for ADHD: A review of current evidence. *Child Adolesc. Psychiatr. Clin. N. Am.* **2014**, *23*, 807–824. [CrossRef] [PubMed]
23. Cortese, S.; Ferrin, M.; Brandeis, D.; Buitelaar, J.; Daley, D.; Dittmann, R.W.; Holtmann, M.; Santosh, P.; Stevenson, J.; Stringaris, A.; et al. Cognitive training for attention-deficit/hyperactivity disorder: Meta-analysis of clinical and neuropsychological outcomes from randomized controlled trials. *J. Am. Acad. Child Adolesc. Psychiatry* **2015**, *54*, 164–174. [CrossRef] [PubMed]
24. Melby-Lervåg, M.; Redick, T.S.; Hulme, C. Working Memory Training Does Not Improve Performance on Measures of Intelligence or Other Measures of "Far Transfer": Evidence From a Meta-Analytic Review. *Perspect. Psychol. Sci.* **2016**, *11*, 512–534. [CrossRef] [PubMed]
25. Bechara, A.; Martin, E.M. Impaired decision making related to working memory deficits in individuals with substance addictions. *Neuropsychology* **2004**, *18*, 152–162. [CrossRef]
26. Lawrence, A.J.; Luty, J.; Bogdan, N.A.; Sahakian, B.J.; Clark, L. Problem gamblers share deficits in impulsive decision-making with alcohol-dependent individuals. *Addiction* **2009**, *104*, 1006–1015. [CrossRef]
27. Malloy-Diniz, L.; Fuentes, D.; Leite, W.B.; Correa, H.; Bechara, A. Impulsive behavior in adults with attention deficit/hyperactivity disorder: Characterization of attentional, motor and cognitive impulsiveness. *J. Int. Neuropsychol. Soc.* **2007**, *13*, 693–698. [CrossRef]

28. Ibanez, A.; Cetkovich, M.; Petroni, A.; Urquina, H.; Baez, S.; Gonzalez-Gadea, M.L.; Kamienkowski, J.E.; Torralva, T.; Torrente, F.; Strejilevich, S.; et al. The Neural Basis of Decision-Making and Reward Processing in Adults with Euthymic Bipolar Disorder or Attention-Deficit/Hyperactivity Disorder (ADHD). *PLoS ONE* **2012**, *7*, e37306. [CrossRef]
29. Drechsler, R.; Rizzo, P.; Steinhausen, H.C. Decision-making on an explicit risk-taking task in preadolescents with attention-deficit/hyperactivity disorder. *J. Neural Transm. (Vienna)* **2008**, *115*, 201–209. [CrossRef]
30. Duarte, N.A.; Woods, S.P.; Rooney, A.; Atkinson, J.H.; Grant, I.; Translational Methamphetamine AIDS Research Center Group. Working memory deficits affect risky decision-making in methamphetamine users with Attention-Deficit/Hyperactivity Disorder. *J. Psychiatr. Res.* **2012**, *46*, 492–499. [CrossRef]
31. Coghill, D.R.; Seth, S.; Matthews, K. A comprehensive assessment of memory, delay aversion, timing, inhibition, decision making and variability in attention deficit hyperactivity disorder: Advancing beyond the three-pathway models. *Psychol. Med.* **2014**, *44*, 1989–2001. [CrossRef] [PubMed]
32. Barkley, R.A.; Fischer, M. The unique contribution of emotional impulsiveness to impairment in major life activities in hyperactive children as adults. *J. Am. Acad. Child Adolesc. Psychiatry* **2010**, *49*, 503–513. [PubMed]
33. Matthies, S.; Philipsen, A.; Svaldi, J. Risky decision making in adults with ADHD. *J. Behav. Ther. Exp. Psychiatry* **2012**, *43*, 938–946. [CrossRef] [PubMed]
34. Brand, M.; Kalbe, E.; Labudda, K.; Fujiwara, E.; Kessler, J.; Markowitsch, H.J. Decision-making impairments in patients with pathological gambling. *Psychiatry Res.* **2005**, *133*, 91–99. [CrossRef] [PubMed]
35. Potenza, M.N. The neurobiology of pathological gambling and drug addiction: An overview and new findings. *Philos. Trans. R. Soc. Lond. B Biol. Sci.* **2008**, *363*, 3181–3189. [CrossRef] [PubMed]
36. Fridberg, D.J.; Gerst, K.R.; Finn, P.R. Effects of working memory load, a history of conduct disorder, and sex on decision making in substance dependent individuals. *Drug Alcohol. Depend.* **2013**, *133*, 654–660. [CrossRef]
37. Cui, J.F.; Wang, Y.; Shi, H.S.; Liu, L.L.; Chen, X.J.; Chen, Y.H. Effects of working memory load on uncertain decision-making: Evidence from the Iowa Gambling Task. *Front. Psychol.* **2015**, *6*, 162. [CrossRef] [PubMed]
38. Gehricke, J.G.; Kruggel, F.; Thampipop, T.; Alejo, S.D.; Tatos, E.; Fallon, J.; Muftuler, L.T. The brain anatomy of attention-deficit/hyperactivity disorder in young adults—A magnetic resonance imaging study. *PLoS ONE* **2017**, *12*, e0175433. [CrossRef]
39. Lilienthal, L.; Tamez, E.; Shelton, J.T.; Myerson, J.; Hale, S. Dual n-back training increases the capacity of the focus of attention. *Psychon. Bull. Rev.* **2013**, *20*, 135–141. [CrossRef]
40. Schweizer, S.; Leung, J.; Kievit, R.; Speekenbrink, M.; Trender, W.; Hampshire, A.; Blakemore, S. Protocol for an app-based affective control training for adolescents: Proof-of-principle double-blind randomized controlled trial [version 2; peer review: 4 approved]. *Wellcome Open Res.* **2019**, *4*, 91. [CrossRef] [PubMed]
41. Mesrobian, S.K.; Villa, A.E.P.; Bader, M.; Götte, L.; Lintas, A. Event-Related Potentials during a Gambling Task in Young Adults with Attention-Deficit/Hyperactivity Disorder. *Front. Hum. Neurosci.* **2018**, *12*, 79. [CrossRef] [PubMed]
42. World Medical Association. World Medical Association Declaration of Helsinki: Ethical principles for medical research involving human subjects. *JAMA* **2000**, *284*, 3043–3045. [CrossRef]
43. American Psychiatric Association. *Diagnostic and Statistical Manual of Mental Disorders*, 4th ed.; American Psychiatric Association: Washington, DC, USA, 2000.
44. Conners, C.K.; Erhardt, D.; Sparrow, E. *Conner's Adult ADHD Rating Scales: Technical Manual*; Multi-Health Systems Incorporated (MHS): North Tonawanda, NY, USA, 1999.
45. Kessler, R.C.; Adler, L.; Ames, M.; Demler, O.; Faraone, S.; Hiripi, E.; Howes, M.J.; Jin, R.; Secnik, K.; Spencer, T.; et al. The World Health Organization Adult ADHD Self-Report Scale (ASRS): A short screening scale for use in the general population. *Psychol. Med.* **2005**, *35*, 245–256. [CrossRef] [PubMed]
46. Fumeaux, P.; Mercier, C.; Roche, S.; Iwaz, J.; Bader, M.; Stéphan, P.; Ecochard, R.; Revol, O. Validation of the French Version of Conners' Parent Rating Scale Revised, Short Version: Factorial Structure and Reliability. *Can. J. Psychiatry* **2016**, *61*, 236–242. [CrossRef]
47. Jaeggi, S.M.; Buschkuehl, M.; Jonides, J.; Perrig, W.J. Improving fluid intelligence with training on working memory. *Proc. Natl. Acad. Sci. USA* **2008**, *105*, 6829–6833. [CrossRef] [PubMed]
48. Mesrobian, S.K. Does working memory training affect decision making? A neuroeconomic study. Ph.D. Thesis, Faculty of Medicine and Biology, University of Lausanne, Lausanne, Switzerland, 2015.

49. Wechsler, D. *Wechsler Adult Intelligence Scale–Fourth Edition (WAIS–IV)*; NCS Pearson: San Antonio, TX, USA, 2008.
50. Kessels, R.P.; van Zandvoort, M.J.; Postma, A.; Kappelle, L.J.; de Haan, E.H. The Corsi Block-Tapping Task: Standardization and normative data. *Appl. Neuropsychol.* **2000**, *7*, 252–258. [CrossRef]
51. Fan, J.; McCandliss, B.D.; Sommer, T.; Raz, A.; Posner, M.I. Testing the efficiency and independence of attentional networks. *J. Cogn. Neurosci.* **2002**, *14*, 340–347. [CrossRef]
52. Gneezy, U.; Potters, J. An experiment on risk taking and evaluation periods. *Q. J. Econ.* **1997**, *112*, 631–645. [CrossRef]
53. Luck, S.J. *An Introduction to Event-Related Potentials and Their Neural Origins*; Massachusetts Institute of Technology: Cambridge, MA, USA, 2005.
54. Brunet, D.; Murray, M.M.; Michel, C.M. Spatiotemporal analysis of multichannel EEG: CARTOOL. *Comput. Intell. Neurosci.* **2011**, *2011*, 813870. [CrossRef]
55. Bland, J.M.; Altman, D.G. Multiple significance tests: the Bonferroni method. *BMJ* **1995**, *310*, 170. [CrossRef]
56. Venables, W.N.; Ripley, B.D. *Modern Applied Statistics with S*, 4th ed.; Statistics and Computing; Springer: New York, NY, USA, 2002; p. 498.
57. Castellanos, F.X.; Tannock, R. Neuroscience of Attention-Deficit/Hyperactivity Disorder: The search for endophenotypes. *Nat. Rev. Neurosci.* **2002**, *3*, 617–628. [CrossRef]
58. Keshavan, M.S.; Vinogradov, S.; Rumsey, J.; Sherrill, J.; Wagner, A. Cognitive training in mental disorders: Update and future directions. *Am. J. Psychiatry* **2014**, *171*, 510–522. [CrossRef]
59. Ansari, S. The therapeutic potential of working memory training for treating mental disorders. *Front. Hum. Neurosci.* **2015**, *9*, 481. [CrossRef] [PubMed]
60. Salomone, S.; Fleming, G.R.; Shanahan, J.M.; Castorina, M.; Bramham, J.; O'Connell, R.G.; Robertson, I.H. The effects of a Self-Alert Training (SAT) program in adults with ADHD. *Front. Hum. Neurosci.* **2015**, *9*, 45. [CrossRef] [PubMed]
61. Lambez, B.; Harwood-Gross, A.; Golumbic, E.Z.; Rassovsky, Y. Non-pharmacological interventions for cognitive difficulties in ADHD: A systematic review and meta-analysis. *J. Psychiatr. Res.* **2020**, *120*, 40–55. [CrossRef] [PubMed]
62. Woltering, S.; Gu, C.; Liu, Z.X.; Tannock, R. Visuospatial Working Memory Capacity in the Brain After Working Memory Training in College Students With ADHD: A Randomized Controlled Trial. *J. Atten. Disord.* **2019**, 1087054719879487. [CrossRef] [PubMed]
63. Salminen, T.; Frensch, P.; Strobach, T.; Schubert, T. Age-specific differences of dual n-back training. *Neuropsychol. Dev. Cogn. B Aging Neuropsychol. Cogn.* **2016**, *23*, 18–39. [CrossRef]
64. Matysiak, O.; Kroemeke, A.; Brzezicka, A. Working Memory Capacity as a Predictor of Cognitive Training Efficacy in the Elderly Population. *Front. Aging Neurosci.* **2019**, *11*, 126. [CrossRef]
65. Au, J.; Sheehan, E.; Tsai, N.; Duncan, G.J.; Buschkuehl, M.; Jaeggi, S.M. Improving fluid intelligence with training on working memory: A meta-analysis. *Psychon. Bull. Rev.* **2015**, *22*, 366–377. [CrossRef]
66. Blacker, K.J.; Negoita, S.; Ewen, J.B.; Courtney, S.M. N-back versus Complex Span Working Memory Training. *J. Cogn. Enhanc.* **2017**, *1*, 434–454. [CrossRef]
67. Theiling, J.; Petermann, F. Neuropsychological Profiles on the WAIS-IV of Adults With ADHD. *J. Atten. Disord.* **2016**, *20*, 913–924. [CrossRef] [PubMed]
68. van Ewijk, H.; Heslenfeld, D.J.; Luman, M.; Rommelse, N.N.; Hartman, C.A.; Hoekstra, P.; Franke, B.; Buitelaar, J.K.; Oosterlaan, J. Visuospatial working memory in ADHD patients, unaffected siblings, and healthy controls. *J. Atten. Disord.* **2014**, *18*, 369–378. [CrossRef] [PubMed]
69. Wang, Z.; Jing, J.; Igarashi, K.; Fan, L.; Yang, S.; Li, Y.; Jin, Y. Executive function predicts the visuospatial working memory in autism spectrum disorder and attention-deficit/hyperactivity disorder. *Autism Res.* **2018**, *11*, 1148–1156. [CrossRef] [PubMed]
70. Cohen, E.; Kalanthroff, E. Visuospatial processing bias in ADHD: A potential artifact in the Wechsler Adult Intelligence Scale and the Rorschach Inkblots Test. *Psychol. Assess.* **2019**, *31*, 699–706. [CrossRef] [PubMed]
71. Lawlor-Savage, L.; Goghari, V.M. Dual N-Back Working Memory Training in Healthy Adults: A Randomized Comparison to Processing Speed Training. *PLoS ONE* **2016**, *11*, e0151817. [CrossRef] [PubMed]
72. Minear, M.; Brasher, F.; Guerrero, C.B.; Brasher, M.; Moore, A.; Sukeena, J. A simultaneous examination of two forms of working memory training: Evidence for near transfer only. *Mem. Cognit.* **2016**, *44*, 1014–1037. [CrossRef]

73. Soveri, A.; Antfolk, J.; Karlsson, L.; Salo, B.; Laine, M. Working memory training revisited: A multi-level meta-analysis of n-back training studies. *Psychon. Bull. Rev.* **2017**, *24*, 1077–1096. [CrossRef]
74. Holmes, J.; Woolgar, F.; Hampshire, A.; Gathercole, S.E. Are Working Memory Training Effects Paradigm-Specific? *Front. Psychol.* **2019**, *10*, 1103. [CrossRef]
75. Mesrobian, S.K.; Lintas, A.; Jacquerod, M.; Bader, M.; Götte, L.; Villa, A.E. An ERP Study Reveals How Training with Dual N-Back Task Affects Risky Decision Making in a Gambling Task in ADHD Patients. In *Advances in Cognitive Neurodynamics (VI)*; Delgado-García, J.M., Pan, X., Sánchez-Campusano, R., Wang, R., Eds.; Springer: Singapore, 2018; chapter 34, pp. 271–277.
76. Liston, C.; Malter Cohen, M.; Teslovich, T.; Levenson, D.; Casey, B.J. Atypical prefrontal connectivity in attention-deficit/hyperactivity disorder: pathway to disease or pathological end point? *Biol. Psychiatry* **2011**, *69*, 1168–1177. [CrossRef]
77. Helenius, P.; Laasonen, M.; Hokkanen, L.; Paetau, R.; Niemivirta, M. Impaired engagement of the ventral attentional pathway in ADHD. *Neuropsychologia* **2011**, *49*, 1889–1896. [CrossRef]
78. Cheung, C.H.M.; Rijsdijk, F.; McLoughlin, G.; Brandeis, D.; Banaschewski, T.; Asherson, P.; Kuntsi, J. Cognitive and neurophysiological markers of ADHD persistence and remission. *Br. J. Psychiatry* **2016**, *208*, 548–555. [CrossRef]
79. Brydges, C.R.; Ozolnieks, K.L.; Roberts, G. Working memory—Not processing speed—Mediates fluid intelligence deficits associated with attention deficit/hyperactivity disorder symptoms. *J. Neuropsychol.* **2017**, *11*, 362–377. [CrossRef]
80. Pollak, Y.; Shalit, R.; Aran, A. Risk taking and adult attention deficit/hyperactivity disorder: A gap between real life behavior and experimental decision making. *Psychiatry Res.* **2018**, *259*, 56–62. [CrossRef]
81. Cui, J.F.; Chen, Y.H.; Wang, Y.; Shum, D.H.K.; Chan, R.C.K. Neural correlates of uncertain decision making: ERP evidence from the Iowa Gambling Task. *Front. Hum. Neurosci.* **2013**, *7*, 776. [CrossRef] [PubMed]
82. Yang, J.; Zhang, Q. Electrophysiological correlates of decision-making in high-risk versus low-risk conditions of a gambling game. *Psychophysiology* **2011**, *48*, 1456–1461. [CrossRef] [PubMed]
83. San Martín, R.; Appelbaum, L.G.; Pearson, J.M.; Huettel, S.A.; Woldorff, M.G. Rapid brain responses independently predict gain maximization and loss minimization during economic decision making. *J. Neurosci.* **2013**, *33*, 7011–7019. [CrossRef] [PubMed]
84. Kimura, K.; Kimura, M.; Iwaki, S. Temporal prediction modulates the evaluative processing of "good" action feedback: An electrophysiological study. *Psychophysiology* **2016**, *53*, 1552–1559. [CrossRef]
85. West, R.; Bailey, K.; Anderson, S. Transient and sustained ERP activity related to feedback processing in the probabilistic selection task. *Int. J. Psychophysiol.* **2018**, *126*, 1–12. [CrossRef]
86. Abouzari, M.; Oberg, S.; Tata, M. Theta-band oscillatory activity differs between gamblers and nongamblers comorbid with attention-deficit hyperactivity disorder in a probabilistic reward-learning task. *Behav. Brain Res.* **2016**, *312*, 195–200. [CrossRef]
87. Coleman, B.; Marion, S.; Rizzo, A.; Turnbull, J.; Nolty, A. Virtual Reality Assessment of Classroom - Related Attention: An Ecologically Relevant Approach to Evaluating the Effectiveness of Working Memory Training. *Front. Psychol.* **2019**, *10*, 1851. [CrossRef]
88. Costa, D.d.S.; Paula, J.J.d.; Alvim-Soares Júnior, A.M.; Diniz, B.S.; Romano-Silva, M.A.; Malloy-Diniz, L.F.; Miranda, D.M.d. ADHD inattentive symptoms mediate the relationship between intelligence and academic performance in children aged 6-14. *Braz. J. Psychiatry* **2014**, *36*, 313–321. [CrossRef] [PubMed]
89. Perchet, C.; Revol, O.; Fourneret, P.; Mauguière, F.; Garcia-Larrea, L. Attention shifts and anticipatory mechanisms in hyperactive children: An ERP study using the Posner paradigm. *Biol. Psychiatry* **2001**, *50*, 44–57. [CrossRef]
90. Barry, R.J.; Clarke, A.R.; Johnstone, S.J. A review of electrophysiology in Attention-Deficit/Hyperactivity Disorder: I. Qualitative and quantitative electroencephalography. *Clin. Neurophysiol.* **2003**, *114*, 171–183. [CrossRef]
91. Sable, J.J.; Knopf, K.L.; Kyle, M.R.; Schully, L.T.; Brooks, M.M.; Parry, K.H.; Thompson, I.A.; Suna, E.B.; Stowe, R.; Flink, L.A.; et al. Attention-deficit hyperactivity disorder reduces automatic attention in young adults. *Psychophysiology* **2013**, *50*, 308–313. [CrossRef]
92. Baijot, S.; Cevallos, C.; Zarka, D.; Leroy, A.; Slama, H.; Colin, C.; Deconinck, N.; Dan, B.; Cheron, G. EEG Dynamics of a Go/Nogo Task in Children with ADHD. *Brain Sci.* **2017**, *7*. [CrossRef]

93. Hillyard, S.A.; Vogel, E.K.; Luck, S.J. Sensory gain control (amplification) as a mechanism of selective attention: Electrophysiological and neuroimaging evidence. *Philos. Trans. R. Soc. Lond. B Biol. Sci.* **1998**, *353*, 1257–1270. [CrossRef]
94. Zani, A.; Proverbio, A.M. Is that a belt or a snake? Object attentional selection affects the early stages of visual sensory processing. *Behav. Brain Funct.* **2012**, *8*, 6. [CrossRef]
95. Lavie, N. Distracted and confused? Selective attention under load. *Trends Cogn. Sci.* **2005**, *9*, 75–82. [CrossRef] [PubMed]
96. Cosman, J.D.; Mordkoff, J.T.; Vecera, S.P. Stimulus recognition occurs under high perceptual load: Evidence from correlated flankers. *J. Exp. Psychol. Hum. Percept. Perform.* **2016**, *42*, 2077–2083. [CrossRef]
97. Singhal, A. Differentiating between spatial and object-based working memory using complex stimuli: An erp study. *Int. J. Neurosci.* **2006**, *116*, 1457–1469. [CrossRef]
98. Bomba, M.D.; Singhal, A. ERP evidence of early cross-modal links between auditory selective attention and visuo-spatial memory. *Brain Cogn.* **2010**, *74*, 273–280. [CrossRef] [PubMed]
99. Quak, M.; Langford, Z.D.; London, R.E.; Talsma, D. Contralateral delay activity does not reflect behavioral feature load in visual working memory. *Biol. Psychol.* **2018**, *137*, 107–115. [CrossRef] [PubMed]
100. Klimesch, W. Evoked alpha and early access to the knowledge system: The P1 inhibition timing hypothesis. *Brain Res.* **2011**, *1408*, 52–71. [CrossRef] [PubMed]
101. Zani, A.; Proverbio, A.M. Endogenous attention to object features modulates the ERP C1 component. *Cogn. Neurosci.* **2018**, *9*, 66–67. [CrossRef]
102. Crick, F. Function of the thalamic reticular complex: The searchlight hypothesis. *Proc. Natl. Acad. Sci. USA* **1984**, *81*, 4586–4590. [CrossRef]
103. Villa, A.E.P.; Tetko, I.V.; Dutoit, P.; De Ribaupierre, Y.; De Ribaupierre, F. Corticofugal modulation of functional connectivity within the auditory thalamus of rat, guinea pig and cat revealed by cooling deactivation. *J. Neurosci. Methods* **1999**, *86*, 161–178. [CrossRef]
104. Lintas, A.; Schwaller, B.; Villa, A.E.P. Visual thalamocortical circuits in parvalbumin-deficient mice. *Brain Res.* **2013**, *1536*, 107–118. [CrossRef]
105. Johansson, M.; Mecklinger, A. The late posterior negativity in ERP studies of episodic memory: Action monitoring and retrieval of attribute conjunctions. *Biol. Psychol.* **2003**, *64*, 91–117. [CrossRef]
106. Gui, P.; Ku, Y.; Li, L.; Li, X.; Bodner, M.; Lenz, F.A.; Wang, L.; Zhou, Y.D. Neural correlates of visuo-tactile crossmodal paired-associate learning and memory in humans. *Neuroscience* **2017**, *362*, 181–195. [CrossRef] [PubMed]
107. Paller, K.A.; Kutas, M. Brain Potentials during Memory Retrieval Provide Neurophysiological Support for the Distinction between Conscious Recollection and Priming. *J. Cogn. Neurosci.* **1992**, *4*, 375–392. [CrossRef]
108. Ranganath, C.; Paller, K.A. Neural correlates of memory retrieval and evaluation. *Brain Res. Cogn. Brain Res.* **2000**, *9*, 209–222. [CrossRef]
109. Wilding, E.L. In what way does the parietal ERP old/new effect index recollection? *Int. J. Psychophysiol.* **2000**, *35*, 81–87. [CrossRef]
110. Nessler, D.; Mecklinger, A.; Penney, T.B. Event related brain potentials and illusory memories: The effects of differential encoding. *Brain Res. Cogn. Brain Res.* **2001**, *10*, 283–301. [CrossRef]
111. Nikolaidis, A.; Voss, M.W.; Lee, H.; Vo, L.T.K.; Kramer, A.F. Parietal plasticity after training with a complex video game is associated with individual differences in improvements in an untrained working memory task. *Front. Hum. Neurosci.* **2014**, *8*, 169. [CrossRef] [PubMed]
112. Jaeggi, S.M.; Buschkuehl, M.; Shah, P.; Jonides, J. The role of individual differences in cognitive training and transfer. *Mem. Cognit.* **2014**, *42*, 464–480. [CrossRef]
113. Mawjee, K.; Woltering, S.; Tannock, R. Working Memory Training in Post-Secondary Students with ADHD: A Randomized Controlled Study. *PLoS ONE* **2015**, *10*, e0137173. [CrossRef]
114. Hale, T.S.; Kane, A.M.; Tung, K.L.; Kaminsky, O.; McGough, J.J.; Hanada, G.; Loo, S.K. Abnormal Parietal Brain Function in ADHD: Replication and Extension of Previous EEG Beta Asymmetry Findings. *Front. Psychiatry* **2014**, *5*, 87. [CrossRef]

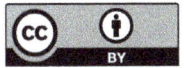

© 2020 by the authors. Licensee MDPI, Basel, Switzerland. This article is an open access article distributed under the terms and conditions of the Creative Commons Attribution (CC BY) license (http://creativecommons.org/licenses/by/4.0/).

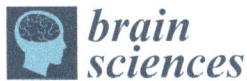

Article

Behavioral and Electrophysiological Correlates of Performance Monitoring and Development in Children and Adolescents with Attention-Deficit/Hyperactivity Disorder

Yanni Liu [1,*], Gregory L. Hanna [1], Barbara S. Hanna [1], Haley E. Rough [1], Paul D. Arnold [2] and William J. Gehring [3]

[1] Department of Psychiatry, University of Michigan, Ann Arbor, Michigan, MI 48109, USA; ghanna@med.umich.edu (G.L.H.); hannab@med.umich.edu (B.S.H.); hrough@med.umich.edu (H.E.R.)
[2] Mathison Centre for Mental Health Research & Education and Department of Psychiatry, University of Calgary, Calgary, Alberta, AB T2N 4Z6, Canada; paul.arnold@ucalgary.ca
[3] Department of Psychology, University of Michigan, Ann Arbor, Michigan, MI 48109, USA; wgehring@umich.edu
* Correspondence: yanniliu@umich.edu; Tel.: +1-734-936-9275; Fax: +1-734-936-7868

Received: 14 January 2020; Accepted: 31 January 2020; Published: 2 February 2020

Abstract: The pathophysiology of attention-deficit/hyperactivity disorder (ADHD) involves deficits in performance monitoring and adaptive adjustments. Yet, the developmental trajectory and underlying neural correlates of performance monitoring deficits in youth with ADHD remain poorly understood. To address the gap, this study recruited 77 children and adolescents with ADHD and 77 age- and gender-matched healthy controls (HC), ages 8–18 years, who performed an arrow flanker task during electroencephalogram recording. Compared to HC, participants with ADHD responded more slowly and showed larger reaction time variability (RTV) and reduced post-error slowing; they also exhibited reduced error-related negativity (ERN) and error positivity effects, and reduced N2 and P3 congruency effects. Age effects were observed across groups: with increasing age, participants responded faster, with less variability, and with increased post-error slowing. They also exhibited increased ERN effects and increased N2 and P3 congruency effects. Increased RTV and reduced P3 amplitude in incongruent trials were associated with increased ADHD Problems Scale scores on the Child Behavior Checklist across groups. The altered behavioral and ERP responses in ADHD are consistent with the pattern associated with younger age across groups. Further research with a longitudinal design may determine specific aspects of developmental alteration and deficits in ADHD during performance monitoring.

Keywords: ADHD; performance monitoring; error processing; event-related potentials

1. Introduction

Attention-deficit/hyperactivity disorder (ADHD) is a neurodevelopmental disorder with symptoms including sustained attention problems, impulsivity, and hyperactivity, affecting ~5% of children and adolescents [1]. Several studies have shown deficits of performance monitoring and adaptive adjustment in children and adults with ADHD [2–4]. While some ADHD symptoms may decline from childhood to adulthood in a subset of children [5], the developmental trajectory of performance monitoring and adaptive adjustment along with their underlying neural correlates of the deficits in youth with ADHD remain poorly understood.

Previous research has shown that children with ADHD perform poorly in a wide range of tasks involving conflict monitoring and inhibitory control (e.g., Go/No-go, flanker, and stop-signal tasks [6]).

In general, their behavioral responses in these high cognitive demand tasks tended to be slower, more variable, and more error-prone, and they showed deficits in adaptation to task demands and following error responses [7–9]. Post-error slowing, or an increase in RT on trials following an error, is a common behavioral indicator of adaptive control [10]. A failure to slow responding on post-error trials has been interpreted as reflecting a deficit in adaptive control. Diminished post-error slowing was found in children with ADHD, relative to controls [11,12]; however, other studies [13,14] reported intact post-error slowing in children with ADHD compared to typically developing children using a flanker task.

In studies using event-related potential (ERP) measures, children with ADHD have also shown deficits in neurocognitive processes of response inhibition and performance monitoring. Error-related negativity (ERN) and error positivity (Pe) are two reliable ERP indices of performance monitoring. Both components are time-locked to responses. The ERN has been observed in a variety of tasks; its onset coincides with response initiation, and it peaks 50–100 milliseconds (msec) thereafter [15]. The ERN has a fronto-central distribution, and is believed to be generated in the anterior cingulate cortex and nearby medial frontal regions involved in self-regulation and performance monitoring [15]. The ERN increases with age after early childhood and reflects the activity of a system that detects errors, increases cognitive control, and adjusts behaviors [15]. Following the ERN, the Pe occurs about 200–400 msec after an error and has a centro-parietal distribution, reflecting error awareness, motivational significance of errors, and initiation of adaptive control processes [16]. Some ADHD studies reported reduced ERN in children and adults with ADHD relative to healthy controls (HC) [17,18]; others reported null findings [19,20], and still another reported increased ERN in ADHD [21] (see review papers [6,22]). Pe results in ADHD studies are also mixed: some studies reported diminished Pe [11,13,23,24] (see review [6]), suggesting deficient error valuation or conscious error processing in ADHD, but others reported no difference [21,25] between participants with ADHD and HC.

In addition to the response-locked ERN and Pe, the N2 and P3 are two main ERP components elicited during stimulus processing, reflecting processes involved in stimulus evaluation and response selection. Specifically, the N2 is a fronto-central negative voltage deflection peaking between 200 and 400 msec after stimulus onset; in cognitive control tasks, a larger N2 is elicited by high conflict trials (e.g., No-go trials in Go/No-go tasks, incongruent trials in flanker tasks) relative to low cognitive conflict trials (e.g., Go trials in Go/No-go tasks and congruent trials in flanker tasks), reflecting adaptive conflict monitoring [26–28]. The P3 is a central-parietal positive voltage deflection peaking between 300 and 500 msec after stimulus onset, first observed in an auditory oddball task, which reflects processes related to attention and working memory [29]; it is also observed in cognitive control tasks, following the N2, relating to resource allocation necessary for task performance. Several studies have reported impairments of processes associated with N2 and P3 in ADHD, but the direction in which participants with ADHD differ from HC in these studies was inconsistent. For instance, some studies reported, compared to HC, participants with ADHD showed reduced N2 on successful inhibition trials in a stop-signal task [30] and a Go/No-go task [31], and reduced N2 congruency effect in a flanker task [25]; others did not find N2 differences in stop-signal tasks [32] or reported an increased N2 effect in No-go vs. Go trials in a Go/No-go task [33,34]. Reduced P3 in ADHD has been reported in Go/No-go tasks (see meta-analyses paper [34,35]), a flanker task [36], and an attention network test [37], but not in some other studies (see review paper [38]).

Variability of behavioral and ERP findings might be accounted for by several factors, including participant heterogeneity, sample size, age range, task paradigms and analysis strategies across laboratories [6]. Many studies have failed to report ADHD subtypes and comorbidity; some studies may have been underpowered to detect group differences in behavioral and ERP correlates of performance monitoring. More work is needed to explore whether the inconsistent results can be accounted for by sampling and methodological differences across studies. Moreover, examining how behavior and ERP correlates of performance monitoring correlate with ADHD symptomatology, and whether the relationship may change with age in youth with ADHD, may improve our understanding of performance monitoring processes and their development in ADHD [6]. Few studies have investigated the relationship of behavioral and ERP correlates with symptom severity in children with ADHD. In adults, Marquardt et al. [18] observed that P3 amplitude in high conflict trials was inversely correlated with symptom severity in the ADHD group; Wiersema et al. [20] reported reduced Pe in error trials and P3 amplitude in high conflict trials were associated with more ADHD symptoms; Herrmann et al. [8] compared individuals with low- and high-ADHD symptom scores in a non-clinical population, and observed lower Pe in the group with higher symptoms scores. In adolescents and adults, Michelini et al. [17] found that ADHD symptoms were correlated with congruent errors, reaction time variability, and Pe. Using magnetic resonance imagining, a brain development study of ADHD suggested a brain structural developmental delay in ADHD; this structural development study may be associated with a functional delay [39]. While conflict processing and performance monitoring developed with age in healthy youth, few ERP studies have had a large enough sample size and age range to examine the developmental trajectory of performance monitoring in ADHD [25].

In the present study, we tested a relatively large (number of participants $n = 77$ in each group) sample of children and adolescents with ADHD with a broad age range (8–18 years), and age- and gender-matched HC in an arrow flanker task. Participants' behavioral performance and ERP correlates of performance monitoring and conflict processing were compared between groups, and these measures were related to ADHD symptom severity measured by the DSM-Oriented ADHD Problems Scale from the Child Behavior Checklist (CBCL) as a continuous measure within and across groups. We hypothesized that youth with ADHD would display slower reaction times, more reaction time variability (RTV), and reduced post-error slowing relative to healthy controls. Considering the inconsistent findings in the ERN, Pe, N2, and P3 in ADHD, we reported ERN and Pe on both error and correct trials and N2 and P3 on both congruent and incongruent trials [6,34]. We focused on difference scores between error and correct trials for the ERN and Pe error effects, along with difference scores between incongruent and congruent trials for N2 and P3 congruency effects, when discussing group differences and developmental alterations in ADHD. We hypothesized reductions in the ERN and Pe error effects and reduced N2 and P3 congruency effects in ADHD, compared to HC. We also hypothesized that behavioral and ERP impairments might be greater with increasing symptom severity within groups. In addition, we investigated whether behavioral and ERP alterations in ADHD vary with diagnostic subtype and age; we hypothesized that there might be a developmental delay in behavioral and ERP indices of performance monitoring in ADHD.

2. Materials and Methods

2.1. Participants

There were 77 youth with ADHD (30 female) and 77 age- and gender-matched healthy controls (HC), ranging in age from 8 to 18 years. Patients were recruited through the Section of Child and Adolescent Psychiatry within the Department of Psychiatry at the University of Michigan. Comparison subjects were recruited from the surrounding community. After a complete description of the study, written informed consent was obtained from at least one parent of the participant and written informed assent from the participant. Participants were paid for their interviews and psychophysiological recordings. All tasks and procedures were approved by the University of Michigan Medical School Institutional Review Board.

All participants were interviewed with the Kiddie Schedule for Affective Disorders and Schizophrenia for School-Aged Children-Present and Lifetime Version (K-SAD-PL) [40] and the Schedule for Obsessive-Compulsive and Other Behavioral Syndromes [41]. Parents completed the Child Behavior Checklist/6–18 (CBCL) [42] and Social Communication Questionnaire (SCQ) [43] about their children. Best-estimate diagnoses were made according to *DSM-5* criteria [44] using all sources of information, including two semi-structured interviews, two parent-report rating scales, four self-report rating scales, and all available clinical records [45]. The clinical records often included outpatient clinic notes, psychological testing results, and teacher rating scales. All participants were evaluated with the Wechsler Abbreviated Scale of Intelligence, Version II (WASI-II), which is normed for individuals ages 6 to 90 [46]. The WASI-II provides a global estimate of overall cognitive abilities with full-scale IQ. The ADHD subtype groups consisted of 23 children with the combined type, six children with the hyperactive-impulsive type, and 48 children with the inattentive type. Eighteen ADHD patients had a comorbid anxiety disorder, eleven patients had comorbid major depression disorder, twelve patients had comorbid oppositional defiant disorder (ODD) and one patient had motor tics that did not interfere with the EEG recording. Participants were excluded if they had a history of intellectual disability, head injury with loss of consciousness, a chronic neurological disorder, or SCQ scores higher than 14. Patients were excluded if they had a lifetime diagnosis of schizophrenia, other psychotic disorder, bipolar disorder, substance-related disorder, conduct disorder, obsessive-compulsive disorder, or anorexia nervosa. HC had no history of a specific axis I disorder. DSM-Oriented ADHD Problems Scale t-scores from the CBCL were used as a continuous measure of ADHD symptoms within and across groups. Symptom counts from the K-SAD-PL (ADHD total score, inattention score, and hyperactive/impulsive score), were used to assess symptom severity in ADHD patients only. Participants with ADHD taking a stimulant ($n = 43$) were asked to stop taking the medication for 48 hours prior to the EEG. Cases and HC were taking no other psychotropic medications. For the error analyses, two participants with ADHD and one healthy control were excluded due to commission of fewer than six errors, leaving a total of 151 participants.

2.2. Procedure

Participants performed a modified Eriksen flanker task in which arrows appeared on a personal computer display with congruent (e.g., →→→→→) and incongruent (e.g., →→←→→) conditions [47]. They were instructed to respond to the central arrow target, while ignoring the adjacent arrows, by pressing one of two buttons indicating the direction of the middle arrow (i.e., right versus left). The stimuli remained on the screen for 250 msec, with an interval of 1500 msec between consecutive trials.

Each participant was seated 65 centimeters directly in front of the computer monitor and told to place equal emphasis on speed and accuracy in responding. Following 40 practice trials, each subject completed eight blocks of 64 trials for a total of 512 trials. Performance feedback was provided after every block to yield an error rate of approximately 10%, with encouragement to focus on speed if there were fewer than four errors or to focus on accuracy if there were more than 10 errors [48].

2.3. Electrophysiological Methods

The electroencephalogram (EEG) was recorded from 64 Ag/AgCl scalp electrodes embedded in a nylon mesh cap, two mastoid electrodes, and two vertical and two horizontal electro-oculographic electrodes using the BioSemi ActiveTwo system (Amsterdam, The Netherlands). Data were digitized at 512 Hz, referenced to a ground formed from a common mode sense active electrode and driven right leg passive electrode (http://www.biosemi.com/ faq/ cms&drl.htm), and re-referenced offline to the average of the two mastoid electrodes. Data were bandpass filtered 0.1–30 Hz using zero-phase shift filters. EEG data were screened using automated algorithms that rejected epochs in which the absolute voltage exceeded 500 µV and epochs containing peak to peak activity greater than 500 µV within 200 msec, with a 100 msec moving window, for midline channels (Fz, FCz, Cz, CPz, and Pz). Ocular movement artifacts were then corrected using a regression-based algorithm [49]. After ocular correction, individual trials were rejected if they contained absolute amplitudes greater than 100 µV, a change greater than 50 µV measured from one data point to the next point, or a maximum voltage difference less than 0.5 µV within a trial in any of the midline electrodes.

2.4. Analyses

Behavioral measures included accuracy and mean reaction times (RT) for each participant. Premature responses faster than 150 ms, slow responses longer than 3000 ms, and reaction times beyond three standard deviations from the mean were not considered in the ERP and behavioral analyses. Intra-individual reaction times variability was estimated as the standard deviation across congruent and incongruent trials. Reaction times after errors were evaluated to determine if there were group differences in post-error behavioral adjustments. Accuracy and mean reaction times on correct trials were further analyzed using analysis of variance (ANOVA) with group (ADHD vs. HC) as a between-subject factor and stimulus type (congruent vs. incongruent) as a within-subject factor.

The ERN was quantified using mean amplitude relative to a pre-response baseline (of −200 to −50 msec). The mean amplitude of the ERN was computed on error trials in a window from 0 to 80 msec following the incorrect response. The correct response negativity (CRN) consisted of the same measure computed on correct trials. The ERN effect was defined as the difference between the ERN and CRN (dERN), calculated by subtracting the CRN from the ERN, since it may isolate activity unique to error processing from activity more broadly related to response monitoring [50]. The Pe was quantified using mean amplitude computed on error trials in a window from 200 to 400 msec following the incorrect response, relative to a pre-response baseline of −200 to −50 msec. The correct Pe consisted of the same measure computed on correct trials. The Pe effect was defined by difference between Pe and Pc (dPe), calculated by subtracting the correct waveform (Pc) from the incorrect (Pe). Both N2 and P3 were quantified using mean amplitude relative to a pre-stimulus baseline of −100 to 0 msec. The mean amplitude of the N2 and P3 were computed on congruent and incongruent correct trials in a window from 300 to 400 ms, and from 400 to 600 msec respectively, following the stimulus onset. N2 and P3 congruency effect were defined by ERP difference between incongruent and congruent trials within corresponding windows. Statistics of ERN, Pe, N2, and P3 were reported at FCz, CPz, FCz, and Pz, respectively, where the maximal mean amplitudes were found, and which were also consistent with previous literature. ERN and Pe amplitude were analyzed respectively with group as a between-subject factor and response type (error vs. correct) as a within-subject factor. N2 and P3 amplitude on correct trials were analyzed with group as a between-subject factor and stimulus type (congruent vs. incongruent) as a within-subject factor.

One-way ANOVAs were conducted to compare group difference on behavioral and ERP measures. Regression analyses were used to examine (1) correlations of behavioral, ERP measures, and age; (2) group difference on correlations of behavioral, ERP measures and age; (3) behavioral and ERP predictors of ADHD symptom severity. All statistical tests were two-tailed with the alpha level set at 0.05 if not otherwise specified.

3. Results

3.1. Behavioral Data in Patients with ADHD and Healthy Controls

Participants' reaction times and accuracy data are presented in Table 1. Participants with ADHD responded more slowly ($p < 0.01$) but as accurately ($p = 0.77$) as HC. Two (congruency: congruent vs. incongruent) by two (group: ADHD vs. HC) repeated-measures ANOVA on correct RT and accuracy revealed main effects of congruency (RT: F (1,152) = 352.4, $p < 0.001$; accuracy: F (1,152) = 470.4, $p < 0.001$) and a trend-level significance of interaction between congruency and group for reaction times (F (1,152) = 3.22, $p = 0.08$), but no such interaction in accuracy (F (1,152) = 0.88, $p = 0.35$). Incongruent trials were completed more slowly and less accurately than congruent trials in both groups. Participants with ADHD tended to have a larger RT congruency effect (86.3 msec vs. 69.5 msec, $p = 0.08$). Moreover, participants with ADHD exhibited smaller post-error slowing ($p = 0.006$) and larger RTV ($p = 0.005$) than HC (Table 1).

Table 1. Demographic, Behavioral and event-related potential (ERP) measures in participants with attention-deficit/hyperactivity disorder (ADHD) compared to healthy controls (HC).

	Mean ADHD	Mean HC	Group Difference F	Group Difference p	Age Correlation (r) ADHD	Age Correlation (r) HC	CBCL ADHD Problems Scale Correlation (r), Covarying Age
			Demographic and Clinical Data				
Age	13.6 ± 3.2	13.6 ± 3.1	0.00	0.982			
IQ	106.3 ± 13.4	110.6 ± 10.2	4.38	0.038			
SCQ	4.0 ± 3.5	1.8 ± 1.8	22.76	0.000			
CBCL_ADHD	65.3 ± 8.3	51.3 ± 3.2	191.71	0.000			
ADHD Symptom Counts from K-SAD-PL							
Hyperactive/Impulsive	3.8 ± 2.8						
Inattentive	7.1 ± 1.6						
Total	10.9 ± 3.1						
			Behavioral Data				
Overall RT (msec)	580.2 ± 176.0	503.0 ± 142.6	8.92	0.003	−0.668 **	−0.668 **	0.330 **
Overall RTV (msec)	185.6 ± 114.4	135.6 ± 101.7	8.20	0.005	−0.677 **	−0.591 **	0.329 **
Overall Accuracy	90.7% ± 5.9%	90.4% ± 5.6%	0.09	0.769	0.208 @	0.325 **	0.041
Post-error Slowing (msec)	14.5 ± 119.4	57.5 ± 62.9	7.80	0.006	0.338 **	0.034	−0.218 **
Conflict RT (msec)	86.3 ± 62.1	69.5 ± 42.9	3.81	0.075	−0.160	−0.321 *	0.161 *
Conflict Accuracy	10.6% ± 8.0%	10.8% ± 7.6%	0.88	0.350	0.102	−0.056	−0.063
			ERP Data				
ERN at FCz	−3.20 ± 5.11	−3.78 ± 4.88	0.42	0.474	−0.346 **	−0.223	0.025
CRN at FCz	0.93 ± 4.77	2.41 ± 3.69	4.53	0.035	0.108	0.248 *	−0.205 *
dERN at FCz	−4.13 ± 6.20	−6.19 ± 5.44	4.72	0.031	−0.369 **	−0.368 **	0.179 *
Pe at CPz	8.99 ± 8.82	12.57 ± 9.66	5.62	0.019	0.014	0.047	−0.208 *
Pc at CPz	−5.40 ± 6.50	−6.10 ± 6.19	0.45	0.506	0.268 *	0.095	−0.052
dPe at CPz	14.40 ± 9.37	18.66 ± 8.75	8.37	0.004	−0.173	−0.017	−0.176 *
N2 con at FCz(μV)	0.36 ± 5.57	0.80 ± 5.25	0.23	0.630	0.242 *	0.563 **	−0.003
N2 inc at FCz(μV)	−0.49 ± 5.14	−0.92 ± 4.81	0.30	0.583	0.229 *	0.458 **	0.073
dN2 at FCz(μV)	−0.84 ± 2.17	−1.72 ± 2.55	5.00	0.027	−0.084	−0.297 **	0.148 @
P3 con at Pz(μV)	8.85 ± 5.47	11.58 ± 6.06	8.63	0.004	−0.086	−0.220 @	−0.266 **
P3 inc at Pz(μV)	10.56 ± 6.16	14.57 ± 6.25	16.10	0.000	0.091	0.010	−0.291 **
dP3 at Pz(μV)	1.71 ± 3.20	3.00 ± 3.16	6.27	0.013	0.323 **	0.443 **	−0.113

ERP, event-related potentials; ADHD, attention deficits/hyperactive disorder; HC, healthy controls; SCQ, score from the Social Communication Questionnaire; CBCL_ADHD, the DSM-Oriented ADHD Problems Scale from the Child Behavior Checklist (CBCL); K-SAD-PL, the Kiddie Schedule for Affective Disorders and Schizophrenia for School-Aged Children-Present and Lifetime Version; RT, reaction times; RTV, reaction time variability; Conflict RT, incongruent RT minus congruent RT; Conflict Accuracy, congruent accuracy minus incongruent accuracy; ERN, error-related negativity; CRN, correct-related negativity; dERN, ERN minus CRN; con, congruent; inc, incongruent; dN2, incongruent N2 minus congruent N2; dP3, incongruent P3 minus congruent P3. ** $p < 0.01$, * $p < 0.05$, @ $p < 0.10$.

Age in all subjects was negatively associated with overall RT (r = −0.647, p < 0.001), RTV (r = −0.620, p < 0.001) and RT congruency effect (incongruent minus congruent RT, r = −0.215, p = 0.007), and was positively correlated with post-error slowing (r = 0.220, p = 0.006) and overall accuracy (r = 0.264, p = 0.001). With age increasing, participants responded faster and more accurately, and showed smaller RT congruency effects and RTV. A correlation of age with post-error slowing was evident in ADHD but not in HC (ADHD: r = 0.339, p = 0.003; HC: r = 0.034, p = 0.767; ADHD vs. HC, p = 0.012). There was no correlation of age with the accuracy congruency effect. Correlation of age with behavioral measures in individual groups is presented in Table 1.

3.2. ERP Data in Patients with ADHD and Healthy Controls

3.2.1. Response-Locked ERN

The two (response type: error vs. correct) by two (group: ADHD vs. HC) repeated-measures ANOVA revealed a main effect of response type (F (1,149) = 118.46, p < 0.001) and an interaction between response type and group (F (1,149) = 4.72, p = 0.031). Error trials elicited a larger ERN (more negative) than correct trials; the ERN effect (i.e., dERN) was smaller in participants with ADHD than in HC (Table 1; Figure 1). There was no main effect of group (F < 1, p = 0.449).

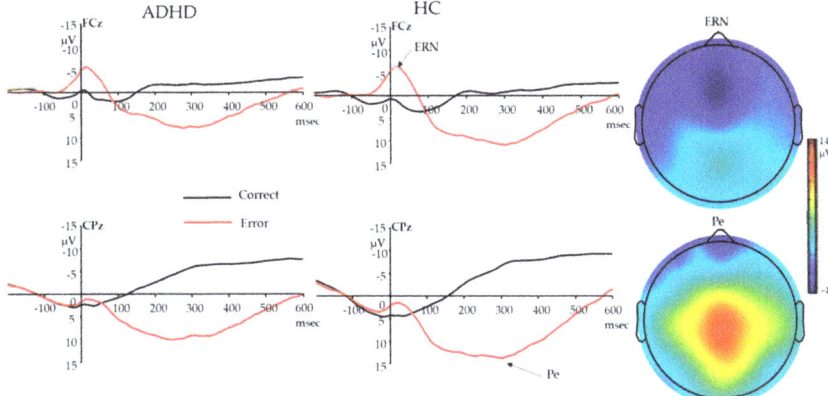

Figure 1. ERN and Pe waveforms for participants with ADHD and HC, and topography for error response (ERN: 0–80 ms; Pe: 200–400 ms; Baseline: −200–−50 ms) in all participants. Responses occurred at 0 msec. ADHD, attention deficits/hyperactive disorder; HC, healthy controls; ERN, error-related negativity; Pe, error positivity.

Age was negatively correlated with ERN amplitude (r = −0.286, p < 0.001) and dERN (r = −0.364, p < 0.001), and positively correlated with CRN (r = 0.167 p = 0.040) across all subjects. There was no significant group difference in correlations with age. With age increasing, participants showed a larger ERN, smaller CRN, and larger ERN effect. When covarying age, CRN was negatively correlated with overall RT (r = −0.318, p < 0.001), RTV (r = −0.263, p = 0.001), accuracy (r = −0.162, p = 0.047), and positively correlated with post-error slowing (r = −0.204, p = 0.012); the ERN effect was positively correlated with overall RT (r = 0.311, p < 0.001) and RTV (r = 0.212, p = 0.009) and negatively correlated with post-error slowing (r = −0.276, p = 0.001). There was no ERN correlation with behavioral performance and no group difference in the correlation between ERN/CRN/dERN and behavioral performance.

3.2.2. Response-Locked Pe

The two (response type: error vs. correct) by two (group: ADHD vs. HC) repeated-measures ANOVA revealed a main effect of response type (F (1, 149) = 502.62, $p < 0.001$) and interaction between response type and group (F (1, 149) = 8.37, $p = 0.004$). Error trials elicited a larger Pe than did correct trials (Pc); the Pe effect (i.e., dPe) was smaller in participants with ADHD than in HC (Table 1; Figure 1). There was no main effect of group (F = 1.826, $p = 0.179$).

Age was positively correlated with Pc on correct trials ($r = 0.182$ $p = 0.026$); there was no significant correlation of age with the Pe or the Pe effect, and there was no group difference in these correlations with age. When covarying age, the Pe and Pe effect were negatively correlated with overall RT (Pe: $r = -0.471$, $p < 0.001$; dPe: $r = -0.386$, $p < 0.001$), RTV (Pe: $r = -0.431$, $p < 0.001$; dPe: $r = -0.413$, $p < 0.001$), positively correlated with accuracy (Pe: $r = 0.213$, $p = 0.009$; dPe: $r = 0.313$, $p < 0.001$) and post-error slowing (Pe: $r = 0.249$, $p = 0.002$; dPe: $r = 0.202$, $p = 0.013$). There was no Pc correlation with behavioral performance or group difference in correlation between Pe/Pc/Pe effect and behavioral performance.

3.2.3. Stimulus-Locked N2

The two (congruency: congruent vs. incongruent) by two (group: ADHD vs. HC) repeated-measures ANOVA revealed a main effect of congruency (F (1,152) = 46.23, $p < 0.001$) and an interaction between congruency and group (F (1,152) = 4.99, $p = 0.027$). Incongruent trials elicited a larger N2 (more negative) than congruent trials; the N2 congruency effect was smaller in participants with ADHD than in HC (Table 1; Figure 2). There was no main effect of group (F < 1, $p = 0.992$).

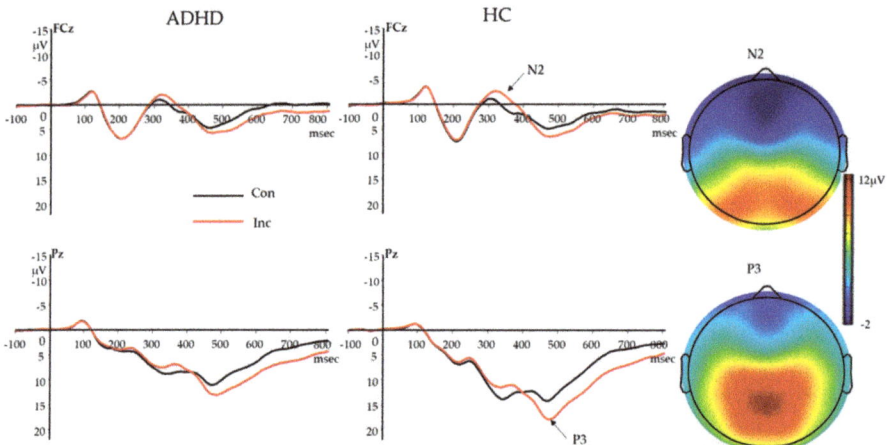

Figure 2. N2 and P3 waveforms for participants with ADHD and HC, and topography for incongruent correct trials (N2: 300–400 ms mean amplitude; P3: 400–600 ms mean amplitude; Baseline: −100–0 ms) in all participants. Stimuli onset occurred at 0 msec. Con, congruent correct trials; Inc, incongruent correct trials; ADHD, attention deficits/hyperactive disorder; HC, healthy controls.

Age was positively correlated with N2 on both congruent ($r = 0.395$, $p < 0.001$) and incongruent trials ($r = 0.338$, $p < 0.001$), and negatively correlated with the N2 congruency effect ($r = -0.194$, $p = 0.016$). There was no significant group difference in correlations with age. With age increasing, participants showed larger N2 congruency effect (more negative), which was evident in HC but not in ADHD cases (HC, $r = -0.297$, $p = 0.009$; ADHD, $r = -0.084$, $p = 0.469$; ADHD vs. HC, $p = 0.118$). When covarying age, there was no significant correlation or group difference in the correlation between N2 and behavioral performance (all $ps > 0.09$).

3.2.4. Stimulus-Locked P3

The two (congruency: congruent vs. incongruent) by two (group: ADHD vs. HC) repeated-measures ANOVA revealed main effects of congruency (F (1,152) = 84.24, $p < 0.001$) and group (F (1,152) = 13.12, $p < 0.001$), a significant interaction between congruency and group (F (1,152) = 6.26, $p = 0.013$). Incongruent trials elicited larger P3 than congruent trials. Participants with ADHD had smaller P3 amplitudes, and also showed smaller P3 congruency effects than HC (Table 1; Figure 2).

Age was not correlated with congruent ($r = -0.151$, $p = 0.062$) or incongruent P3 ($r = 0.049$, $p = 0.544$) amplitudes, but was positively correlated with the P3 congruency effect ($r = 0.375$, $p < 0.001$). There was no significant group difference in the correlation of age with P3 congruency effect. With age increasing, participants showed larger P3 congruency effects. When covarying age, RT on congruent and incongruent trials were negatively correlated with P3 at congruent ($r = -0.404$, $p < 0.001$) and incongruent trials ($r = -0.432$, $p < 0.001$) respectively. The RT congruency effect was negatively correlated with the P3 congruency effect ($r = -0.171$, $p = 0.034$). There was no significant association between accuracy and P3, and there was no group difference in the correlation of P3 with behavioral performance.

3.3. The Association of Behavioral and ERP Measures with ADHD Symptoms and ADHD Subtype

3.3.1. The Association of Behavioral and ERP Measures with K-SAD-PL ADHD Symptoms

In ADHD, age was negatively correlated with ADHD total score ($r = -0.385$, $p = 0.001$) and hyperactivity/impulsive score ($r = -0.443$, $p < 0.001$). Older youth with ADHD in our sample had reduced symptom severity in total and hyperactivity/impulsive scores; there was no correlation of age with the inattention score ($r = 0.043$, $p = 0.710$). When covarying age, there was no correlation between any ADHD symptom scores (including ADHD total score, inattention score, or hyperactive/impulsive score) and behavioral performance (all $ps > 0.1$). There was no correlation between ADHD symptom scores and ERP measures, except that the P3 congruency effect was found positively correlated with the inattention subscale ($r = 0.336$, $p = 0.003$).

3.3.2. The Association of Behavioral and ERP Measures with CBCL ADHD Problems Scale Scores

Across all subjects, age was negatively correlated with CBCL ADHD Problems Scale scores ($r = -0.179$, $p = 0.028$). The age correlation with symptom severity was more significant in ADHD patients than in HC (ADHD: $r = -0.329$, $p = 0.004$; HC: $r = 0.194$, $p = 0.090$; ADHD vs. HC: $t = 2.13$, $p = 0.035$). When covarying age, ADHD Problems Scale scores were correlated with overall RT ($r = 0.330$, $p < 0.001$), RTV ($r = 0.329$, $p < 0.001$), post-error slowing ($r = -0.218$, $p = 0.007$) and the RT congruency effect ($r = 0.161$, $p = 0.049$). When age and these significant behavioral measures were included in a backward stepwise regression model, only RTV was found positively correlated with ADHD Problems Scale scores ($b = 0.031$, $p < 0.001$). When covarying age, ADHD Problems Scale scores were correlated with the CRN ($r = -0.205$, $p = 0.013$), ERN effect ($r = 0.179$, $p = 0.030$), Pe ($r = -0.208$, $p = 0.011$), Pe effect ($r = -0.176$, $p = 0.033$), and P3 on congruent ($r = -0.266$, $p = 0.001$) and incongruent ($r = -0.291$, $p = 0.001$) trials. When age and these significant ERP measures were included in a backward stepwise regression model, only P3 on incongruent trials was found negatively correlated with ADHD Problems Scale scores ($b = -0.339$, $p = 0.004$). In the ADHD or HC group alone, there was no correlation of ADHD Problems Scale scores with any behavioral or ERP measures when covarying age.

3.3.3. Behavioral and ERP Measures Among Different ADHD Subtypes

For patients included in our sample, participants with ADHD inattentive type (14.7 ± 2.8 years) were older than patients with combined type (11.6 ± 2.9, $p < 0.001$), and patients with the hyperactive/impulsive type (12.6 ± 3.9, $p < 0.001$). When controlling age, there were no group differences on any behavioral or ERP measures among the three subtypes of ADHD (all $ps > 0.1$).

4. Discussion

We investigated behavioral and electrophysiological indices of performance monitoring and the association of these indices with age in children and adolescents with ADHD and healthy controls, using an EEG arrow-flanker task. Overall, with age increasing, participants responded faster, more accurately, and less variably, and they showed an increased post-error slowing effect. In addition, they exhibited an increased ERN effect and increased N2 and P3 congruency effects. Children and adolescents with ADHD showed impaired behavioral performance, attenuated error awareness and conflict monitoring. Specifically, participants with ADHD responded more slowly, more variably and had reduced post-error slowing; they showed reduced ERN and Pe effects in error monitoring, and reduced N2 and P3 congruency effects. Impaired behavioral and ERP indices of performance monitoring are consistent with the pattern associated with younger age across groups. Moreover, increased reaction time variability and reduced P3 amplitude in incongruent trials were associated with increased ADHD Problems Scale scores measured by CBCL across all participants.

The developmental effects on behavioral performance across groups, including faster reaction times, increased accuracy, decreased reaction time conflict, and decreased reaction time variability, are consistent with the literature [51,52]. With increased age and brain maturation, children increase their response speed and improve their attention and ability to resolve conflict. As expected, relative to HC, participants with ADHD responded more slowly, with increased reaction time variability; they also tended to show a larger RT congruency effect. Impairments in these behavioral measures are thought to result from lapses in attention and failures in executive control [17]; the pattern of performance deficits in ADHD is in line with the pattern shown in younger ages across study participants, consistent with the developmental lag model for ADHD [53]. Regarding post-error processes, there was a lack of post-error slowing in ADHD, while HC slowed their response after errors. However, the post-error slowing was positively correlated with age in ADHD, suggesting that the post-error slowing effect in ADHD was not developed until later in adolescence, which further suggests that impairment of performance monitoring in ADHD may be associated with a developmental delay. We did not observe a reduced accuracy among children with ADHD, which may be related to our speed-accuracy instructions to respond quickly enough to maintain a certain number of error trials. Consistently with the previous literature, RTV is found to be larger in ADHD than in HC; among several behavioral indices showing group differences between ADHD and HC, RTV is uniquely associated with continuous measures of ADHD Problems Scale scores, suggesting RTV is a robust marker of ADHD symptoms.

Error responses elicited a larger ERN and Pe than did correct responses. ERN and Pe effects were larger with faster reaction times, reduced RTV and greater post-error adjustments, suggesting that increased ERN and Pe effects may reflect better performance monitoring and compensatory processing. Consistent with the literature, ERN effects increased with age and Pe effects did not change with age in children and adolescents [54,55]. The reduced ERN effect found in ADHD compared to healthy controls is consistent with most pediatric and adult studies on ADHD [22,56], suggesting an error detection deficit in ADHD. Following early error detection, participants with ADHD showed a reduced Pe effect compared to healthy controls, suggesting alterations in the evaluation of error responses and their motivational significance. Individuals with ADHD may fail to initiate adaptive control processes after errors to make adjustment in the next trial, as demonstrated by diminished post-error slowing. Together with evidence of a larger ERN effect with increasing age, and larger ERN and Pe effects with better performance, the alteration of ERN and Pe effects in ADHD may be associated with a developmental delay in ADHD.

Incongruent compared with congruent stimuli yielded the typical N2 and P3 amplitude enhancement across groups. Both effects were stronger when participants were older across groups, suggesting larger N2 and P3 effects may reflect enhancements of conflict monitoring with age. While N2 was not associated with behavioral performance, a larger P3 effect was associated with a reduced RT congruency effect. Participants with ADHD showed reduced N2 and P3 effects, indicating problems with conflict monitoring and attention resource allocations. Specially, the attenuated N2 congruency effect in ADHD is consistent with previous findings that N2 is reduced in ADHD and unaffected siblings [25], and in line with the notion that N2 is an index for a general conflict monitoring process. In ADHD, the reduced P3 congruency effect and the reduced P3 amplitude on both congruent and incongruent trials are consistent with previous findings of a general deficit in attention resource allocation [37]. Meanwhile, P3 amplitude on incongruent trials was negatively correlated with CBCL ADHD Problems Scale scores as a continuous measure across groups, further suggesting the cognitive process underlying P3 may serve as a target of intervention to reduce ADHD symptoms. Reduced congruency effects indicated by N2 and P3 in ADHD, together with stronger N2 and P3 effects with age increasing across groups, could also imply a developmental delay in ADHD.

The current study investigated performance monitoring and its development in ADHD. Our study used a larger sample size ($n = 77$ per group) and broader age range (ages 8–18) than has been typical in the literature, and in addition, our control group was closely matched in age and matched in gender. While the broad age range allowed us to investigate age effects on performance monitoring, the sample was less homogenous and sample size was small for any given age, preventing us from analyzing the effects of other factors, such as gender, comorbidity and medication [6]. Moreover, the current study included participants ranging in age from 8 to 18 years old, though the development of performance monitoring begins earlier and continues later into the life course [49]; further work should evaluate the relationship between brain activation and ADHD across a wider age range. We have interpreted developmental results using a cross-sectional design, which needs to be verified through a longitudinal design. Another limitation of our study is that we included patients with comorbid anxiety, depression and ODD in ADHD group to increase sample size. While comorbid anxiety may have increased ERN in the ADHD group [57], effects of anxiety, depression and ODD comorbidity on different measures of ERPs call for further investigation.

5. Conclusions

This study using ERPs to investigate performance monitoring and its development in ADHD adds to our knowledge of alterations and developmental delays in conflict processing and error monitoring in children with ADHD. Future research should be longitudinal and should include participants across the life span to determine developmental course of performance monitoring and its neural correlates in ADHD. It will also be important to identify behavioral and neural targets for intervention, both for clinical benefit as well as to develop better causal models of the development of ADHD symptoms.

Author Contributions: Conceptualization, Y.L., G.L.H., P.D.A and W.J.G.; Methodology, Y.L., G.L.H., and W.J.G.; Formal analysis, Y.L.; Data curation, Y.L., G.L.H., B.S.H, H.E.R.; Writing—original draft preparation, Y.L., G.L.H., W.J.G.; writing—review and editing, G.L.H., W.J.G, P.D.A., H.E.R.; visualization, Y.L.; project administration, G.H., B.S.H., H.E.R.; funding acquisition, G.L.H., P.D.A and W.J.G. All authors have read and agreed to the published version of the manuscript.

Funding: This research was supported by National Institute of Mental Health grantR01 MH101493 (G.L.H., P.D.A., and W.J.G.). P.D.A. also receives support from the Alberta Innovates Translational Health Chair in Child and Youth Mental Health.

Conflicts of Interest: The authors declare no conflict of interest.

References

1. Willcutt, E.G. The prevalence of DSM-IV attention-deficit/hyperactivity disorder: a meta-analytic review. *Neurotherapeutics* **2012**, *9*, 490–499. [CrossRef] [PubMed]
2. Willcutt, E.G.; Doyle, A.E.; Nigg, J.T.; Faraone, S.V.; Pennington, B.F. Validity of the executive function theory of attention-deficit/hyperactivity disorder: a meta-analytic review. *Boil. Psychiatry* **2005**, *57*, 1336–1346. [CrossRef] [PubMed]
3. Castellanos, F.X.; Tannock, R. Neuroscience of attention-deficit/hyperactivity disorder: the search for endophenotypes. *Nat. Rev. Neurosci.* **2002**, *3*, 617–628. [CrossRef] [PubMed]

4. Ehlis, A.-C.; Deppermann, S.; Fallgatter, A.J. Performance monitoring and post-error adjustments in adults with attention-deficit/hyperactivity disorder: an EEG analysis. *J. Psychiatry Neurosci.* **2018**, *43*, 396–406. [CrossRef] [PubMed]
5. Faraone, S.V.; Biederman, J.; Mick, E. The age-dependent decline of attention deficit hyperactivity disorder: A meta-analysis of follow-up studies. *Psychol. Med.* **2006**, *36*, 159–165. [CrossRef]
6. Shiels, K.; Hawk, L.W., Jr. Self-regulation in ADHD: The role of error processing. *Clin. Psychol. Rev.* **2010**, *30*, 951–961. [CrossRef]
7. Klein, C.; Wendling, K.; Huettner, P.; Ruder, H.; Peper, M. Intra-subject variability in attention-deficit hyperactivity disorder. *Boil. Psychiatry* **2006**, *60*, 1088–1097. [CrossRef] [PubMed]
8. Herrmann, M.J.; Mader, K.; Schreppel, T.; Jacob, C.; Heine, M.; Boreatti-Hümmer, A.; Ehlis, A.-C.; Scheuerpflug, P.; Pauli, P.; Fallgatter, A.J. Neural correlates of performance monitoring in adult patients with attention deficit hyperactivity disorder (ADHD). *World J. Boil. Psychiatry* **2010**, *11*, 457–464. [CrossRef]
9. Balogh, L.; Czobor, P. Post-error slowing in patients with ADHD: a meta-analysis. *J. Atten. Disord.* **2016**, *20*, 1004–1016. [CrossRef] [PubMed]
10. Dutilh, G.; Vandekerckhove, J.; Forstmann, B.U.; Keuleers, E.; Brysbaert, M.; Wagenmakers, E.J. Testing theories of post-error slowing. *Atten. Percept. Psychophys.* **2012**, *74*, 454–465. [CrossRef] [PubMed]
11. Wiersema, J.R.; Van Der Meere, J.J.; Roeyers, H. ERP correlates of impaired error monitoring in children with ADHD. *J. Neural Transm.* **2005**, *112*, 1417–1430. [CrossRef] [PubMed]
12. Schachar, R.J.; Chen, S.; Logan, G.D.; Ornstein, T.J.; Crosbie, J.; Ickowicz, A.; Pakulak, A. Evidence for an error monitoring deficit in attention deficit hyperactivity disorder. *J. Abnorm. Child Psychol.* **2004**, *32*, 285–293. [CrossRef] [PubMed]
13. Jonkman, L.; Van Melis, J.J.; Kemner, C.; Markus, C.R. Methylphenidate improves deficient error evaluation in children with ADHD: An event-related brain potential study. *Boil. Psychol.* **2007**, *76*, 217–229. [CrossRef] [PubMed]
14. Van Meel, C.S.; Heslenfeld, D.J.; Oosterlaan, J.; Sergeant, J.A. Adaptive control deficits in attention-deficit/hyperactivity disorder (ADHD): The role of error processing. *Psychiatry Res.* **2007**, *151*, 211–220. [CrossRef] [PubMed]
15. Gehring, W.J.; Liu, Y.; Orr, J.M.; Carp, J. *The error-related negativity (ERN/Ne)*; Luck, S.J., Kappenman, E.S., Eds.; The Oxford Handbook of Event-Related Potential Components; Oxford University Press: New York, NY, USA, 2012.
16. Ullsperger, M.; Danielmeier, C.; Jocham, G. Neurophysiology of performance monitoring and adaptive behavior. *Physiol. Rev.* **2014**, *94*, 35–79. [CrossRef] [PubMed]
17. Michelini, G.; Kitsune, G.L.; Cheung, C.H.; Brandeis, D.; Banaschewski, T.; Asherson, P.; McLoughlin, G.; Kuntsi, J. Attention-deficit/hyperactivity disorder remission is linked to better neurophysiological error detection and attention-vigilance processes. *Boil. Psychiatry* **2016**, *80*, 923–932. [CrossRef] [PubMed]
18. Marquardt, L.; Eichele, H.; Lundervold, A.J.; Haavik, J.; Eichele, T. Event-related-potential (ERP) correlates of performance monitoring in adults with attention-deficit/hyperactivity disorder (ADHD). *Front. Psychol.* **2018**, *9*, 485. [CrossRef]
19. Groom, M.J.; Cahill, J.D.; Bates, A.T.; Jackson, G.M.; Calton, T.G.; Liddle, P.F.; Hollis, C. Electrophysiological indices of abnormal error-processing in adolescents with attention deficit hyperactivity disorder (ADHD). *J. Child. Psychol. Psychiatry.* **2010**, *51*, 66–76. [CrossRef]
20. Wiersema, J.R.; van der Meere, J.J.; Roeyers, H. ERP correlates of error monitoring in adult ADHD. *J. Neural. Transm. (Vienna)* **2009**, *116*, 371–379. [CrossRef]
21. Burgio-Murphy, A.; Klorman, R.; Shaywitz, S.E.; Fletcher, J.M.; Marchione, K.E.; Holahan, J.; Stuebing, K.K.; Thatcher, J.E.; Shaywitz, B.A. Error-related event-related potentials in children with attention-deficit hyperactivity disorder, oppositional defiant disorder, reading disorder, and math disorder. *Biol. Psychol.* **2007**, *75*, 75–86. [CrossRef]
22. Meyer, A.; Hajcak, G. A review examining the relationship between individual differences in the error-related negativity and cognitive control. *Int. J. Psychophysiol.* **2019**, *144*, 7–13. [CrossRef] [PubMed]
23. Groen, Y.; Wijers, A.A.; Mulder, L.J.; Waggeveld, B.; Minderaa, R.B.; Althaus, M. Error and feedback processing in children with ADHD and children with Autistic Spectrum Disorder: An EEG event-related potential study. *Clin. Neurophysiol.* **2008**, *119*, 2476–2493. [CrossRef] [PubMed]

24. Van De Voorde, S.; Roeyers, H.; Wiersema, J.R. Error monitoring in children with ADHD or reading disorder: An event-related potential study. *Boil. Psychol.* **2010**, *84*, 176–185. [CrossRef] [PubMed]
25. Albrecht, B.; Brandeis, D.; Uebel, H.; Heinrich, H.; Mueller, U.C.; Hasselhorn, M.; Steinhausen, H.C.; Rothenberger, A.; Banaschewski, T. Action monitoring in boys with attention-deficit/hyperactivity disorder, their nonaffected siblings, and normal control subjects: Evidence for an endophenotype. *Biological Psychiatry* **2008**, *64*, 615–625. [CrossRef]
26. Kopp, B.; Rist, F.; Mattler, U. N200 in the flanker task as a neurobehavioral tool for investigating executive control. *Psychophysiology* **1996**, *33*, 282–294. [CrossRef]
27. Nieuwenhuis, S.; Yeung, N.; Wildenberg, W.V.D.; Ridderinkhof, K.R. Electrophysiological correlates of anterior cingulate function in a go/no-go task: effects of response conflict and trial type frequency. *Cogn. Affect. Behav. Neurosci.* **2003**, *3*, 17–26. [CrossRef]
28. Van Veen, V.; Carter, C.S. The anterior cingulate as a conflict monitor: fMRI and ERP studies. *Physiol. Behav.* **2002**, *77*, 477–482. [CrossRef]
29. Polich, J. Updating P300: An integrative theory of P3a and P3b. *Clin. Neurophysiol.* **2007**, *118*, 2128–2148. [CrossRef]
30. Johnstone, S.J.; Barry, R.J.; Clarke, A.R. Behavioural and ERP indices of response inhibition during a Stop-signal task in children with two subtypes of Attention-Deficit Hyperactivity Disorder. *Int. J. Psychophysiol.* **2007**, *66*, 37–47. [CrossRef]
31. Groom, M.J.; Bates, A.T.; Jackson, G.M.; Calton, T.G.; Liddle, P.F.; Hollis, C. Event-related potentials in adolescents with schizophrenia and their siblings: a comparison with attention-deficit/hyperactivity disorder. *Boil. Psychiatry* **2008**, *63*, 784–792. [CrossRef]
32. Shen, I.-H.; Tsai, S.-Y.; Duann, J.-R. Inhibition control and error processing in children with attention deficit/hyperactivity disorder: An event-related potentials study. *Int. J. Psychophysiol.* **2011**, *81*, 1–11. [CrossRef] [PubMed]
33. Smith, J.L.; Johnstone, S.J.; Barry, R.J. Inhibitory processing during the Go/NoGo task: an ERP analysis of children with attention-deficit/hyperactivity disorder. *Clin. Neurophysiol.* **2004**, *115*, 1320–1331. [CrossRef] [PubMed]
34. Johnstone, S.J.; Barry, R.J.; Clarke, A.R. Ten years on: A follow-up review of ERP research in attention-deficit/hyperactivity disorder. *Clin. Neurophysiol.* **2013**, *124*, 644–657. [CrossRef] [PubMed]
35. Szuromi, B.; Czobor, P.; Komlosi, S.; Bitter, I. P300 deficits in adults with attention deficit hyperactivity disorder: A meta-analysis. *Psychol. Med.* **2011**, *41*, 1529–1538. [CrossRef]
36. Johnstone, S.J.; Barry, R.J.; Markovska, V.; Dimoska, A.; Clarke, A.R. Response inhibition and interference control in children with AD/HD: A visual ERP investigation. *Int. J. Psychophysiol.* **2009**, *72*, 145–153. [CrossRef]
37. Kratz, O.; Studer, P.; Malcherek, S.; Erbe, K.; Moll, G.H.; Heinrich, H. Attentional processes in children with ADHD: An event-related potential study using the attention network test. *Int. J. Psychophysiol.* **2011**, *81*, 82–90. [CrossRef]
38. Barry, R.J.; Johnstone, S.J.; Clarke, A.R. A review of electrophysiology in attention-deficit/hyperactivity disorder: II. Event-related potentials. *Clin. Neurophysiol.* **2003**, *114*, 184–198. [CrossRef]
39. A Friedman, L.; Rapoport, J.L. Brain development in ADHD. *Curr. Opin. Neurobiol.* **2015**, *30*, 106–111. [CrossRef]
40. Kaufman, J.; Birmaher, B.; Brent, D.; Rao, U.; Flynn, C.; Moreci, P.; Williamson, D.; Ryan, N. Schedule for affective disorders and schizophrenia for school-age children-present and lifetime version (K-SADS-PL): Initial Reliability and Validity Data. *J. Am. Acad. Child Adolesc. Psychiatry* **1997**, *36*, 980–988. [CrossRef]
41. Hanna, G.L. *Schedule for obsessive-compulsive and other behavioral syndromes (SOCOBS)*; University of Michigan: Ann Abor, MI, USA, 2013.
42. Achenbach, T.M.; Rescorla, L.A. *Manual for the ASEBA school-age forms & profiles*; University of Vermont, Research Center for Children, Youth, and Families: Burlington, VT, USA, 2001.
43. Berument, S.K.; Rutter, M.; Lord, C.; Pickles, A.; Bailey, A. Autism screening questionnaire: diagnostic validity. *Br. J. Psychiatry* **1999**, *175*, 444–451. [CrossRef]
44. American Psychiatric Association Diagnostic and Statistical Manual of Mental Disorders. *Diagn. Stat. Man. Ment. Disord.* 2013.

45. Leckman, J.F.; Sholomskas, D.; Thompson, W.D.; Belanger, A.; Weissman, M.M. Best estimate of lifetime psychiatric diagnosis: a methodological study. *Arch. Gen. Psychiatry* **1982**, *39*, 879–883. [CrossRef] [PubMed]
46. Wechsler, D. *Wechsler Abbreviated Scale of Intelligence (WASI-II)*; Psychological Corporation: San Antonio, TX, USA, 2011.
47. Eriksen, B.A.; Eriksen, C.W. Effects of noise letters upon the identification of a target letter in a nonsearch task. *Percep. Psychophysics* **1974**, *16*, 143–149. [CrossRef]
48. Hanna, G.L.; Liu, Y.; Isaacs, Y.E.; Ayoub, A.M.; Torres, J.J.; O'Hara, N.B.; Gehring, W.J. Withdrawn/depressed behaviors and error-Related brain activity in youth With Obsessive-Compulsive Disorder. *J. Am. Acad. Child Adolesc. Psychiatry* **2016**, *55*, 906–913.e2. [CrossRef]
49. Gratton, G.; Coles, M.G.; Donchin, E. A new method for off-line removal of ocular artifact. *Electroencephalogr. Clin. Neurophysiol.* **1983**, *55*, 468–484. [CrossRef]
50. Simons, R.F. The way of our errors: theme and variations. *Psychophysiology* **2010**, *47*, 1–14. [CrossRef]
51. Best, J.R.; Miller, P.H. A developmental perspective on executive function. *Child Dev.* **2010**, *81*, 1641–1660. [CrossRef]
52. Davidson, M.C.; Amso, D.; Anderson, L.C.; Diamond, A. Development of cognitive control and executive functions from 4 to 13 years: evidence from manipulations of memory, inhibition, and task switching. *Neuropsychologia* **2006**, *44*, 2037–2078. [CrossRef]
53. Doehnert, M.; Brandeis, D.; Imhof, K.; Drechsler, R.; Steinhausen, H.-C. Mapping attention-deficit/hyperactivity disorder from childhood to adolescence—no neurophysiologic evidence for a developmental lag of attention but some for Inhibition. *Boil. Psychiatry* **2010**, *67*, 608–616. [CrossRef]
54. Tamnes, C.K.; Walhovd, K.B.; Torstveit, M.; Sells, V.T.; Fjell, A.M. Performance monitoring in children and adolescents: a review of developmental changes in the error-related negativity and brain maturation. *Dev. Cogn. Neurosci.* **2013**, *6*, 1–13. [CrossRef]
55. Wiersema, J.R.; Van Der Meere, J.J.; Roeyers, H. Developmental changes in error monitoring: an event-related potential study. *Neuropsychologia* **2007**, *45*, 1649–1657. [CrossRef] [PubMed]
56. Geburek, A.; Rist, F.; Gediga, G.; Stroux, D.; Pedersen, A. Electrophysiological indices of error monitoring in juvenile and adult attention deficit hyperactivity disorder (ADHD)—a meta-analytic appraisal. *Int. J. Psychophysiol.* **2013**, *87*, 349–362. [CrossRef] [PubMed]
57. Moser, J.S.; Moran, T.P.; Schroder, H.S.; Donnellan, M.B.; Yeung, N. On the relationship between anxiety and error monitoring: a meta-analysis and conceptual framework. *Front. Hum. Neurosci.* **2013**, *7*, 466. [CrossRef] [PubMed]

© 2020 by the authors. Licensee MDPI, Basel, Switzerland. This article is an open access article distributed under the terms and conditions of the Creative Commons Attribution (CC BY) license (http://creativecommons.org/licenses/by/4.0/).

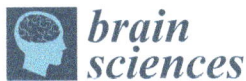

Article

Electrophysiological Markers of Visuospatial Attention Recovery after Mild Traumatic Brain Injury

Julie Bolduc-Teasdale [1,2], Pierre Jolicoeur [2] and Michelle McKerral [1,2,*]

1. Centre for Interdisciplinary Research in Rehabilitation (CRIR), IURDPM, CIUSSS du Centre-Sud-de-l'Île-de-Montréal, Montreal, QC H3S 1M9, Canada; juliebolduct@me.com
2. Department of Psychology, Université de Montréal, Montreal, QC H3C 3J7, Canada; pierre.jolicoeur@umontreal.ca
* Correspondence: michelle.mckerral@umontreal.ca; Tel.: +1-514-343-6503

Received: 21 October 2019; Accepted: 22 November 2019; Published: 27 November 2019

Abstract: Objective: Attentional problems are amongst the most commonly reported complaints following mild traumatic brain injury (mTBI), including difficulties orienting and disengaging attention, sustaining it over time, and dividing attentional resources across multiple simultaneous demands. The objective of this study was to track, using a single novel electrophysiological task, various components associated with the deployment of visuospatial selective attention. Methods: A paradigm was designed to evoke earlier visual evoked potentials (VEPs), as well as attention-related and visuocognitive ERPs. Data from 36 individuals with mTBI (19 subacute, 17 chronic) and 22 uninjured controls are presented. Postconcussion symptoms (PCS), anxiety (BAI), depression (BDI-II) and visual attention (TEA Map Search, DKEFS Trail Making Test) were also assessed. Results: Earlier VEPs (P1, N1), as well as processes related to visuospatial orientation (N2pc) and encoding in visual short-term memory (SPCN), appear comparable in mTBI and control participants. However, there appears to be a disruption in the spatiotemporal dynamics of attention (N2pc-Ptc, P2) in subacute mTBI, which recovers within six months. This is also reflected in altered neuropsychological performance (information processing speed, attentional shifting). Furthermore, orientation of attention (P3a) and working memory processes (P3b) are also affected and remain as such in the chronic post-mTBI period, in co-occurrence with persisting postconcussion symptomatology. Conclusions: This study adds original findings indicating that such a sensitive and rigorous ERP task implemented at diagnostic and follow-up levels could allow for the identification of subtle but complex brain activation and connectivity deficits that can occur following mTBI.

Keywords: mTBI; event-related potentials; visual–attentional processing; brain connectivity; neuropsychological measures; postconcussion symptoms

1. Introduction

In recent years, an increasing number of studies have shown the impact of mild traumatic brain injury (mTBI) on cognitive functions. The fact that mTBIs are considered a major health issue involving long-term health risks raises questions as to how their impact can be best identified and measured in order to be treated and managed optimally.

A TBI is produced by a large transfer of energy generated by a direct impact of the head against a hard surface, or by forces (acceleration, deceleration, rotation) created during the impact [1]. In the case of mTBI, these forces are responsible for stretching of the axons and microbleeds, which lead to a complex neurometabolic cascade [2]. There is now growing and reproducible evidence that following mTBI microstructural damage and neurochemical imbalances occur in a number of brain regions (e.g., frontal, temporal, motor cortex) and in white matter integrity (e.g., corpus callosum) [3–8]. These alterations have been related to the known post-mTBI physical (e.g., headaches, drowsiness, fatigue, dizziness), cognitive (e.g., attention and memory problems, bradyphrenia), and affective (e.g., irritability, depression, anxiety) symptoms [1,9,10]. These symptoms are more intense in the first days and weeks following the injury and slowly decrease during the subacute recovery period, which has been described as the first three months post-trauma. However, in a non-negligible proportion of individuals these symptoms are at risk of becoming chronic [11].

Attentional problems such as difficulties orienting and disengaging attention [12], sustaining it over time, and/or dividing attentional resources across multiple simultaneous demands [13,14] are amongst the most common complaints reported by individuals after a mTBI. On a behavioural level, these deficits usually disappear over a period of seven to 10 days [10,12,15]. However, mTBI can have negative long-term neuropsychological impacts on subtle aspects of complex attention and working memory [16,17], even with normal behavioural performances, where some individuals report the persistence of attentional difficulties that interfere with the demands of their daily life and social participation. The need for a more sensitive functional measure of the impact of mTBI on distinct steps involved in the deployment of attention thus remains.

Event-related brain potentials (ERPs) can represent a relatively simple, inexpensive, and precise answer to that question because they allow us to assess the integrity (reflected by the amplitude of a component) and efficiency (reflected by its latency) of specific and complex cognitive processes [1,18]. With excellent temporal resolution, ERPs possess an advantage over reaction time measures because they provide measures of multiple stages of cognitive processing, instead of the summation of the duration of all the intervening mechanisms involved in the generation of a response [18].

Experimental paradigms have historically been designed to study precise cognitive processes along with their event-related components. For instance, oddball paradigms have been used to evoke the P3, a component reflecting a target stimulus upgrade in working memory [19]. Such paradigms have been shown to be sensitive following mTBI [20–24]. However, since mTBI can present with deficits at different levels within the deployment of attention, one needs to be able to rapidly track the steps of the process that are distinctly affected.

The objective of this study was to track, with the help of a single task, the deployment of visuospatial attentional mechanisms and to identify underlying deficits at different recovery time points after mTBI. The task we used allowed us to measure the integrity of the different visual and cognitive processes involved in the deployment of visuospatial selective attention. We studied components reflecting earlier visual–attentional processing, such as the N1 (discrimination processes within the focus of visual attention and central attention) [25,26], P1 (facilitation effect for stimuli presented at an attended localisation) [27], and P2 (early attentional modulation) [28] components, which we expected would not be different between the mTBI and control groups. We also investigated later attention-related and visuocognitive mechanisms such as the N2pc (deployment and orientation of visuospatial attention) [28], Ptc (target isolation once identified among distractors) [29], SPCN (encoding in visual short-term memory, working memory capacity) [30], P3a (disengaging of attention to re-orient toward novel stimuli) [31], and P3b (tracking of task-relevant stimuli during updating in working memory) [19] components, which were expected to be affected, at least for later components.

2. Materials and Methods

2.1. Participants

Three groups of participants were enrolled in the study: 24 uninjured controls, 24 individuals in the subacute phase of mTBI (first three months post-mTBI), and 24 individuals in the chronic phase of mTBI (six months to one year post-trauma).

The uninjured control participants were recruited through publicity posted in a community centre. Exclusion criteria consisted of any neurological (history of brain trauma, seizures, attention deficit disorder, or learning disability) or psychiatric (depression, anxiety disorder, or other) antecedents. The mTBI participants had sustained their injury during an accident involving a motor vehicle or a fall. Diagnostic criteria for mTBI were: 1) Glasgow Coma Scale, on presentation at emergency room, between 13 and 15 (on a maximum total of 15); 2) having had any alteration in consciousness not lasting more 30 min or a post-traumatic amnesia duration of less than 24 h [32]. All participants with mTBI had been diagnosed by a rehabilitation medicine physician and were recruited from either a local trauma hospital or a rehabilitation centre. Exclusion criteria were the same as for the control participants. Additionally, participants with muscular–skeletal lesions or whiplash injuries sustained during or prior to the accident that caused the mTBI were excluded. The chronic mTBI group included eight participants from the subacute group who were re-tested. Also, according to event-related potential guidelines [18], all participants had to be at least 48 h removed from any alcohol or drug intake, and those under psychoactive medication were not included in the study. All participants had normal or corrected-to-normal vision.

Data from some participants had to be excluded from the analysis because of loss of trials (more than 50% of trials) due to eye blinks, movements, excessive sweating, or very large alpha oscillations that were mainly related to temporary temperature control issues in the testing environment. Analyses were performed on data from 22 participants in the control group (12 males, mean age 26.8 years, SD 6.6), 19 in the subacute mTBI group (17 males, mean age 36.6 years, SD 13.5, mean postinjury time 57 days, SD 19), and 17 in the chronic mTBI group (11 males, mean age 39.2 years, SD 13.5, mean postinjury time 271 days, SD 87). Groups were not quite equivalent for age ($F(2,55) = 3.29$, $p = 0.045$), with the control group being slightly younger, and there were more males ($X^2(2, n = 58) = 6.02$, $p = 0.049$).

2.2. Procedure

A consent form, previously approved by the institutional ethics committee, was signed by the participants before their participation in the study. Neuropsychological and ERP testing lasted approximately 90 min, including electrode preparation/removal and frequent breaks. Participants received a financial compensation of 80 Canadian dollars for their participation.

2.2.1. Neuropsychological Testing

To quantify the presence of self-reported symptoms, participants rated the Postconcussion Symptoms scale (PCS; 22 items, rated 0—asymptomatic to 6—severely symptomatic, for a maximum score of 132) [33]. Participants also completed the Beck Anxiety Inventory Scale (BAI; 21 items, rated 0—symptoms absent to 3—severe symptoms, for a maximum score of 63) [34] and the Beck Depression Inventory Scale–II (BDI-II; 21 items, rated 0—symptoms absent to 3—severe symptoms, for a maximum score of 63) [35]. Visual attention was tested with the Map Search subtest (number of target symbols circled among distractors within 1 and 2 min, maximum 80) of the Test of Everyday Attention (TEA) [36], and by the Delis-Kaplan Executive Function System (DKEFS) Trail Making Test (time to completion for conditions 1 to 5: Visual Scanning, Number Sequencing, Letter Sequencing, Number–Letter Sequencing, Motor Speed) [37].

2.2.2. ERP Paradigm

The paradigm used in this study, which is presented in Figure 1, was first described by Bolduc-Teasdale, Jolicoeur & McKerral [38], where the detailed procedure, which was based on previously published paradigms [19,39,40], can be found.

2.2.3. EEG recording and Analysis

We used a widely accepted EEG recording and analysis method, with a 64 Ag/AgCL scalp-electrodes montage, along with VEOG and HEOG electrodes and mastoid reference [38]. Number of trials included in EEG averaging were similar across conditions and groups, with a minimum of 35 trials per task condition.

Brain Sci. **2019**, 9, 343

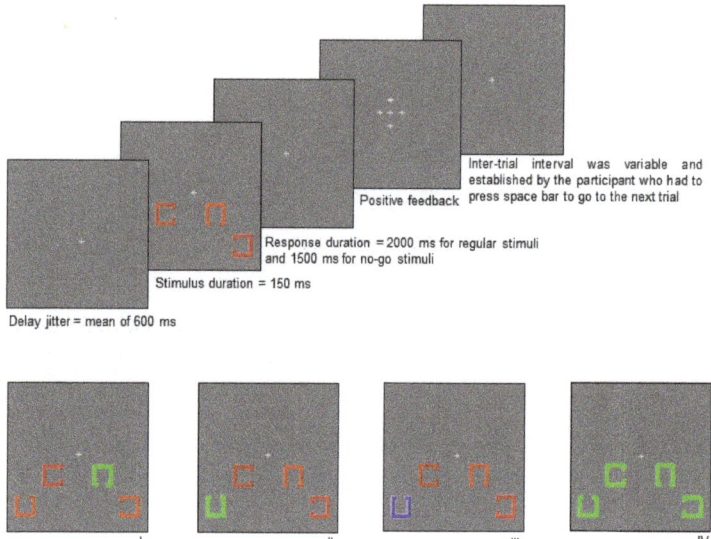

Figure 1. Experimental paradigm. *Top panel*: Experimental design. Each of the four squares subtended a visual angle of 1° × 1° with an opening of 0.33° on one side. Two squares were presented on each side of the fixation point. The centre of the squares nearest to the fixation point was 1.5° below and 3.5° to the left or the right of the fixation point. The centre of the farthest squares was 3° below and 5° to the left or right of the fixation point. The target square was presented equally often at each of the four possible positions (near left of fixation, near-right of fixation, far-left of fixation, far-right of fixation). The squares were in one of three different colours; blue, red, or green. The ERPs were evoked by manipulating the position of the opening of target squares, their colour, and the frequency of their occurrence. All these parameters were counterbalanced amongst participants such that the specific colours were not confounded with the various conditions in the experiment (the colours illustrated in Figure 1 represent the colour assignments for one of the many counterbalanced conditions). The intensity of the different colours of squares was calibrated to be equiluminant with a chroma meter (Minolta CS100) in order to control for low-level sensory responses. *Lower panel*: Stimuli. I. Frequent position of the square opening (standard stimulus), II. Infrequent position of the square opening (target stimulus), III. Infrequent colour of the target stimulus, IV. Same colour stimulus. Colour of different type of stimuli was counterbalanced among participants.

Epochs were baseline-corrected based on mean amplitude of activity recorded over a period of 200 ms prestimulus. Subtraction methods were used to isolate specific ERP components. The P3a wave was obtained by averaging waveforms associated with irrelevant infrequent trials and frequent standard trials separately, and then subtracting the frequent standard stimuli activity from the irrelevant infrequent target signal. The latency of the P3a on the Fz electrode site was calculated by measuring the most positive point recorded between 350–540 ms for all groups [41]. The mean amplitude of this component was also quantified over the same time frame. To isolate the P3b component, infrequent response trials and frequent response trials were averaged separately. Activity for frequent stimuli was subtracted from the averaged infrequent target signal. The time window that was then used to quantify the P3b mean amplitude was between 500–615 ms for all groups. The latency of this component was calculated by taking the most positive point recorded within this predefined time window on the Pz electrode site [42].

The N2pc and SPCN components were obtained by separately averaging trials with either right or left visual targets over 1000 ms epochs, including a 200 ms prestimulus baseline. These components were obtained by subtracting ipsilateral neural activity (recorded over the hemisphere on the same side as the stimulated visual field) from contralateral neural activity (recorded over the hemisphere on the opposing side of the stimulated visual field). For all groups, the mean amplitudes were computed in time windows between 245 and 265 ms for the N2pc, and 380–680 ms for the SPCN. Previous work has shown that such lateralized components reached maximum peak amplitudes at the P07 and P08 electrode sites [28,43].

Using the same methodology as that previously described to obtain the N2pc and the SPCN (subtracting ipsilateral neural activity from contralateral neural activity), we also obtained the Ptc (positivity toward temporal electrodes contralateral). The analyses were conducted on the P07-P08 electrodes and the time window analysis was defined between 290–320 ms for all groups. The N2pc-Ptc peak-to-peak amplitude was calculated as a measure of spatiotemporal attentional efficiency.

P1, N1, and P2 waveform analyses were conducted on the Oz electrode site, between 80–90 ms, 140–170 ms, and 215–225 ms, respectively, for all groups.

For each component, maximal mean amplitude was measured in the indicated time window for each peak based on the grand average waveform. The latency was estimated using a semi-automatic peak detection function in the Brain Vision Analyzer program (Brain Products GmbH, Gilching, Germany). The indicated time windows set around the peak of the components and visual inspection assured that the peak detected corresponded with the maximal point of the component.

2.3. Statistical Analysis

Descriptive statistics were used to analyse the latency and amplitude data of each ERP component, behavioural data from the ERP recordings task, and neuropsychological data. Analysis of variance (ANOVA) was subsequently used for hypothesis testing across the three groups.

3. Results

3.1. Neuropsychological Results

Mean scores were computed for each measure, for the three groups, and are shown in Table 1.

Table 1. Neuropsychological test results for the three groups.

Task	Controls Mean (SD)	Subacute mTBI Mean (SD)	Chronic mTBI Mean (SD)	F
PCS Number of symptoms	2.97 (2.78)	8.69 (5.75)	7.37 (5.37)	8.78 *
PCS Total score	5.16 (5.76)	21.62 (18.12)	19.67 (21.04)	6.57 *
BAI	4.57 (3.72)	8.04 (7.60)	7.94 (11.69)	0.25
BDI-II	5.36 (3.97)	11.94 (8.23)	10.41 (10.43)	4.09 *
Map Search 1 min (targets)	59.64 (13.91)	52.58 (12.28)	53.90 (14.93)	1.55
Map Search 2 min (targets)	77.06 (4.85)	74.84 (6.88)	75.60 (7.38)	1.04
Trail 1 (s)	16.59 (2.92)	19.42 (8.20)	18.35 (5.82)	1.19
Trail 2 (s)	27.37 (7.63)	33.94 (9.52)	34.47 (12.93)	3.17 *
Trail 3 (s)	25.94 (7.28)	33.57 (9.89)	30.88 (8.73)	4.14 *
Trail 4 (s)	57.95 (15.70)	75.50 (29.28)	68.71 (15.52)	3.62 *
Trail 5 (s)	23.82 (10.23)	35.79 (32.09)	31.65 (17.84)	1.62

* Significant at $p < 0.05$.

Scores on the PCS for number of symptoms reported and total symptom score were submitted to a between-groups ANOVA. Results showed significant differences across groups for both number of reported symptoms ($F(2,49) = 8.40$, $p = 0.001$, $\eta^2 = 0.23$) and total symptom score ($F(2,49) = 6.61$, $p = 0.003$, $\eta^2 = 0.19$). Post hoc analysis showed that subacute and chronic mTBI groups reported more symptoms than controls (number of symptoms: $p < 0.05$; total score: $p < 0.05$). There was no significant difference between subacute and chronic mTBI (number of symptoms and total score: $p > 0.05$).

Analyses for the BAI and BDI-II were conducted on the total score for each group. There were no significant group differences for anxiety scores on the BAI ($F(2,55) = 1.41$, $p = 0.25$). There was a significant difference for depression scores on the BDI-II ($F(2,55) = 4.10$, $p = 0.02$, $\eta^2 = 0.13$), with post hoc analysis showing that the subacute mTBI group reported higher levels of depressive symptoms than the control group ($p < 0.03$), although not reaching the clinical criteria for depression (Beck, Sterr, and Garbin, 1988).

TEA Map Search analyses were conducted on the 1 min and 2 min conditions. There were no significant between-group differences for these two conditions (1 min: $F(2,55) = 1.55$, $p = 0.22$), 2 min: $F(2,55) = 1.04$, $p = 0.36$).

The D-KEFS Trails (conditions 1 to 5) analyses showed significant between group differences for Trail 2 (number sequencing) ($F(2,55) = 3.17$, $p = 0.05$, $\eta^2 = 0.10$), Trail 3 (letter sequencing) ($F(2,55) = 4.14$, $p = 0.02$, $\eta^2 = 0.13$) and Trail 4 (number-letter sequencing, switching condition) ($F(2,55) = 3.62$, $p = 0.03$, $\eta^2 = 0.12$). There were no between-group differences for Trail 1 (detection condition) ($F(2,55) = 1.2$, $p > 0.31$) or Trail 5 (motor control condition) ($F(2,55) = 1.62$, $p = 0.21$). Also, the three groups had equivalent number of errors ($F(2,55) = 0.21$, $p = 0.82$). Post hoc analyses showed that subacute mTBI participants had slower completion times than the control group for Trail 2 ($p < 0.09$), Trail 3 ($p < 0.02$) and Trail 4 ($p < 0.03$).

3.2. Task Performance

Mean percentage of accuracy was computed for each condition (same colour trials, infrequent position or colour, frequent position or colour, right hemifield, left hemifield), for the three groups. The first 400 trials were included in the analysis in order to eliminate possible practice and fatigue effects. Mean percentage of accuracy in the visuospatial attention task for each condition and for all groups are presented in Table 2. Results show that control as well as mTBI participants showed valid and reproducible behavioural data on the task. Groups were equivalent on all the conditions of the task ($F_s < 1$).

Table 2. Accuracy (percent) for each task condition, for the three groups.

Task Condition	Controls Mean (SD)	Subacute mTBI Mean (SD)	Chronic mTBI Mean (SD)
Same colour	96.3 (4.8)	95.7 (9.7)	92.8 (23.6)
Infrequent target position	90.3 (6.0)	83.1 (19.9)	90.2 (9.2)
Frequent target position	96.3 (4.3)	94.6 (4.3)	95.4 (5.7)
Infrequent target colour	95.8 (3.5)	89.7 (9.6)	90.3 (13.6)
Frequent target colour	94.6 (5.1)	92.3 (6.5)	95.1 (4.9)
Right	95.1 (3.7)	91.7 (7.4)	93.3 (7.2)
Left	94.5 (4.8)	91.8 (7.1)	94.9 (4.4)

Mean reaction times for correct responses were computed for each condition (same colour trials, infrequent position or colour, frequent position or colour, right hemifield, left hemifield), for each group. Results are presented in Table 3. For all individual conditions tested, there was a significant between group difference on mean reaction times ($F_s(2,55) \geq 3.7$, $p_s < 0.05$), where subacute mTBI participants were slower than controls ($p < 0.05$).

Table 3. Reaction time (ms) for each task condition, for correct trials, for the three groups.

Task Condition	Controls Mean (SD)	Subacute mTBI Mean (SD)	Chronic mTBI Mean (SD)
Same colour	No-go trial	No-go trial	No-go trial
Infrequent target position	769 (122)	876 (150)	801 (99)
Frequent target position	754 (129)	832 (143)	776 (138)
Infrequent target colour	778 (114)	878 (164)	830 (155)
Frequent target colour	752 (132)	832 (141)	771 (115)
Right	746 (123)	839 (144)	782 (137)
Left	769 (131)	842 (141)	781 (110)

3.3. Electrophysiological Results

Results showed no significant amplitude or latency differences between groups for P1 ($F(2,55) = 1.737$, $p = 0.186$; $F(2,55) = 0.679$, $p = 0.52$) and N1 components ($F(2,55) = 0.232$, $p = 0.79$; $F(2,55) = 0.605$, $p = 0.55$). Although it did not reach the significance level, there was a tendency toward a larger P2 amplitude in controls ($F(2,55) = 2.783$, $p = 0.07$). The were no significant latency differences for the P2 component ($F(2,55) = 2.312$, $p = 0.11$) (see Figure 2).

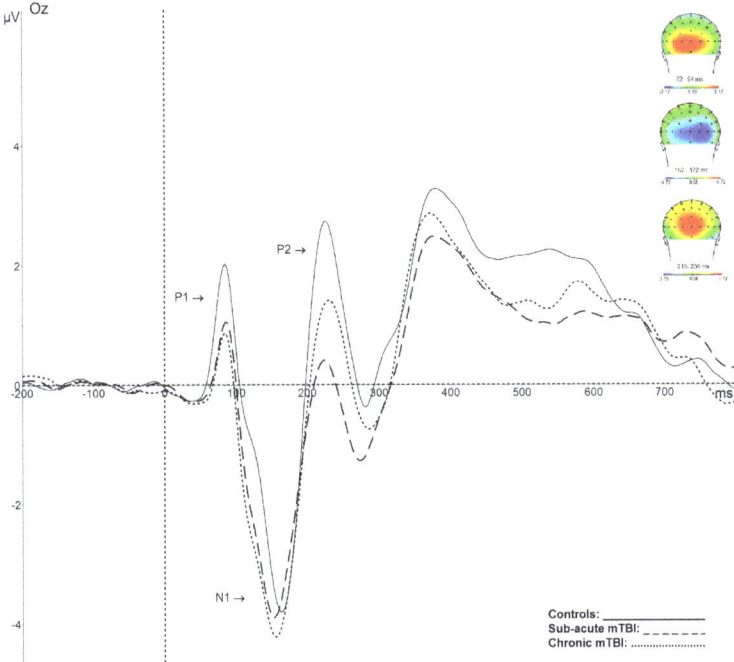

Figure 2. Grand average waveforms at Oz showing the visual P1, N1, and P2 components, and corresponding topographical maps, for controls (plain line), subacute mTBI (dashed line), and chronic mTBI (dotted line) participants. There is a tendency towards a larger P2 amplitude in controls.

N2pc results show that there were no significant differences between groups for the amplitude of the N2pc ($F(2,55) = 0.960$, $p = 0.39$), nor for its latency ($F(2,55) = 1.368$, $p = 0.26$) (see Figure 3). The same was found for the amplitude of the Ptc component ($F(2,55) = 1.07$, $p = 0.35$), and its latency ($F(2,55) = 2.616$, $p = 0.08$). When comparing peak-to-peak amplitude shifts from the N2pc to the next-positive peak, the Ptc, the result was significant ($F(2,55) = 4.25$, $p = 0.02$, $\eta^2 = 0.13$), with a smaller amplitude shift between these components for subacute mTBI participants compared to controls ($p < 0.05$). Figure 3 also depicts averaged SPCN waveforms obtained on pooled electrodes PO7-PO8. There were no significant between-group differences for SPCN amplitude ($F(2,55) = 0.7$, $p = 0.5$).

There were significant differences between groups for the amplitude of the P3a ($F(2,55) = 5.571$, $p = 0.01$, $\eta^2 = 0.17$). Post hoc analysis showed that P3a was significantly larger for mTBI groups (subacute and chronic compared to controls: $p < 0.05$). There were no significant differences between groups for P3a latency ($F(2,55) = 1.483$, $p = 0.24$) (see Figure 4).

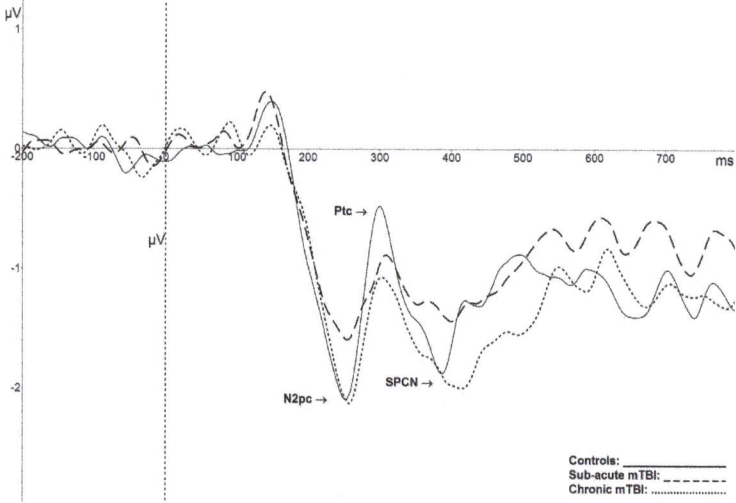

Figure 3. Grand average N2pc, Ptc, and SPCN components, evoked by lateralized stimuli, recorded at P07-P08 for controls (plain line), subacute mTBI (dashed line), and chronic mTBI (dotted line) groups. The N2pc-Ptc peak-to-peak amplitude shift is significantly smaller in the subacute mTBI group than in controls.

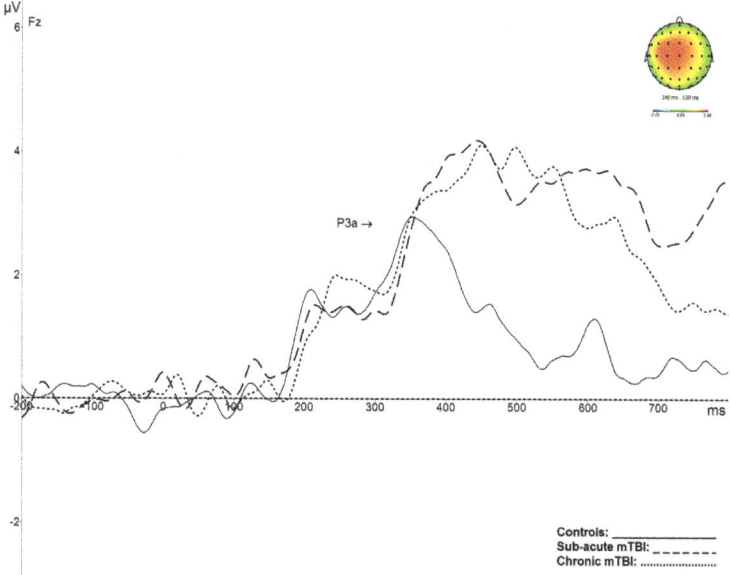

Figure 4. Average P3a components, obtained after the subtraction of activity evoked by same colour target and frequent colour standard stimuli, recorded at Fz, and corresponding topographical maps. The amplitude of the P3a component is significantly enhanced for subacute mTBI (dashed line) and chronic mTBI (dotted line) participants, in comparison with controls (plain line).

P3b results are shown in Figure 5. P3b amplitude was significantly smaller in both groups of mTBI participants ($p < 0.05$) relative to control participants ($F(2,55) = 7.214$, $p < 0.002$, $\eta^2 = 0.21$).

The latency of the P3b was also significantly delayed in the mTBI groups ($p < 0.05$) compared to controls ($F(2,55) = 7.839, p < 0.001, \eta^2 = 0.22$).

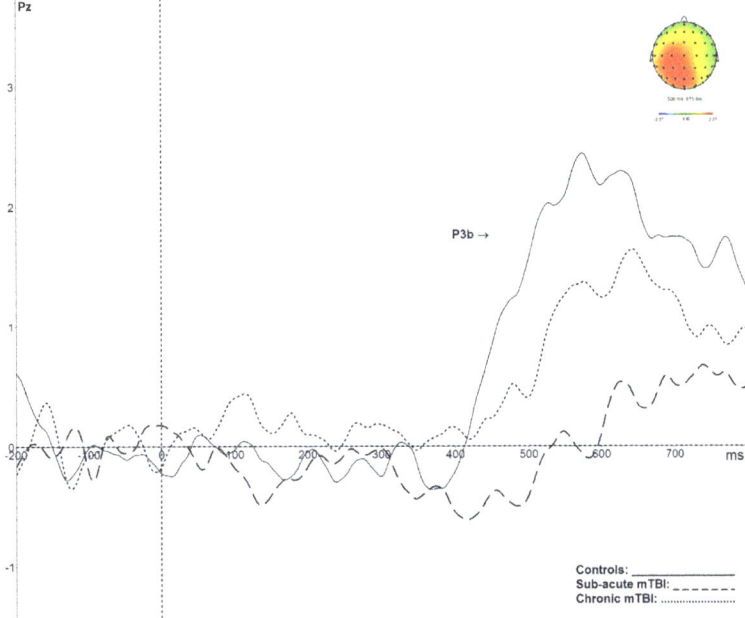

Figure 5. Grand average P3b components, obtained after the subtraction of activity evoked by infrequent position target stimuli and frequent position standard stimuli, recorded at Pz, and corresponding topographical maps. The P3b is significantly reduced and delayed in the subacute mTBI group (dashed line) and reduced in the chronic mTBI group (dotted line) in comparison with controls (plain line).

4. Discussion

The electrophysiological paradigm implemented in the present study allowed us to measure several visuoperceptual and cognitive functions in a single session, resulting in a detailed examination and in original findings regarding the possible functional consequences of mTBI.

First, this study agrees with previous results by showing that, after a mTBI, earlier visual potentials are comparable to data from uninjured control participants [22]. It is, however, worth mentioning that there was a strong tendency for P2 amplitude reduction in mTBI compared to controls. This could suggest early attentional modulation difficulties in the form of less efficient visual search following mTBI [44].

Neuropsychological testing is recognized as an important part of the evaluation and follow-up of possible sequalae caused by mTBI [45]. It is now well known that, while symptoms sometimes recover within the few days after an injury, cognitive deficits may persist for longer [46]. The results obtained in this study are in accordance with the literature demonstrating that neuropsychological measures can be sensitive after a mTBI, at least in the subacute phase. Participants tested in the first three months post-mTBI showed slower processing speed in a visual attention task. While their basic selective visual attention abilities (TEA Map search, DKEFS Trail 1) appeared intact, they were negatively affected on a condition requiring rapid visuospatial processing (DKEFS: Trails 2 and 3), as well as in a condition known to target attentional and cognitive flexibility (DKEFS: Trail 4).

The chronic mTBI participants in this study did not show significant neuropsychological deficits. This result is in accordance with the literature, which often failed to demonstrate long-term effects on clinical neuropsychological testing after a single mTBI [47]. However, studies using more sensitive neurocognitive tasks measuring information processing speed and working memory have been able to show persisting cognitive impacts following mTBI [17,48]. Also, some studies have shown some neuropsychological deficits after two or more mTBIs [49,50].

In this study, the electrophysiological paradigm used revealed several statistically significant impacts, with large effect sizes, on neurocognition following a single mTBI. Previous work has found decreased amplitudes and increased latencies of the P3b component after mTBI [20,22,49,51]. Our results replicate such a pattern, where participants who sustained a mTBI showed significantly decreased amplitudes and increased latencies on the P3b component. Animal models have suggested that these impacts could be explained by the fragility of the hippocampic cells and of their related brain circuits, which are involved in updating the stimulus representation within working memory during an oddball paradigm and are thus reflected in the P3b component [52].

Neurometabolic and microstructural changes taking place after a mTBI were thus evidenced using the present ERP paradigm and can explain the decrease in efficiency and speed of associated cognitive processes. Indeed, participants who sustained a mTBI and were tested during the subacute phase (less than three months post-trauma) did have slower response times than uninjured controls and individuals with chronic mTBI during the ERP task, as well as on the neuropsychological tests requiring deployment of visuospatial attentional and executive processes. Another indicator that these cognitive processes were impacted by mTBI and were not as efficient as those of uninjured control participants is the fact that, while neuropsychological measures in the chronic mTBI group were comparable to those of the control group, P3b results showed persisting amplitude attenuation, even six months postinjury. This finding is in accordance with studies reporting the longer-term impact of mTBI on the P3b [21]. While the study of de Beaumont and al. [21] showed this type of result after multiple concussions, the present study demonstrates that such impairments can occur after a single mTBI.

Based on a study published by Halterman et al. [12], we assumed that orienting visuospatial attention would be affected in the subacute phase after mTBI. Indeed, they showed that individuals with mTBI were slower than controls in an orientation task, especially on the executive components of the task. In our ERP task, the N2pc component reflects these mechanisms, more precisely the attentional filter that allows the orientation of attention toward the target. Results obtained in this study did not show a significant impact of mTBI on the N2pc, although, as shown in Figure 3, visual inspection of the component appears to indicate an amplitude reduction in mTBI compared to controls at a more acute stage. This result is consistent with a previous study by de Beaumont et al. [49], who found no significant effect on that component at nine months post-trauma in athletes who sustained multiple concussions. The N2pc is a component of relatively small amplitude (often less than 3 µV) obtained from a subtraction (contralateral minus ipsilateral), and thus the difference score has the combined variance of the contralateral and ipsilateral waves. It is possible that more participants could have allowed a significant difference to emerge. Indeed, even a small decrease in the amplitude of the N2pc could be clinically significant without being statistically significant. The same pattern of results was obtained with the SPCN, which represents the coding of visual information in visual short-term memory. As the N2pc, the SPCN is of very small amplitude, so at this point, it is not possible to exclude the possibility that this component could be affected by a mTBI in larger groups of participants.

Further observation of the results allows the identification of the latency shift between the N2pc and the following positivity Ptc peak, which significantly differs between the control and subacute mTBI groups. The Ptc component is thought to reflect the process used to isolate the target once it is identified among distractors [29]. The shorter N2pc-Ptc peak-to-peak amplitude shift in the subacute mTBI group is another aspect that points to a disruption in the spatiotemporal dynamics of attentional processes following mTBI. This mechanism appears to be affected in the subacute phase but seems to recover among chronic mTBI participants. Such a fluctuation in these spatiotemporal processes could have important implications, especially when clinicians contribute to return to play decisions for athletes. Indeed, contact sports rely heavily on visual-attentional abilities and require one to be alert and respond rapidly in order to avoid re-injury. Knowing that another mTBI within a short time frame could ultimately result in a second impact syndrome, causing massive brain swelling and sometimes death [53], returning an athlete to play before the recovery of such neurophysiological alterations could have major impacts on the health of the player.

While these mechanisms appear to recover within a few months after mTBI, the results of the P3b differ in the way that the amplitude decrease and latency increase shown for this component, as well as postconcussion symptoms, remain significantly present in the chronic stage of mTBI. The results obtained for the P3a also show a long-term impact on the orientation of attention. Indeed, it appears that the mTBI participants (both subacute and chronic) had difficulties in disengaging their attention (as reflected in a much larger and sustained amplitude) once it had been directed toward the target. Such a result was also obtained for the subacute mTBI group on the neuropsychological task tapping into this process (D-KEFS: trail 4). Indeed, it measures cognitive flexibility, a process that allows one to disengage attention to be able to switch between different stimuli. While this task was affected in mTBI in the subacute phase, P3a results show that this disengaging process was still impaired after more than six months postinjury. These original results, which are along the same line as others obtained with different methodologies [13,14,17], underscore the importance of carefully monitoring, with appropriate tools, individuals with mTBI who need to go back to activities that require maintaining high attentional levels or multitasking (e.g., operation of heavy machinery, contact sports, driving).

The main limitation of this study is the small number of participants in each group and the cross-sectional design. Indeed, we were confronted with different recruitment and participation retention issues because of the nature of this clinical population. Also, some of the participants had to be removed from the analyses because they showed too many artefacts on their EEG. Performance accuracy rates were, however, very high in all groups. Among the participants included in the analyses, we noticed a relatively high degree of inter- and intra-individual variability. Nonetheless, effect sizes for significant results were large.

Future studies with a greater number of subjects will help to determine the optimal conditions for clinical use of this paradigm. This is especially relevant as this new task allowed us to track the deployment of visuospatial attention as reflected in several ERP components, ultimately providing a rich possible set of biomarkers for mTBI. For example, in some individuals with mTBI, we were able to observe a clear decrease of the N2pc, with a normal P3b and SPCN. For other participants, the P3b was decreased, while the N2pc and the SPCN were normal. These specific patterns were lost in the averaging process required for ERP analyses. It appears that the clinical interest of this ERP task lies in the gathering of normative data that could bring to light these different individual clinical neurocognitive patterns of visual–attentional processing after a mTBI.

5. Conclusions

It thus appears that such a complete, sensitive and rigorous task [38] implemented at the diagnostic level can provide a clear and specific window into brain functions and connectivity, allowing the identification of multiple and complex alterations in attention following mTBI. This highlights the necessity of measuring various aspects of information processing before drawing an early conclusion of complete recovery on the basis of a single variable or of postconcussion symptomatology alone.

Author Contributions: Conceptualization, J.B.-T., P.J. and M.M.; Data curation, J.B.-T.; Formal analysis, J.B.-T., P.J. and M.M.; Funding acquisition, J.B.-T., P.J. and M.M.; Investigation, J.B.-T. and P.J.; Methodology, J.B.-T., P.J. and M.M.; Project administration, J.B.-T. and M.M.; Resources, P.J. and M.M.; Software, P.J. and M.M.; Supervision, P.J. and M.M.; Validation, P.J.; Visualization, J.B.-T. and P.J.; Writing—original draft, J.B.-T.; Writing—review and editing, P.J. and M.M.

Funding: This work was supported by the Canadian Institutes of Health Research (scholarship to J.B.-T.), by research funds (awarded to M.M.) from the Natural Sciences and Engineering Research Council (N.S.E.R.C.) of Canada and the Quebec Rehabilitation Research Network, and funding from the N.S.E.R.C., the Canada Foundation for Innovation and the Canada Research Chairs program awarded to P.J., and finally by infrastructure support to the Centre for Research in Neuropsychology and Cognition, and the Centre for Interdisciplinary Research in Rehabilitation from the Fonds de Recherche du Québec—Santé (F.R.Q.S.).

Acknowledgments: The authors wish to thank Elaine de Guise, Nicolas Robitaille, Christine Lefebvre, and Stéphane Denis for their help and support at various levels of this project.

Conflicts of Interest: The authors declare no conflict of interest.

References

1. Gaetz, M. The neurophysiology of brain injury. *Clin. Neurophysiol.* **2004**, *115*, 4–18. [CrossRef]
2. Giza, C.C.; Hovda, D.A. The neurometabolic cascade of concussion. *J. Athl. Train.* **2001**, *36*, 228–235. [CrossRef]
3. Rizzo, M.; Tranel, D. Overview of head injury and postconcussive syndrome. In *Head Injury and Postconcussive Syndrome*; Rizzo, M., Tranel, D., Eds.; Churchill Livingstone: New York, NY, USA, 1996.
4. Mathias, J.L.; Bigler, E.D.; Jones, N.R.; Bowden, S.C.; Barrett-Woodbridge, M.; Brown, G.C.; Taylor, D.J. Neuropsychological and information processing performance and its relationship to white matter changes following moderate and severe traumatic brain injury: A preliminary study. *Appl. Neuropsychol.* **2004**, *11*, 134–152. [CrossRef] [PubMed]
5. Henry, L.C.; Tremblay, S.; Boulanger, Y.; Ellemberg, D.; Lassonde, M. Neurometabolics changes in the acute phase after sports concussions correlate with symptoms severity. *J. Neurotrauma* **2010**, *27*, 65–76. [CrossRef]
6. Yeo, R.A.; Gasparovic, C.; Merideth, F.; Ruhl, D.; Doezema, D.; Mayer, A.R. A longitudinal proton magnetic resonance spectroscopy study of mild traumatic brain injury. *J. Neurotrauma* **2011**, *28*, 1–11. [CrossRef]
7. Beauchamp, M.H.; Ditchfield, M.; Babl, F.E.; Kean, M.; Catroppa, C.; Yeates, K.O.; Anderson, V. Detecting traumatic brain lesions in children: CT versus MRI versus susceptibility weighted imaging (SWI). *J. Neurotrauma* **2011**, *28*, 915–927. [CrossRef]
8. Wu, X.; Kirov, I.I.; Gonen, O.; Ge, Y.; Grossman, R.I.; Lui, Y.W. MR Imaging Applications in Mild Traumatic Brain Injury: An Imaging Update. *Radiology* **2016**, *279*, 693–707. [CrossRef]
9. Alexander, M.P. Mild traumatic brain injury: Pathophysiology, natural history, and clinical management. *Neurology* **1995**, *45*, 1253–1260. [CrossRef]
10. Katz, D.I.; Cohen, S.I.; Alexander, M.P. Mild Traumatic Brain Injury. *Handb. Clin. Neurol.* **2015**, *127*, 131–156.
11. Dikmen, S.; Machamer, J.; Fann, J.R.; Temkin, N.R. Rates of symptoms reporting following traumatic brain injury. *J. Int. Neuropsychol. Soc.* **2010**, *16*, 401–411. [CrossRef]
12. Halterman, C.I.; Langan, J.; Drew, A.; Rodriguez, E.; Osternig, L.R.; Chou, L.S.; van Donkelaar, P. Tracking the recovery of visuospatial attention deficits in mild traumatic brain injury. *Brain* **2006**, *129*, 747–753. [CrossRef] [PubMed]
13. Kwok, F.Y.; Lee, T.M.; Leung, C.H.; Poon, W.S. Changes of cognitive functioning following mild traumatic brain injury over a 3-month period. *Brain Inj.* **2008**, *22*, 740–751. [CrossRef] [PubMed]
14. Paré, N.; Rabin, L.A.; Fogel, J.; Pépin, M. Mild traumatic brain injury and its sequelae: Characterisation of divided attention deficits. *Neuropsychol. Rehabil.* **2009**, *19*, 110–137.
15. Echemendia, R.J.; Cantu, R.C. Return to play following sports-related mild traumatic brain injury: The role for neuropsychology. *Appl. Neuropsychol.* **2003**, *10*, 48–55. [CrossRef] [PubMed]
16. Vanderploeg, R.D.; Curtiss, G.; Belanger, H.G. Long-term neuropsychological outcomes following mild traumatic brain injury. *J. Int. Neuropsychol. Soc.* **2005**, *11*, 228–236. [CrossRef]
17. McInnes, K.; Friesen, C.L.; MacKenzie, D.E.; Westwood, D.A.; Boe, S.G. Mild Traumatic Brain Injury (mTBI) and chronic cognitive impairment: A scoping review. *PLoS ONE* **2017**, *12*, e0174847. [CrossRef]
18. Luck, S.J. *An Introduction to the Event-Related Potential Technique*; MIT Press: Cambridge, MA, USA, 2005.
19. Comerchero, M.D.; Polich, J. P3a and P3b from typical auditory and visual stimuli. *Clin. Neurophysiol.* **1999**, *11*, 24–30. [CrossRef]
20. Broglio, S.P.; Moore, R.D.; Hillman, C.H. A history of sport-related concussion on event-related brain potentials correlates of cognition. *Int. J. Psychophysiol.* **2011**, *82*, 16–23. [CrossRef]
21. De Beaumont, L.; Théoret, H.; Mongeon, D.; Messier, J.; Leclerc, S.; Tremblay, S.; Ellemberg, D.; Lassonde, M. Brain function decline in healthy retired athletes who sustained their last concussion in early adulthood. *Brain* **2009**, *132*, 695–708. [CrossRef]
22. Lachapelle, J.; Bolduc-Teasdale, J.; Ptito, A.; McKerral, M. Deficits in complex visual information processing after mild TBI: Electrophysiological markers and vocational outcome prognosis. *Brain Inj.* **2008**, *22*, 265–274. [CrossRef]

23. Gosselin, N.; Bottari, C.; Chen, J.K.; Huntgeburth, S.C.; de Beaumont, L.; Petrides, M.; Cheung, B.; Ptito, A. Evaluating the cognitive consequences of mild traumatic brain injury and concussion by using electrophysiology. *Neurosurg. Focus* **2012**, *33*, 1–7. [CrossRef]
24. Rapp, P.E.; Keyser, D.O.; Albano, A.; Hernandez, R.; Gibson, D.B.; Zambon, R.A.; Hairston, W.D.; Hughes, J.D.; Krystal, A.; Nichols, A.S. Traumatic brain injury detection using electrophysiological methods. *Front. Hum. Neurosci.* **2015**, *9*, 11. [CrossRef] [PubMed]
25. Brisson, B.; Jolicoeur, P. A psychological refractory period in access to visual short-term memory and the deployment of visual-spatial attention: Multitasking processing deficits revealed by event-related potentials. *Psychophysiology* **2007**, *44*, 323–333. [CrossRef] [PubMed]
26. Vogel, E.K.; Luck, S.J. The visual N1 component as an index of a discrimination process. *Psychophysiology* **2000**, *37*, 190–203. [CrossRef]
27. Luck, S.J.; Heinze, H.J.; Mangun, G.R.; Hillyard, S.A. Visual event-related potentials index focused attention within bilateral stimulus arrays. II. Functional dissociation of P1 and N1 components. *Electroencephalogr. Clin. Neurophysiol.* **1990**, *75*, 528–542. [CrossRef]
28. Luck, S.J.; Hillyard, S.A. Spatial filtering during visual search: Evidence from human electrophysiology. *J. Exp. Psychol. Hum. Percept. Perform.* **1994**, *20*, 1000–1014. [CrossRef]
29. Hilimire, M.R.; Mounts, J.R.W.; Parks, N.A.; Corballis, P.M.H. Event-Related Potentials Dissociate Effects of Salience and Space in Biased Competition for Visual Representation. *PLoS ONE* **2010**, *5*, e12677. [CrossRef]
30. Vogel, E.K.; Machizawa, M.G. Neural activity predicts individual differences in visual working memory capacity. *Nature* **2004**, *428*, 748–751. [CrossRef]
31. Arlinghaus, K.A.; Shoaib, A.M.; Price, T.R.P. Neuropsychiatric assessment. In *Textbook of Traumatic Brain Injury*; Silver, J., McAllister, T.W., Yudofsky, S., Eds.; American Psychiatric Publishing: Washington, DC, USA, 2007; pp. 59–78.
32. Hagen, G.F.; Gatherwright, J.R.; Lopez, B.A.; Polich, J. P3a from visual stimuli: Task difficulty effects. *Int. J. Psychophysiol.* **2006**, *59*, 8–14. [CrossRef]
33. Lovell, M.R.; Iverson, G.L.; Collins, M.W.; Podell, K.; Johnston, K.M.; Pardini, D.; Pardini, J.; Norwig, J.; Maroon, J.C. Measurement of Symptoms Following Sports-Related Concussion: Reliability and Normative Data for the Post-Concussion Scale. *Appl. Neuropsychol.* **2006**, *13*, 166–174. [CrossRef]
34. Beck, A.T.; Epstein, N.; Brown, G.; Steer, R.A. An inventory for measuring clinical anxiety: Psychometric properties. *J. Consult. Clin. Psychol.* **1988**, *56*, 893–897. [CrossRef] [PubMed]
35. Beck, A.T.; Steer, R.A.; Brown, G.K. *Manual for the Beck Depression Inventory-II*; Psychological Corporation: San Antonio, TX, USA, 1996.
36. Robertson, I.H.; Ward, T.; Ridgeway, V.; Nimmo-Smith, I. The structure of normal human attention: The test of everyday attention. *J. Int. Neuropsychol. Soc.* **1996**, *2*, 525–534. [CrossRef] [PubMed]
37. Delis, D.C.; Kramer, J.H.; Kaplan, E.; Holdnack, J. Reliability and validity of the Delis-Kaplan Executive Function System: An Update. *J. Int. Neuropsychol. Soc.* **2004**, *10*, 301–303. [CrossRef] [PubMed]
38. Bolduc Teasdale, J.; Jolicoeur, P.; McKerral, M. Multiple electrophysiological markers of visual attentional processing in a novel task directed toward clinical use. *J. Ophthalmol.* **2012**, *2012*, 618654. [CrossRef] [PubMed]
39. Donchin, E. Surprise! Surprise? *Psychophysiology* **1981**, *18*, 493–513. [CrossRef] [PubMed]
40. Luck, S.J.; Girelli, M.; McDermott, M.T.; Ford, M.A. Bridging the gap between monkey neurophysiology and human perception: An ambiguity resolution theory of visual selective attention. *Cogn. Psychol.* **1997**, *33*, 64–87. [CrossRef]
41. Polich, J. Neuropsychology of P3a and P3b: A theoretical Overview. In *Brainwaves and Mind: Recent Developments*; Moore, N.C., Arikan, K., Eds.; Kjellberg Inc.: Wheaton, IL, USA, 2004.
42. Sessa, P.; Luria, R.; Verleger, R.; Dell'Acqua, R. P3 latency shifts in the attentional blink: Further evidence for second target processing postponement. *Brain Res.* **2007**, *1137*, 131–139. [CrossRef]
43. Brisson, B.; Jolicoeur, P. Cross-modal multitasking processing deficits prior to the central bottleneck revealed by event-related potentials. *Neuropsychologia* **2007**, *45*, 3038–3053. [CrossRef]
44. Qian, C.; Al-Aidroos, N.; West, G.; Abrams, R.A.; Pratt, J. The visual P2 is attenuated for attended objects near the hands. *Cogn. Neurosci.* **2012**, *3*, 98–104. [CrossRef]

45. McCrory, P.; Meeuwisse, W.; Dvorak, J.; Aubry, M.; Bailes, J.; Broglio, S.; Cantu, R.C.; Cassidy, D.; Echemendia, R.J.; Castellani, R.J.; et al. Consensus statement on concussion in sport–the 5th international conference on concussion in sport held in Berlin, October 2016. *Br. J. Sports Med.* **2018**, *51*, 838–847.
46. Vagnozzi, R.; Signoretti, S.; Cristofori, L.; Alessandrini, F.; Floris, R.; Isgro, E.; Ria, A.; Marziale, S.; Zoccatelli, G.; Tavazzi, B.; et al. Assessment of metabolic brain damage and recovery following mild traumatic brain injury: A multicentre, proton magnetic resonance spectroscopic study in concussed patients. *Brain* **2010**, *133*, 3232–3234. [CrossRef] [PubMed]
47. Lange, R.T.; Brickell, T.A.; French, L.M.; Merritt, V.C.; Bhagwat, A.; Pancholi, S.; Iverson, G.L. Neuropsychological outcome from uncomplicated mild, complicated mild and moderate traumatic brain injury in US military personnel. *Arch. Clin. Neuropsychol.* **2012**, *27*, 480–494. [CrossRef] [PubMed]
48. Dean, P.; Sterr, A. Long-term effects of mild traumatic brain injury on cognitive performance. *Front. Hum. Neurosci.* **2013**, *7*, 30. [CrossRef] [PubMed]
49. De Beaumont, L.; Brisson, B.; Lassonde, M.; Jolicoeur, P. Long-term electrophysiological changes in athletes with a history of multiple concussions. *Brain Inj.* **2007**, *21*, 631–644. [CrossRef] [PubMed]
50. Thériault, M.; de Beaumont, L.; Tremblay, S.; Lassonde, M.; Jolicoeur, P. Cumulative effects of concussions in athletes revealed by electrophysiological abnormalities on visual working memory. *J. Clin. Exp. Neuropsychol.* **2011**, *33*, 30–41. [CrossRef] [PubMed]
51. Thériault, M.; de Beaumont, L.; Gosselin, N.; Filipinni, M.; Lassonde, M. Electrophysiological abnormalities in well functioning multiple concussed athletes. *Brain Inj.* **2009**, *23*, 899–906. [CrossRef] [PubMed]
52. McAllister, T.W.; Sparling, M.B.; Flashman, L.A.; Guerin, S.J.; Mamourian, A.C.; Saykin, A.J. Differential working memory load effects after mild traumatic brain injury. *Neuroimage* **2001**, *14*, 1004–1012. [CrossRef]
53. McCrory, P.; Davis, G.; Makdissi, M. Second impact syndrome or cerebral swelling after sporting head injury. *Curr. Sports Med. Rep.* **2012**, *11*, 21–23. [CrossRef]

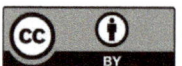

© 2019 by the authors. Licensee MDPI, Basel, Switzerland. This article is an open access article distributed under the terms and conditions of the Creative Commons Attribution (CC BY) license (http://creativecommons.org/licenses/by/4.0/).

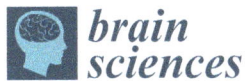

Article

Evaluating Preschool Visual Attentional Selective-Set: Preliminary ERP Modeling and Simulation of Target Enhancement Homology

Amedeo D'Angiulli [1,2,*], Dao Anh Thu Pham [2,3], Gerry Leisman [4] and Gary Goldfield [5,6]

1. Department of Neuroscience, Carleton University, Ottawa, ON K1S 5B6, Canada
2. Neuroscience of Imagination, Cognition & Emotion Research (NICER) Lab, Carleton University, Ottawa, ON K1S 5B6, Canada; DaoAnhThuPham@cmail.carleton.ca
3. Department of Systems and Computer Engineering, Carleton University, Ottawa, ON K1S 5B6, Canada
4. Faculty of Social Welfare and Health Sciences, University of Haifa, Haifa 3498838, Israel; g.leisman@edu.haifa.ac.il
5. Department of Pediatrics, University of Ottawa, Ottawa, ON K1N 6N5, Canada; ggoldfield@cheo.on.ca
6. Children's Hospital of Eastern Ontario, Ottawa, ON K1H 5B2, Canada
* Correspondence: amedeo.dangiulli@carleton.ca

Received: 29 December 2019; Accepted: 19 February 2020; Published: 22 February 2020

Abstract: We reanalyzed, modeled and simulated Event-Related Potential (ERP) data from 13 healthy children (Mean age = 5.12, Standard Deviation = 0.75) during a computerized visual sustained target detection task. Extending an ERP-based ACT–R (Adaptive Control of Thought–Rational) neurocognitive modeling approach, we tested whether visual sustained selective-set attention in preschool children involves the enhancement of neural response to targets, and it shows key adult-like features (neurofunctional homology). Blinded automatic peaks analysis was conducted on vincentized binned grand ERP averages. Time-course and distribution of scalp activity were detailed through topographic mapping and paths analysis. Reaction times and accuracy were also measured. Adult Magnetic Resonance Imaging-based mapping using ACT–R dipole source modeling and electric-field spiking simulation provided very good fit with the actual ERP data ($R^2 > 0.70$). In most electrodes, between 50 and 400 ms, ERPs concurrent with target presentation were enhanced relative to distractor, without manual response confounds. Triangulation of peak analysis, ACT–R modeling and simulation for the entire ERP epochs up to the moment of manual response (~700 ms, on average) suggested converging evidence of distinct but interacting processes of enhancement and planning for response release/inhibition, respectively. The latter involved functions and structures consistent with adult ERP activity which might correspond to a large-scale network, implicating Dorsal and Ventral Attentional Networks, corticostriatal loops, and subcortical hubs connected to prefrontal cortex top-down working memory executive control. Although preliminary, the present approach suggests novel directions for further tests and falsifiable hypotheses on the origins and development of visual selective attention and their ERP correlates.

Keywords: event-related potentials; visual sustained selective attention; voluntary control; self-regulation; executive functions; preschool children; ACT–R; Dipole analysis; spiking simulation

1. Introduction

Relative to goal-directed actions (manifested with behavioral responses), *selective-set* (as defined by Kahneman and Triesman [1]) is a mechanism of selective attention which underlies the ability of detecting task-relevant target information while ignoring (temporally simultaneous or separate) irrelevant information within a sequence of stimuli [1]. In many variations of the selective-set paradigm, speed and accuracy of behavioral response generally improve with age (for review see [2]), and one consistently replicated finding is a sharp developmental transition observed in children between 3 and 5 years of age—he developmental period usually known as "preschool". This transition is often implied as a critical period for detailing neurofunctional mapping [3,4], and for understanding typical and atypical development of executive attention during the lifespan [5].

The preschool transition has also been reported in studies in which event-related potentials (ERPs) were measured concurrently with different variants of the selective-set paradigm. An important component of selective-set detection is *response inhibition*, which has been studied in the laboratory by using deviant target detection tasks such as the go/no-go task, continuous performance task (CPT) and the stop-signal task [4–6]. Specifically, in ERP studies, predominantly in the auditory modality, larger amplitudes of the N2 with (200–300 ms) component have been found for successful responses to no-go trials compared to go trials, which are similar to those found in adults [6–8]. However, the N2 component of young children is usually observed between 250 and 500 ms after stimulus onset [9,10] and the no-go N2 effect is larger and more widely distributed across the fronto-parietal electrodes [9,11]. Similar findings in both morphology and latency differences have been reported for other visual processing and visual search tasks [12,13] and in a body of converging findings on error monitoring during visual go/no-go tasks related to error positivity (Pe) and negativity (ERN) components [14–16].

To date, Ridderinkhof and van der Stelt [17] conducted the most exhaustive review (including reviews of older studies) of adult and children's ERP data, which shows that signatures such as the N200 and P300-like (especially the P3b component) were reported in experiments using deviant target detection paradigms such as visual oddball tasks. Importantly, these studies included small convenience samples of 5–6 year-old children (sometimes in groups of broader age ranges, i.e., 4–7 year-olds). Late negative Nc (410 ms) and positive Pc (900 ms) waves (see [18]) as well as Slow Waves were observed in the young participants, and further in conditions where targets were novel stimuli. During the preschool and kindergarten years, the timing of the P300 is significantly slower, peaking on average around 700 ms and ranging between about 600 and 900 ms. Both children and young adults show greater P3 amplitudes to target, attended stimuli relative to non-target, unattended stimuli, and their topographical organizations are qualitatively similar in distribution across posterior electrodes [18].

Based on a modeling analysis of the reviewed studies, Ridderinkhof and Van der Stelt [17] concluded that attentional selective-set is essentially "adult-like" in preschool children, but the age differences in ERP wave morphology and latency may indicate that processing speed and efficiency undergo developmental improvement. Thus, their conclusion implies a form of developmental homology, i.e., an equivalence of structure and functions at two different developmental moments [19]—preschool and adulthood—capturing some neurocognitive aspects of selective-set, but not others (such as, for instance, those related to the execution of response). How this correspondence may practically translate to specific neural mechanisms is still an open question.

According to an influential interpretation [20,21], preschool transition involves a shift from involuntary detection and response towards novelty, to voluntary control of attention and of response to target (including withholding response or attenuating distractors' interference, or inhibitory control, in favor of more appropriate target response). The shift to voluntary control is usually attributed to the relatively early development of response inhibition and linked with the functional maturation of the frontal system, which is assumed to reflect key changes in the connectivity of the prefrontal cortex (PFC) during the preschool period [22–24]. Indeed, the preschool period shows a dramatic maturation of axonal density and myelination of structures supporting visuomotor functions in the frontal-striatum and fronto-basal ganglia networks, and in the fast propagating fibers of the callosal connections of the motor corticospinal system [25–34].

Voluntary control of visual selective attention has been most recently defined as "top-down" driven (i.e., "regulated by the working memory central executive") neuronal activity, which is directed to selectively enhance relevant target information and attenuate potential distractors [35]. *Enhancement* is generally associated with larger neuronal and significantly higher electrophysiological activity (see review in [36]) or eye-movement activity [37] concurrent to targets as compared to distractors.

In the present study, we tested the twofold hypothesis that voluntary selective-set detection in preschool children may be associated specifically with enhancement of neural response to target (enhancement hypothesis). Furthermore, we tested the hypothesis that in preschool children this mechanism can be described by some of the similar features, structural and functional, which are attributed to adults (neurofunctional homology).

In the first and second part of the study, we reanalyzed and modeled ERP data from preschool children on a sustained visual detection task, specifically probing set-selection. We expected to find converging evidence that children's ERP activity concurrent with the target would generally show higher amplitudes, as compared to ERP activity concurrent with the distractor.

In the third part of the study, we extended an ERP-based neurocognitive modeling approach to test the extent to which: 1) The pattern and timing of the preschoolers' actual ERP responses to target and distractor could be explained by a simulated adult model of ERP activity (functional homology); and 2) the dipoles estimated from preschool children's ERP activity could approximate the adult spatiotemporal simulation of estimated ERP generators (structural homology).

For periods of the task examined here, the ERP correlates of the selective-set process were confounded with those of the execution of manual response. Nonetheless, by triangulating peak analysis, source dipole modeling, simulation, and spiking modeling, we sought to partition distinct temporal intervals in which we could discriminate with reasonable degree of probability the neural processes recruited predominantly for target enhancement from those recruited for the planning of release/inhibition of response.

2. Materials and Methods

2.1. Part 1: Reanalysis of Children's ERP Data

In the first part of this study, we reanalyzed ERP data collected from preschool children who were tested on an adapted computerized version of Akshomoff's visual sustained detection task [38]. First, using a binning-averaging technique (vincentization), we tested whether ERP amplitudes for targets could be characterized as enhanced activity compared to the ERP amplitudes for distractors. Data vincentization made sure these differences were parametrized; namely, they did not depend on phase or time delays between the two conditions' waveforms, and neither on other individual's distribution variations from the grand average distribution.

2.1.1. Participants

Participants were 13 children (9 males, mean age = 5.12, Standard Deviation = 0.75 years) after data additional three children were discarded due to excessive EEG artefacts or inadequate response accuracy level (<75%). Children were recruited as part of an optional follow up to a separate large epidemiological early childhood developmental study [39]. Children were screened with a computerized adapted version of the Peabody Picture Vocabulary Test (PPVT; [40]). Parents completed two standardized age-normed screening assessments: Behavior Rating Inventory of Executive Function®–Preschool Version (BRIEF®-P; [41]), and the Child Behaviour Checklist for Ages $1\frac{1}{2}$-5(CBCL/1.5-5; [42]). All children lived in the same neighborhood and came from middle to high socio-economic status families. Participants had normal or corrected to normal vision and had no known, auditory, sensory or cognitive deficits. All participants were typically developing children with no history of medication or referral to disability assessment or services, as ascertained from parental reports and the day care center records. Participants' scores on all screening measures were within norm.

2.1.2. Visual Sustained Selective-set Attention Task (VSSAT)

The VSSAT (see Figure 1) was originally selected because: (1) it was validated on samples of similar age and with similar background to the one we previously tested, affording direct comparisons;

(2) differently than in most of the typical versions of go/no go tasks, it involves a continuous stream of picture stimuli in short blocks, which allows to determine whether participants are continuously attentive to the target throughout the trial (on correct trials) or when participants cease to attend to the target (on incorrect trials); (3) relative to older subject groups preschoolers can perform it with similar accuracy and engagement levels but show delay in responding to targets, therefore, reaction time measures embedded in this task can be modelled so as to reliably differentiate between the processing stage of visual target selection and the processing stage of the initiation of response to target; (4) this computerized paradigm can be easily used in combination with EEG recording.

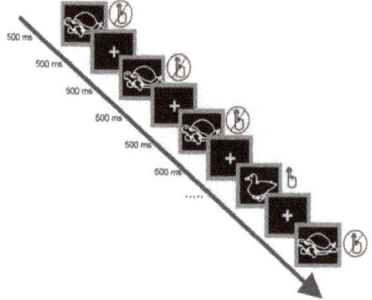

Figure 1. Stimulus presentation and time intervals of each trial in the Visual Sustained Selective-set Attention Task (VSSAT). Adapted from D'Angiulli and Devenyi (2019) [41].

Stimuli were presented through the Neuroscan Stim software program (Neuroscan, North Carolina, USA) and displayed on a 19″ flat screen monitor. Each trial in the VSSAT consisted of a white outline of a duck or a turtle presented in the center of the monitor on black background and remained on the screen for a duration of 500 ms, followed by a fixation cross for a duration of 500 ms (See Figure 2). Participants were instructed to press a button if the outline of a duck appeared and to refrain from pressing the button if any other image appeared.

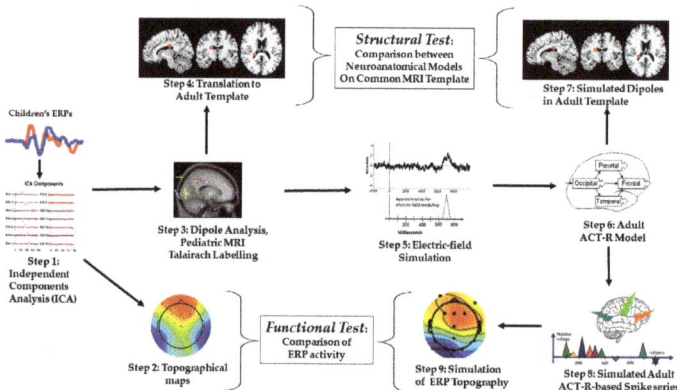

Figure 2. Process flow of the present study. Steps 1–4 describe modeling of actual children's data; Steps 3–9 describe adult simulations.

2.1.3. Procedure

Upon arrival at the research center, each child's active assent and signed parental consent was obtained according to protocols approved by the Research Ethics Boards of all participating institutions. Upon parental completion of the in-take assessments, children were tested in a sound-proof electromagnetically shielded EEG booth. Each child was seated at a distance of 58 cm from a 19″ flat screen monitor. Children were instructed to respond by pressing a button when they saw a duck and to refrain from pressing the button if they saw any other image.

The entire session consisted of several practice blocks followed by the experimental block. In each block, the duck was shown 25% of the time, while the turtle was shown 75% of the time. Participants proceeded to start the experiment once that they attained 100% accuracy on three consecutive practice blocks. In the experimental block, there were 37 target images and 113 distractor images for a total of 150 trials.

2.1.4. Data Collection and Processing

An elastic cap (Quik Cap, Neuroscan, El Paso, TX, USA) adhering to the standard ten–twenty international system of electrode placement, with recessed Ag–AgCl electrodes (10 mm each) was used for the EEG recordings. The cap montage included 12 electrodes corresponding to electrode reference points at Frontal (F3, Fz, F4), Central (Cz), Temporal (T7, T8), Parietal (P7, Pz, P8), and Occipital (O1, Oz, O2) sites. Horizontal and vertical electro-oculograms (EOG) recorded eye movements with two split bipolar electrodes positioned at the outer canthi for the horizontal EOG and on the suborbital ridge of each eye for the vertical EOG. Previous work and pilot studies in children of similar ages [43–47] suggest no critical loss of reliability in source analysis performed with the present set up.

All impedances were kept below 5 kOhms. Low-pass and high-pass filtering (0.5 to 250 Hz) were applied to the signal prior to digitization. Trials from non-ocular electrode sites that were contaminated by excessive peak-to-peak deflection (i.e., >100 μV or <−100 μV) due to non-stereotypical noise were manually excluded. Brain Electric Source Analysis (BESA v.5.4.28; http://www.besa.de/), an electroencephalographic analysis software package was used to analyze EEG recordings and calculate ERP averages for each of the twelve electrode locations (F3, Fz, F4, Cz, T7, T8, P7, Pz, P8, O1, Oz, O2). Ocular correction was performed using the integrated BESA *adaptive artifact correction* [48] and the *surrogate model* [49]. Principal component analysis decomposition was used to correct for ocular artefacts by selecting components for the horizontal and vertical eye movements as well as eye-blinks. The proportion of rejected trials was less than 15% after artefact correction and removal. ERPs were averaged offline separately for each stimulus type (i.e., target and distractor) at each electrode with all epochs time-locked to the onset of the image and ending at 1000 ms after the onset of the image.

2.1.5. ERP Data Analysis

One known issue in customary peak analysis techniques is that the assumed correspondences are based on subjective selections of time windows which are made post hoc, after examining the data [50]; this issue is exacerbated when young children are compared to adults since analyses often rely on many untested a-priori assumptions on alleged morphological correspondences between peaks of ERPs of young children and the adults. An alternative is to standardize time windows by latency and to examine the entire single ERP waveform across the entire epoch by using automatic blinded analysis procedures such as *waveform binning* [40,51–53]. We adopted a hybrid approach in which automatic blinded binning includes traditional peak analysis.

EEGLab [54] was used to analyze EEG recordings and calculate ERP averages for each data point for the twelve electrode locations (F3, Fz, F4, Cz, T7, T8, P7, Pz, P8, O1, Oz, O2). ERPs were averaged offline separately for each stimulus type (i.e., targets and distractors). Each epoch ranged from 200 ms prior to the presentation of the image to 1000 ms preceding the presentation of the image.

EEG sampling rate was 1000 Hz, resulting in a total of 1200 data points for each epoch. Time interval analysis of data points obtained from ERP data were simplified using a standard binning procedure that divided each epoch into bins of equal time intervals. Each epoch was divided into twelve bins of 100 ms time interval. To ensure equivalent data density across bins, the ERP averages across subjects were transformed to vincentized quantile bins [55–57]. The computation of the quantile bins was performed assuming the following empirical distribution for the time series of the averaged ERPs:

$$F_i^{-1}(\alpha) = inf\{-200 < t < +1000; F_i(t) \geq \alpha\}, \text{ with } 0 < \alpha < 1 \quad (1)$$

The Vincent average of the F_is mid-points was then computed as:

$$\sum w_i F_i^{-1}(\alpha), \text{ where } i = 1 \ldots n, \text{ and } w_1 + \ldots + w_n = 1 \quad (2)$$

Due to its shape-preservation property, this procedure minimizes the effects of distortions of individual differences in the distributions of averaged ERP peak mid-points, and given that the skewness in our data was modest, it partially offset biases in parametric testing associated with our relatively small sample size (see [57]). Amplitudes sorted within each bin for each epoch were assessed for each of the twelve electrode sites and averaged separately for target and distractor stimuli. To draw a comparison between ERPs for target and distractor stimuli over time, the number of bins for distractors was kept consistent with the target even though distractors did not require a response.

Vincentized amplitudes were analyzed in a mixed model design with interval bins (12 levels) as a between subjects factor and electrode (12 levels) and condition: (2 levels: target vs. distractor) as within subjects factors. To compare differences between target and distractor, focused ANOVA contrasts between mean amplitudes for each electrode and time interval were conducted to obtain the minimum significant standardized absolute difference using the following formula:

$$\text{Amp diff}_{\mu V} = t_{crit} \left(\sqrt{[\text{MSE}_{within}\Sigma(\lambda_i^2/n_j)]}\right) \quad (3)$$

where Abs Amp diff$_{\mu V}$ indicates the significant difference in amplitude peaks between target and distractor conditions for a given electrode within a given interval bin, t_{crit} represents the t-value corresponding to the critical p-value for determining significance threshold after using a Bonferroni correction for 12 electrodes for multiple comparisons. MSE$_{within}$ represents the error factor for focused t-contrasts across all comparisons. This was the within subjects Mean Square error for the interaction between electrode × condition from the omnibus ANOVA. λ_i represents the contrast weights [58].

2.1.6. ERP Activity Paths

The differences in ERP waveforms between target and distractor conditions can be more easily interpreted via ERP activity path analysis [40,53]. This graphic summary method illustrates the temporal sequence of neural activity between electrode regions while considering differences between target and distractor conditions.

To obtain activity paths, we used the following procedure. All significant average ERP differences for target and distractor conditions observed were compared. The electrode corresponding to the maximum average ERP difference between target and distractor conditions at each interval bin was noted and the brain area corresponding to this electrode was plotted on head maps for target or distractor conditions at each interval bin. If similar (non-significantly different) maximum average ERP differences were observed for two or three electrodes within the same interval bin, areas corresponding to both or all three electrodes were assumed to be simultaneously activated for that interval and were illustrated on the head map.

The principle of *neural wiring minimization* [59] was used as a rationale for plotting the least-path sequence between simultaneous ERP activity electrodes/areas within same interval bin. Accordingly, the following restrictions were applied due to neuroanatomical boundaries: neural activation from occipital electrodes (O1, Oz, O2) could only move forward or laterally, neural activation from frontal electrodes (F3, Fz, F4) could only move backward or laterally. Likewise, lateral activation from left electrodes (F3, T7, P7, O1) could only occur toward the right, whereas lateral activation from right electrodes (F4, T8, P8, O2) could only occur toward the left.

2.2. Part 2: Modeling of Children's ERP Data

In the second part of the study, we run a type of Independent Component Analysis (ICA; [60]) on which we built models of the children's data. Figure 2 describes the steps in the analysis pipeline. ICA (Step 1) was used to build ERP topographical mappings (Step 2), and then to identify the dipoles corresponding to target and distractor ERPs; this information was then mapped on a pediatric structural MRI template from the Talairach coordinate system (Step 3). Using corresponding neuroanatomical labels and a visual matching procedure, we confirmed and translated the pediatric Talairach coordinates into an adult structural MRI template (Step 4).

2.2.1. Independent Component Analysis (Step 1) and Topographic Mapping (Step 2)

A second Independent Component Analysis (ICA) was performed to identify ERP components using the EEGLab FASTICA algorithm [61]. While the ICA method can estimate location and timings of components, it cannot estimate an absolute magnitude for them since there is an inherent ambiguity between the strength of the component and the attenuation from it to the measurement point. Therefore, the results were converted to topographic maps.

EEGLab includes an editing graphic utility which allows to represent the epochs of averaged ERP onto topographic maps as clips of 10 ms, and then it permits to put these together in sequence resulting in a capture of time course of the dynamic ERP activity. The specific single topographic maps selected for further analysis reflected scalp activity at the mid-points of the time intervals corresponding with vincentized bins corresponding to those described in the ERP activity paths.

2.2.2. Dipole Analysis (Step 3)

The DIPFIT component of EEGLab was used to estimate a set of dipoles in the averaged ERP data that would explain the independent components extracted. Each dipole is assumed to be a region of cortex where several thousand neurons act together in parallel so that their combined electric field is responsible for the EEG signal measured at the scalp. The DIPFIT software usually finds one or sometimes two dipoles for each of the specific regions that appear to produce the independent components.

The EEGLab MRI-based spherical head model with standard age-appropriate (pediatric) Talairach coordinates was selected. The labels of the brain regions which the locations corresponded to were found using the most recently updated version of the Talairach database [62]. We used the built-in function of this software which permits searching for the nearest grey matter within concentric cubes (voxels) from a minimum of ±1 mm up to a maximum range within ±5 mm to exact dipole origin. That is, nearest gray searches involve concentric cube searches with varying diameters. In general, it searches consecutively larger cubes until it finds a gray matter label, with the same outer limit of a 11 mm-wide cube, so it is also possible to find no gray matter labels.

2.2.3. Translation to Adult MRI Template (Step 4)

The pediatric MRI coordinates obtained through the Talairach database [62] were converted to the Yale Bioimage Suite [63] by entering the pediatric coordinates and by matching the anatomical labels. This process was confirmed by visual analysis based on consensus among two independent anonymous judges with expertise in pediatric and adult neuroanatomy.

2.3. Part 3: Simulation of Adult ERP Data

In what follows, the descriptions of the components of the analysis pipeline for the third part of the study are organized according to the sequence of steps illustrated in Figure 1. From the information derived from the ICA (Step 1) and the estimated dipoles (Step 3), we derived simple single spiking representations adopting electric-fields estimation modeling (Step 5). Next, the results of Step 5 were used to implement an ERP-based Adaptive Control of Thought—Rational (ACT–R) modeling approach previously validated on the same task [43,44]. We organized the simulated dipoles and the simulated ERP spikes in patterns or chunks of activity corresponding to cortical areas postulated in the adult ACT–R (Step 6). The results of Step 6 allowed us to simulate the sequence of spatiotemporal activity as dipoles mapped onto the same adult structural MRI template as the children's data (Step 7). This was the basis for comparing children's and simulated adult estimated localization, therefore, testing for structural homology.

The results of Steps 6 and 7 were also used for aggregate series of simulated spikes to build polyspiking patterns for the simulated dipoles (Step 8). Finally, in Step 9, the simulated data obtained from Step 8 were converted to ERP topographic maps. This final step made possible to contrast children's and simulated ERP topographic mappings, therefore, testing for functional homology.

2.3.1. Electric-Field Spiking Modeling (Step 5)

To simulate the electrical activity, each module in the neurocognitive model was assumed to be generating one or two dipoles in the location identified in the dipole-fitting stage. The module was assumed to produce its electrical energy in a rising and falling spike. For modeling purposes, a simple triangular wave was assumed, which peaked at the center of the module. The resulting electric field (voltage) was then calculated at the surface of the head for each electrode as the sum of the individual dipole contributions. Elsewhere, we have shown that this method generates reliable, valid and consistent descriptions of actual ERP activity [43,44]. Since the spiking activities of the components occurred at different times in the observed data, it was not necessary to add the effects of more than one dipole at a given time.

The effect of each dipole was estimated in the simulation by following three steps (see Figure 3): (i) The square of the distance r from the dipole to an electrode was calculated by using Pythagoras. Next, (ii) the cosine of the angle θ between the electrode and the dipole was calculated by using vector dot product. Successively, (iii) the electric potential from the dipole at the electrode was derived from Coulomb's law ($=k.p.\cos(\theta)/r^2$), where p is the strength of the dipole and k is a constant. (It was not necessary to know the value of the constant since relative magnitudes were used in the model).

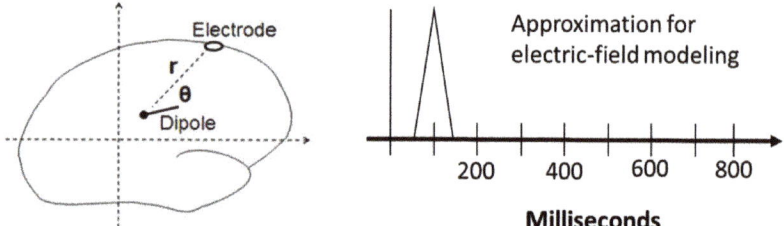

Figure 3. Schematic representation of the calculation of an electric dipole field spiking by simulation; the left panel shows the output of the calculated electric-field potential represented as a simplified spike at fixed timing (determined by the simulated production schedule, here shown at an arbitrary time point for example sake; for the actual simulated timings in the present study see the production schedule shown in Table 1).

Table 1. Simulated locations and predicted timing of spiking occurrence according to the present adapted Python ACT–R architecture.

Function	Brain Region	Time (ms)
Visual processing	Occipital	150
Spatial attention	Parietal	250
Declarative	Temporal	350
Executive	Frontal	450
Procedural	Basal ganglia	550
Manual	Parietal	650

Note: The timings shown in the table include the base constant and the increments from the 50-millisecond cognitive cycle (described in Section 2.3.2) and each of them represent the approximate estimated moment in which a given production process in the ACT–R model is completed.

2.3.2. ACT–R Simulation (Step 6)

To model and simulate our data, we used an adapted version of John R. Anderson's Adaptive (Control of Thought—Rational) ACT–R [64]. In the general architecture, cognition is considered to arise from the parallel interaction of several independent modules. However, top-down processes are directed by the Procedural Module, which is meant to model procedural memory. ACT–R models procedural memory as a production system. Specifically, procedural memory contains production rules (i.e., if/then rules). Communication to and from the Procedural Module is managed by buffers and chunks (see Figure 4). Chunks in ACT–R are lists of predicated information (for example, "duck" could be represented by the chunk: Is-an:animal, Name:duckling, Color:yellow, Size:small).

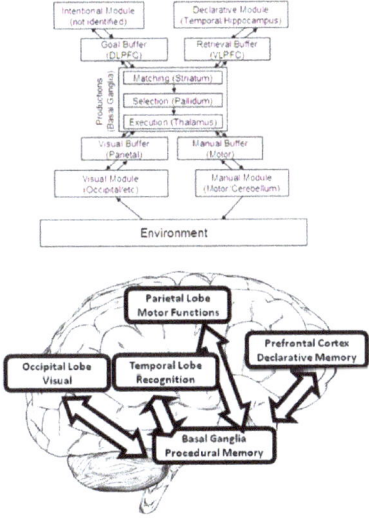

Figure 4. The organization of information in ACT–R (Adaptive Control of Thought–Rational). Adapted with permission from [42].

Each buffer can contain one chunk at a time. Each module has at least one buffer, so there is a visual buffer, a declarative memory buffer, and so on. Modules receive instructions from their buffers and place the results of their activity in their buffers. Collectively, the buffers can be thought of as working memory; they can also be thought of as representing the current context of the task. Productions "fire" when their "*if* condition" matches the contents of the buffers. The "*then*" part of a production then alters the content of the buffers. Productions can only fire one at a time.

In our version of ACT–R, the productions represent electric-field potentials. We programmed the simulation to fit the midpoint of the vincentized bins used to parametrize the ERP data series, so that each production was conditioned to occur at successive steps of approximately t_i + 50 ms, with i = 0, 100 ... , 600. The 50-millisecond cognitive cycle is assumed in many realistic modeling architectures besides ACT–R (for example, Soar, EPIC, GOMS, see [65] for discussion). The neurobiological plausibility of this 50-millisecond cycle has been demonstrated by spiking neural network models simulating well known time constants for the GABA-A receptors in the Basal Ganglia, which in ACT–R (and in various other architectures) is assumed to be responsible for the working memory central executive [66]. Therefore, in the practical implementation of the model we assumed a base production-completion time constant which corresponded to the size of the vincentized bins (100 ms) plus the 50-millisecond cycle constant. Each module contained functions (specifically, ex-gaussian convolutions) to determine activation levels during rest, during the task and the decay rate after firing. Effectively, these functions determined the spiking behavior associated with a given production: Faster productions corresponded to more intense and more quickly decaying spiking.

To implement the simulation, we adopted Python ACT–R [67]. In particular, the present version of the model assumed that the caudate in the basal ganglia acts as the central coordinator (executive) of productions. The hippocampus controls declarative memory while the cingulate cortex controls attention to conflicting stimuli. Frontal cortex supports declarative memory while visual processing takes place in the occipital with further processing in the parietal (see Figure 3). With the time constraints as shown in Table 1, we implemented an ACT–R model which predicted that initially the visual module (occipital) would be activated by the displayed pictures of the target (duck) and turtle (distractor) and would place a representation of the picture in the visual buffer (parietal). Next, the "parietal" representation would be used to retrieve the label of the object and the appropriate instruction about what to do in response to the image of that animal from declarative memory (temporal), which in turn would be placed in the planning buffer (frontal) and initiate the motor program for the manual response, or stop it (basal ganglia).

2.3.3. Adult ACT–R Simulated Dipole Mapping (Step 7)

As in the case of the actual children's dipoles, the ACT–R simulated dipole data was mapped on a standardized MRI template provided by the Yale Bioimage Suite Web [63].

2.3.4. Adult ACT–R Simulated Spike Series (Polyspiking) (Step 8)

In this step, the simulated electric-field spikes were chunked in ordered series corresponding respectively to the standard localizations and predicted timing of spiking assumed in the programmed schedule for the firing of ACT–R productions (see Table 1). The output of this step was a set of polyspiking patterns including a minimum of six spikes for each of the twelve electrodes. Within each pattern, the spike with maximal activation derived from the dipole of interest at a given bin interval, while all other spikes reflected resting or decaying background activations from the other dipoles. The latter configuration permitted to obtain *coarse coding* which could quantify the amplitude of each spike in the aggregated pattern as a color category (see example in Step 8, Figure 1) corresponding to a standard RGB value so that it could be ordered along an intensity scale.

2.3.5. Adult ACT–R Simulated ERP Topographical Mapping (Step 9)

The simulated topographical maps were obtained through the same utility of EEGLab as the one used for the actual ERP data. To feed the simulated data in a compatible format, the values of the color intensities corresponding to the polyspiking patterns were previously converted (in Stage 8) into an arbitrary relative voltage scale (with range from blue/black, −6 µV, to red/orange, 6 µV).

2.3.6. Actual vs. Simulated Data Comparisons: Homology Tests

MRI-mappings and Structural Test

To run the structural comparison, we first estimated the margin of localization error by computing the range differences based on the matches resulting from the search nearest grey area procedure; the measures were in millimeters. Successively, we computed z-scores of these ranges (henceforth called *z-Ranges*) which permitted to compare the extent of variations in localization in the actual children's data against those in the adult simulated estimations.

Topographical Mappings and Functional Test

ERP activity comparison between the actual children's topographic maps and the topographic maps derived from the simulated ERP activity were computed as linear regressions of vincentized averaged ERP amplitudes in the topographic map of children against the corresponding ACT–R simulated data; the fit was assessed by calculating the coefficient of determination, R^2.

3. Results

3.1. Behavioral Performance

Overall accuracy across all trials was high (Mean percent correct = 89.89%, Standard Error = 1.34%). Mean Hit proportion was 77.5%; mean False Alarm proportion was 6.07% ($d' = 2.31$; $c = 0.40$). Mean response time was 685 ms (SE = 35.64 ms). Age was positively correlated with accuracy ($r_{(13)} = 0.61$, $p < 0.05$) but not with response times.

3.2. ERP Data

Figure 5 shows overall average vincentized ERP waveforms (thick lines) and standard errors (thin lines) recorded over twelve electrode locations (F3, Fz, F4, Cz, T7, T8, P7, Pz, P8, O1, Oz, O2) from the time interval of 200 ms prior to onset of the image to 1000 ms after presentation of the image for both target (blue lines) and distractor (red lines) conditions.

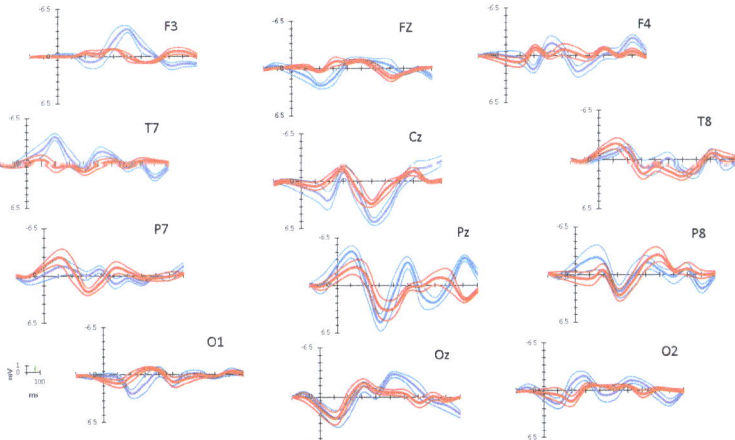

Figure 5. Average vincentized event-related potential (ERP) waveforms for targets (thick blue line) and distractors (thick red line) recorded over twelve electrode locations (F3, Fz, F4, Cz, T7, T8, P7, Pz, P8, O1, Oz, O2) for the epoch ranging from 200 ms prior to onset of each stimulus image to 1000 ms after the stimulus image. Standard errors are represented by thin lines. The microvolt value corresponding to the significance threshold is shown as a green line in scale against the y-axis in μV of observed ERP amplitude range at the bottom left legend.

For all electrodes, within most bin intervals, larger overall ERP peak amplitudes were observed for targets than for distractors. Significant differences in grand peak amplitudes were found (F (1,13068) = 160.124, $p < 0.01$; MSE = 0.468; $\eta^2 = 0.13$), with larger grand amplitudes for targets than distractors. In addition, there was also a three-way interaction between interval bins, electrodes and condition (F (12,13068) = 154.628, $p < 0.01$; MSE = 20.367; $\eta^2 = 0.13$).

Given the three-way interaction, to compare differences between target and distractor conditions across electrode locations and time intervals we then performed Focused ANOVA t-contrasts (see Section 2.1.5). The t-value corresponding to the critical p-value for determining significance threshold after using a Bonferroni correction was t_{crit} (12) = 5.69 ((MSE = 0.132); $p = 0.0001$ (two-tailed); $\eta^2 = 0.71$). Accordingly, the minimum significant amplitude difference between standard and distractor peak amplitudes was computed to be 0.80 µV. The significance threshold is shown in scale against the y-axis µV legend in Figure 5.

We also performed traditional peak analysis, which is presented in the Supplementary Materials. There were no substantial discrepancies between the two analyses.

Table 2 reports the differences of average peak ERP amplitudes in target and distractor conditions (peak amplitude target − peak amplitude distractor) within interval bins of 100 ms for all electrodes. This analysis focused only on bins capturing processes before motor responses, that is, up to the approximate time of the occurrence of manual response for most children (bins including data up to 700 ms) to exclude effects that might be attributed to motor responses (i.e., when participants responded to targets).

Table 2. Differences of average peak ERP amplitudes and corresponding latencies in target and distractor conditions (absolute value of (peak amplitude target − peak amplitude distractor)) within interval bins of 100 ms of epoch range (0 to 700 ms) for all electrodes.

	Interval Bins						
	(0–100 ms)	(101–200 ms)	(201–300 ms)	(301–400 ms)	(401–500 ms)	(501–600 ms)	(601–700 ms)
	Mean Differences in Peak Amplitudes (Target − Distractor) in µV						
	Frontal Network						
Left (F3)	−0.142	1.280 T	0.809 T	−1.198 T	−3.855 T	−2.266 T	−0.686
Midline (Fz)	1.298 T	1.997 T	2.275 T	−0.101	−0.109	−0.876 D	−1.781 D
Right (F4)	−0.550	2.962 T	−1.617 T	−0.024	2.493 T	1.017 T	0.800 T
	Centro-Temporal Network						
Left (T7)	−1.644 T	−4.249 T	0.095	−1.375 T	−0.568	1.067 T	−0.782
Midline (Cz)	0.805 T	2.976 T	0.436	0.371	2.356 T	3.061 T	1.074 T
Right (T8)	1.240 T	−0.646	−0.946 D	−0.148	−1.806 T	−0.749	0.753
	Parietal Network						
Left (P7)	1.366 T	−0.106	−2.172 D	−1.772 D	2.118 T	0.870 T	0.822 T
Midline (Pz)	−2.256 T	0.993 T	2.139 T	−2.181 T	−3.538 T	1.241 T	3.268 T
Right (P8)	−2.720 T	−1.200 T	−0.526	−0.620	0.293	2.100 T	0.846 T
	Occipital Network						
Left (O1)	−0.882 T	2.402 T	2.020 T	0.147	−0.059	−0.677	−0.314
Midline (Oz)	−0.045	0.060	0.561	0.388	−2.287 T	−2.029 T	−1.690 T
Right (O2)	1.196 T	−2.431 T	−1.358 T	1.062 T	0.729	−0.742	−1.466 T

Note: Superscripts indicate significant differences in peak amplitude between target and distractor condition: "T" indicates larger amplitude for target; "D" indicates larger amplitude for distractor.

Inspection of Table 2 confirms that the effects in most of the significant pairwise comparisons (46 out of 84) involved higher amplitudes for targets as compared to distractors. In contrast, larger amplitudes for distractors over targets occurred only for much fewer comparisons (5 out of 84). The difference between the proportions of significant target enhancement (55%) vs. distractor (6%) is substantial ($\chi^2(1) = 45.05$; $p < 0.0001$).

3.3. ERP Activity Paths

The results of the ERP activity paths analysis are shown in Figure 6. Neural paths of maximum mean difference in neural activity for targets are shown in blue and neural paths of maximum mean difference in neural activity for distractors are shown in red. The paths were constructed from the results of Table 2.

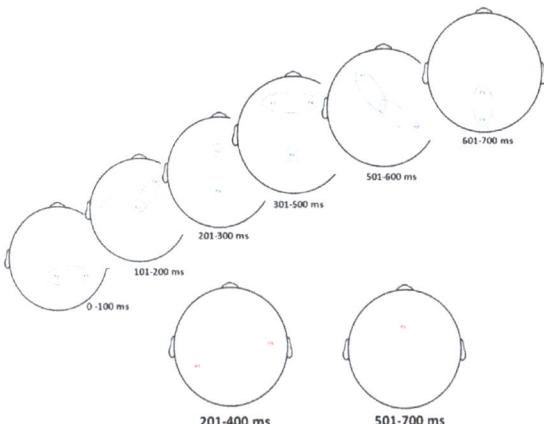

Figure 6. Neural paths of maximum ERP activity over seven interval bins of 100 ms time intervals. Top Panel: Target. Bottom Panel: Distractor.

With reference to the onset of target, ERP paths based on maximum mean differences in peak amplitudes first occurred at the parietal central and right electrodes and moved anteriorly to the left temporal, central and right frontal electrodes. Activation subsequently occurred at the frontal and mid parietal electrodes and finally moved to central parietal and occipital electrodes. For the distractor, ERP pathways based on maximum differences in peak amplitudes were only detected at the left parietal and right temporal electrodes. Neural activation finally moved to the mid-frontal electrode.

3.4. Comparison of ERP Activity and Localization: Preschool Data vs. Adult Simulation

Figures 7 and 8 report the comparison between the localization of dipoles for distractor and target trials. The figures also show the ERP topographical maps of the actual children's data contrasted with the adult simulation data.

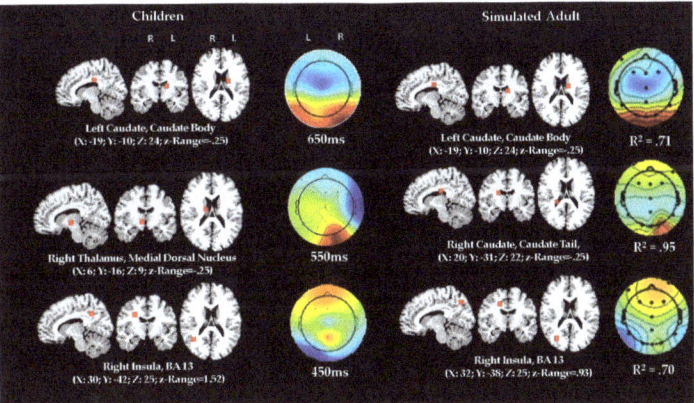

Figure 7. *Cont.*

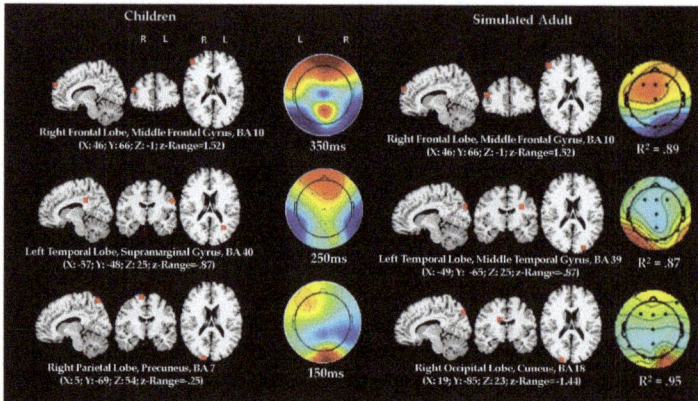

Figure 7. Comparison between dipole source analysis and topographical mappings of actual preschool children ERP data and simulated ERP data by using an ACT–R modeling architecture in the target condition. Timings are set by the ACT–R model module production schedule simulation (given in Figure 3). Coefficient of determinations show fit results for actual and simulated topographic maps comparisons. "R" represents right, and "L" represents left (Please note that lateral side of brain is showed opposite to perspective of the observer in MRI scans). Z-range represents range of normalized Talairach coordinates and is a measure of margin of error expressed as z score; comparisons between the z-ranges in actual and simulated data showed no significant differences.

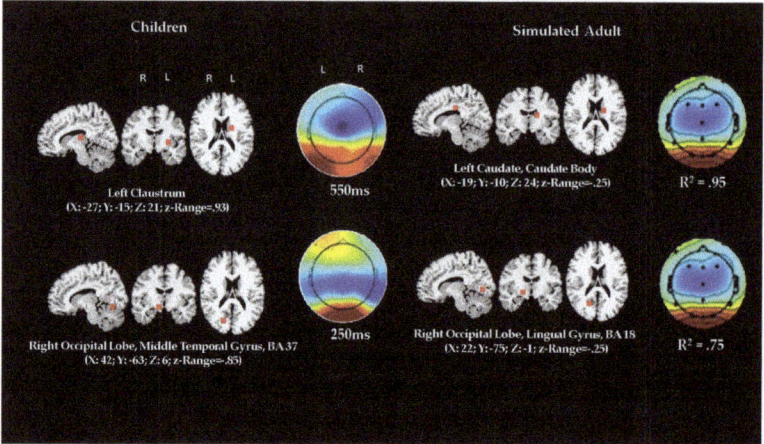

Figure 8. Comparison between dipole source analysis and topographical mappings of actual preschool children ERP data and simulated ERP data by using an ACT–R modeling architecture in the distractor condition. Timings are set by the ACT–R model module production schedule simulation (given in Figure 3). Coefficient of determinations show fit results for actual and simulated topographic maps comparisons. "R" represents right, and "L" represents left (Please note that lateral side of brain is showed opposite to perspective of the observer in MRI scans). Z-range represents range of normalized Talairach coordinates and is a measure of margin of error expressed as z score; comparisons between the z-ranges in actual and simulated data showed no significant differences.

The z-scores of the variation in matched anatomical localizations did not show significant differences between the children's and the adult simulated data. Similarly, there was a strong fit between the topographic maps of the actual observed children's data and the simulated adult data.

For both target and distractor condition, in the regressed data fitting model between actual and simulated data, the coefficients of determination ranged similarly from $R^2 = 0.70$ (F (1,11) = 23.65; $p = 0.0005$) to $R^2 = 0.95$ (F (1,11) = 148.30; $p < 0.0001$), indicating very strong correspondence.

Overall, the results show that the ACT–R model has a very good fit with the actual ERP data, however, two discrepancies are of note. The MRI Talairach coordinates did not match in one instance out of six comparisons concerning the target data, although the spatial coordinate variation was moderate and within satisfactory margins. The match was more imprecise for the distractor data where in both comparisons the Talairach coordinates referred to very proximal but still distinctly different anatomical structures. In addition, differences between ERP time latencies in the actual data and the one derived by simulation might have worsened the fit statistics, since the time of ERP occurrence predicted by ACT–R might actually have not led to sample the most optimal actual data to be fed to the simulation algorithm.

4. Discussion

In the present study, preschool children's performance on VSSAT replicated previous behavioral results [38]; their concurrent ERPs showed that, for most electrodes, the amplitudes were more pronounced in target than distractor trials from about 50 ms to 650 ms post-stimulus presentation. However, response to distractor had relatively higher amplitude than targets in right temporal and left parietal electrodes in the interval ranges of 200–400 ms and in the midfrontal electrode at 500–700 ms. These exceptions concerned a narrow subset of electrodes, for a narrow time range, with relatively smaller effects, and might be interpreted as correlates of *interference control*, namely, resistance to interference from the distractor and suppression of its impact on ongoing selective-set processing aimed at releasing or inhibiting the appropriate (correct) manual response [68].

In the task we used, the ERP correlates of enhancement were confounded with those of the execution of manual response only after 400 ms. The determination of response times within ±2 standard deviations from the grand mean (685 ms) reveals that manual response in most cases could be estimated to occur between 425 and 945 ms. Therefore, selective-set effects were unconfounded by manual motor processing across bin-intervals up to 400 ms. Within this time interval, the peak analysis showed evidence of enhancement of ERP to target except for the two instances mentioned. This analysis also corroborated older findings in showing anteriorly and centrally distributed adult-like N200 and N400 and posteriorly distributed P100 and P300 waveforms. Therefore, we conclude that the present findings support a slightly amended version of the enhancement hypothesis in that a parallel relatively minor and segregated processing may have occurred in a subnetwork in order to suppress the distractor's interference.

By triangulating response times analysis, peak analysis, source dipole modeling, simulation, and spiking modeling, we provided converging evidence separating the selective-set processes as occurring earlier (before 400 ms) than the actual response (at around 700 ms, on average) and showing yet another distinct spatiotemporal pattern of activity from those associated with later processes (between 500 and 650 ms), which presumably reflected the planning and preparation of response.

We also performed activity paths analysis to illustrate plausible sequence of the prominent neural activity over time for target and distractor based on maximum differences in peak amplitudes. The results seem compatible with the interpretation that attending the target while holding in working memory the response plan yielded a neural path starting from the parietal regions, then to right temporal and central regions and finally to the frontal regions. In contrast, withholding responses to distractor seemed associated with punctuated activity at the left parietal and right temporal regions. Importantly, comparison of neural activity between target and distractor reveals that in the initial 400 ms there was less involvement of frontal areas concurrent to the distractor.

Dipole analysis further suggests possible and plausible neurofunctional pathways and dynamics involved at cortical and subcortical level. This analysis (see Left Panels of Figures 7 and 8) estimated that initially, within the first 150 ms, the generators of scalp ERP signals, which are distributed posteriorly at right and mid parietal electrodes, seem to correspond to activity in the precuneus. Subsequently, around 250 ms, the ERP activity, mapped on the scalp at left temporal, central, and right frontal electrodes, seems to correspond to a dipole source in the left supramarginal gyrus of the left temporal cortex. Before what might be reasonably considered the timeframe for implementing the manual response, around 350 ms, ERP activity mapped at mid parietal and frontal electrodes was estimated as being generated at the level of a dipole located in middle frontal gyrus of the right frontal lobe. At approximately 45 ms, ERP activity was then estimated to a source in the right insula. The following ERP activity, at 550 and 650 ms, was associated with dipoles in the medial dorsal nucleus of the right thalamus and the right caudate body, respectively.

In contrast, ERP activity concurrent to the distractor was accounted for by just two dipoles, the first occurring at 250 ms in a source located in the middle temporal gyrus, at the junction of right occipital and temporal cortices, the second occurring at 550 ms in the left claustrum.

The previous analysis converges with the findings of a close fit between the preschool children's ERP topographic as well as derived source data and the adult-based ACT–R functional and structural simulations. This convergence suggests evidence of neurofunctional homology. In addition to providing preliminary validity and reliability to the analysis based on the actual data, the converging results from the ACT–R modeling may provide a framework for interpreting the results in a coherent meaningful way and for a detailed inferential reconstruction of the plausible, possible underlying neurocognitive processes related to the enhancement mechanism.

As modeled through ACT–R, our findings may be interpreted as showing that in the initial phase of the VSSAT, target presentation might have been associated with the involvement of key structures of the dorsal (precuneus, BA 7) and ventral (supramarginal gyrus, BA 40) attentional networks [69–71]. These structures appeared to be activated relatively early, similarly than in adults. Next, activation seemed to follow in two functionally interconnected parts, one in the dorsolateral prefrontal cortex (middle frontal gyrus, BA 10); the other in the frontal part of the dorsal attentional network (insula, BA 13). The literature indicates that these structures seem to be activated during the processing of deviants and standards, and specifically, both structures seem to be involved in voluntary target detection, playing important roles in top-down selective attentional control [72–74]. Successively, activation seems to have involved the thalamic dorsomedial nucleus, which might play a role in the regulation of cortical networks, especially when the maintenance and temporal extension of persistent activity patterns in the frontal lobe areas are required, as in the case of sustained attention [75]. The final stage leading to manual response seemed to be associated with the involvement of a key structure in basal ganglia-striatum network, the caudate body. This "cognitive" part of the caudate seems to participate in the control of action including executive functions such as working memory, set shifting, and inhibitory control [76–78].

The presentation of the distractor seemed to be associated with early engagement of the middle temporal gyrus (BA 37) which is generally deemed to be involved in visual recognition and verbal labeling/categorization [79]. Subsequent late activation seemed to involve the claustrum, a structure thought to participate in the regulation of vigilance and in voluntary allocation of attention [80].

Triangulation of peak analysis, ACT–R modeling and simulation for the entire ERP epochs up to the moment of manual response (~700 ms, on average) suggested converging evidence of distinct but separate interacting processes of enhancement and planning for response release/inhibition, respectively. Thus, the results from the triangulation, considering both target and distractor conditions, overall suggest potentially important interrelations between basal–parietal–temporal–frontal–basal loops and large-scale attentional networks. The feedback loops and functional connectivity originating and ending in the basal ganglia and the striatum, as postulated by the ACT–R architecture, control diverse behaviors largely but not exclusively involved in high-level perception, walking, talking, thinking, language, comprehension, associated with frontal lobes, where the motor strip also sits [81]. As some theories have proposed [82], the aspects which might undergo fine-tuning in young children, in terms of speed and efficiency, most likely may not involve the selective-set in isolation, but rather its voluntary and flexible coordination with high-level perceptual and working memory processes, recruited for selecting, monitoring and executing or inhibiting the appropriate behavioral response.

A brief discussion of the main limitations and caveats of our study is in order. While the number of electrodes and montage set-up we used may be justified for dipole source analysis in young children (as we have detailed in the methods section and especially for practical challenges in collecting EEGs in this population), it may not be sufficient for reliable source analysis in adults. Therefore, the results need to be replicated in further studies which combine real fMRI and possibly eye movement measurements. Furthermore, as we have already noted ACT–R simulation could be refined (or even replaced by a more flexible architecture) to improve fit and predictions in timings and anatomical localization of neurofunctional modules.

Lastly but not least, although our modeling and simulation procedures are grounded in the literature, being validated by separate tests of the most relevant components of ERPs from actual adult samples [83–85], still we did not report data from an actual adult comparison group. While we acknowledge that in this respect our results are preliminary, and indeed this is a desirable priority for future research, adult comparison on this version of the VSSAT might not necessarily augment the strength of the supporting evidence because it presents non-trivial methodological challenges. In particular, we have learned from small pilot studies in our lab that the current VSSAT is not appropriate for adults. This task needs to be adapted to prevent confounds of other spurious aspects (i.e., boredom, engagement level, ceiling effects) occurring in adult participants (but not in preschool children). In other words, this task should be modified significantly to "equate" children's state and age-appropriate task demands. However, as pointed out by others (notably, see [17]), if children and adults are not compared on the same task, data interpretation would still depend on assumptions derived from a priori hypothetical models. Consequently, under such differing conditions, the correspondence defining homology on the basis of comparisons between actual adult and children ERP data would still be based on a type of model-mediated inductive inference. This would be essentially similar to the present approach, therefore, the resulting evidence would not be more "direct" or "realistic" or logically different than the one offered here.

5. Conclusions

In summary, the pattern of results invites the conclusion that preschool children's ERPs associated with visual attentional selective-set were enhanced in response to target as compared to distractor, and may have involved functions and structures consistent with adult ERP activity. The modeling results suggest a large-scale network, including Dorsal and Ventral Attentional Networks, corticostriatal loops, and subcortical hubs connected to prefrontal cortex top-down (working memory) executive control. The present findings are compatible with the claim [17] that the attentional selective-set might be, or become, adult-like by 4–5 years of age. Although preliminary, our approach may contribute to suggest novel directions for further tests and falsifiable hypotheses on the origins and development of visual selective attention and their ERP correlates.

Supplementary Materials: The following are available online at http://www.mdpi.com/2076-3425/10/2/124/s1.

Author Contributions: A.D. is the primary author and contributor responsible for data collection, conceptualization, resources, supervision, funding, analyses, and final preparation and editing of the manuscript. D.A.T.P. was responsible for literature review, data analysis, methodological aspects and assembly and preparation of the first draft. G.G. was responsible for conceptualization, writing-review and editing and funding. G.L. was responsible for conceptualization, writing-review and editing of the revised final versions. All authors have read and agreed to the published version of the manuscript.

Funding: This research was funded by a standard research grant to A.D. and an insight grant to G.G. from Social Sciences and Humanities Research Council of Canada.

Acknowledgments: We thank Patricia Van Roon for assistance with EEG/ERP analysis. We thank Nina Hedayati for curating parts of the project and preliminary writing for conference dissemination. We thank Christine Miller for assistance with data collection. We thank two anonymous pediatric neurology experts affiliated with the University of Ottawa Brain and Mind Research Institute who served as judges for the MRI mapping.

Conflicts of Interest: The authors declare no conflict of interest.

References

1. Kahneman, D.; Treisman, A. Changing views of attention and automaticity. In *Varieties of Attention*; Parasuraman, R., Davies, D.R., Eds.; Academic Press: New York, NY, USA, 1984; pp. 29–61.
2. Fisher, A.V.; Thiessen, E.; Godwin, K.; Kloos, H.; Dickerson, J. Assessing selective sustained attention in 3- to 5-year-old children: Evidence from a new paradigm. *J. Exp. Child Psychol.* **2012**, *114*, 275–294. [CrossRef] [PubMed]
3. Posner, M.; Rothbart, M.K.; Voelker, P. Developing brain networks of attention. *Curr. Opin. Pediatr.* **2016**, *28*, 720–724. [CrossRef] [PubMed]
4. Posner, M.; Rothbart, M.K.; Sheese, B.E.; Voelker, P. Developing Attention: Behavioral and Brain Mechanisms. *Adv. Neurosci.* **2014**, *2014*, 405094. [CrossRef] [PubMed]
5. Jones, L.; Rothbart, M.K.; Posner, M. Development of executive attention in preschool children. *Dev. Sci.* **2003**, *6*, 498–504. [CrossRef]
6. Jodo, E.; Kayama, Y. Relation of a negative ERP component to response inhibition in a Go/No-go task. *Electroencephalogr. Clin. Neurophysiol.* **1992**, *82*, 477–482. [CrossRef]
7. Johnstone, S.J.; Pleffer, C.B.; Barry, R.J.; Clarke, A.R.; Smith, J.L. Development of inhibitory processing during the go/nogo task. *J. Psychophysiol.* **2005**, *19*, 11–23. [CrossRef]
8. Lahat, A.; Todd, R.M.; Mahy, C.E.V.; Lau, K.; Zelazo, P.D. Neurophysiological Correlates of Executive Function: A Comparison of European-Canadian and Chinese-Canadian 5-Year-Old Children. *Front. Hum. Neurosci.* **2010**, *3*, 72. [CrossRef]
9. Lamm, C.; Zelazo, P.D.; Lewis, M.D. Neural correlates of cognitive control in childhood and adolescence: Disentangling the contributions of age and executive function. *Neuropsychology* **2006**, *44*, 2139–2148. [CrossRef]
10. Jonkman, L.M. The development of preparation, conflict monitoring and inhibition from early childhood to young adulthood; a Go/Nogo ERP study. *Brain Res.* **2006**, *1097*, 181–193. [CrossRef]
11. Kaganovich, N.; Ancel, E. Different neural processes underlie visual speech perception in school-age children and adults: An event-related potentials study. *J. Exp. Child Psychol.* **2019**, *184*, 98–122. [CrossRef]
12. Zhang, Q.; Shi, J.; Luo, Y.; Zhao, D.; Yang, J. Intelligence and information processing during a visual search task in children: An event-related potential study. *NeuroReport* **2006**, *17*, 747–752. [CrossRef] [PubMed]
13. Zhao, P.; Zhao, J.; Weng, X.; Li, S. Event-related potential evidence in Chinese children. *Int. J. Behav. Dev.* **2017**, *42*, 311–320. [CrossRef]
14. Kim, S.H.; Buzzell, G.; Faja, S.; Choi, Y.B.; Thomas, H.R.; Brito, N.H.; Shuffrey, L.C.; Fifer, W.P.; Morrison, F.D.; Lord, C.; et al. Neural dynamics of executive function in cognitively able kindergarteners with autism spectrum disorders as predictors of concurrent academic achievement. *Autism* **2019**, *23*. [CrossRef] [PubMed]
15. Grammer, J.K.; Carrasco, M.; Gehring, W.J.; Morrison, F.J. Age-related changes in error processing in young children: A school-based investigation. *Dev. Cogn. Neurosci.* **2014**, *9*, 93–105. [CrossRef]
16. Kim, M.H.; Grammer, J.K.; Marulis, L.M.; Carrasco, M.; Morrison, F.J.; Gehring, W.J. Early math and reading achievement are associated with the error positivity. *Dev. Cogn. Neurosci.* **2016**, *22*, 18–26. [CrossRef]
17. Ridderinkhof, K.R.; Van Der Stelt, O. Attention and selection in the growing child: Views derived from developmental psychophysiology. *Boil. Psychol.* **2000**, *54*, 55–106. [CrossRef]
18. Courchesne, E. Chronology of postnatal human brain development: Event-related potential, positron emission tomography, myelinogenesis, and synaptogenesis studies. In *Related Brain Potentials: Basic Issues and Applications*; Rohrbaugh, J.W., Parasuraman, R., Johnson, R., Eds.; Oxford University Press: New York, NY, USA, 1990; pp. 210–241.
19. Lickliter, R.; Bahrick, L.E. The concept of homology as a basis for evaluating developmental mechanisms: Exploring selective attention across the life-span. *Dev. Psychobiol.* **2012**, *55*, 76–83. [CrossRef]
20. Ruff, H.A.; Rothbart, M.K. Attention in early development. In *Themes and Variations*; Oxford University Press: New York, NY, USA, 2001.
21. Rueda, M.R.; Posner, M.I.; Rothbart, M.K. Attentional control and self-regulation. In *Handbook of Self-Regulation: Research, Theory, and Applications*, 2nd ed.; Baumeister, R.F., Vohs, K.D., Eds.; Guilford Press: New York, NY, USA, 2011; pp. 284–299.

22. Casey, B.; Tottenham, N.; Liston, C.; Durston, S. Imaging the developing brain: What have we learned about cognitive development? *Trends Cogn. Sci.* **2005**, *9*, 104–110. [CrossRef]
23. Tsujimoto, S. The Prefrontal Cortex: Functional Neural Development during Early Childhood. *Neuroscientist* **2008**, *14*, 345–358. [CrossRef]
24. Brown, T.T.; Jernigan, T.L. Brain development during the preschool years. *Neuropsychol. Rev.* **2012**, *22*, 313–333. [CrossRef]
25. Chevalier, N.; Kurth, S.; Doucette, M.R.; Wiseheart, M.; Deoni, S.C.L.; Dean, D.C.; O'Muircheartaigh, J.; Blackwell, K.A.; Munakata, Y.; LeBourgeois, M.K. Myelination Is Associated with Processing Speed in Early Childhood: Preliminary Insights. *PLoS ONE* **2015**, *10*, e0139897. [CrossRef] [PubMed]
26. Deoni, S.C.; O'Muircheartaigh, J.; Elison, J.T.; Walker, L.; Doernberg, E.; Waskiewicz, N.; Dirks, H.; Piryatinsky, I.; Dean, D.C.; Jumbé, N.L. White matter maturation profiles through early childhood predict general cognitive ability. *Brain Struct. Funct.* **2014**, *221*, 1189–1203. [CrossRef] [PubMed]
27. Fields, R.D. Change in the Brain's white matter: The role of the brain's white matter in active learning and memory may be underestimated. *Science* **2010**, *330*, 768–769. [CrossRef] [PubMed]
28. Dubois, J.; Dehaene-Lambertz, G.; Soarès, C.; Cointepas, Y.; Le Bihan, D.; Hertz-Pannier, L. Microstructural Correlates of Infant Functional Development: Example of the Visual Pathways. *J. Neurosci.* **2008**, *28*, 1943–1948. [CrossRef]
29. Jolles, D.; Wassermann, D.; Chokhani, R.; Richardson, J.; Tenison, C.; Bammer, R.; Fuchs, L.; Supekar, K.; Menon, V. Plasticity of left perisylvian white-matter tracts is associated with individual differences in math learning. *Brain Struct. Funct.* **2015**, *221*, 1337–1351. [CrossRef]
30. Nagy, Z.; Westerberg, H.; Klingberg, T. Maturation of White Matter is Associated with the Development of Cognitive Functions during Childhood. *J. Cogn. Neurosci.* **2004**, *16*, 1227–1233. [CrossRef]
31. O'Muircheartaigh, J.; Dean, D.C.; Ginestet, C.E.; Walker, L.; Waskiewicz, N.; Lehman, K.; Dirks, H.; Piryatinsky, I.; Deoni, S.C.; Iii, D.C.D. White matter development and early cognition in babies and toddlers. *Hum. Brain Mapp.* **2014**, *35*, 4475–4487. [CrossRef]
32. Zatorre, R.J.; Fields, R.D.; Johansen-Berg, H. Plasticity in gray and white: Neuroimaging changes in brain structure during learning. *Nat. Neurosci.* **2012**, *15*, 528–536. [CrossRef]
33. Heinen, F.; Glocker, F.-X.; Fietzek, U.; Meyer, B.-U.; Lücking, C.-H.; Korinthenberg, R. Absence of transcallosal inhibition following focal mangnetic stimulation in preschool children. *Ann. Neurol.* **1998**, *43*, 608–612. [CrossRef]
34. Dai, X.; Hadjipantelis, P.; Wang, J.-L.; Deoni, S.C.L.; Müller, H.-G. Longitudinal associations between white matter maturation and cognitive development across early childhood. *Hum. Brain Mapp.* **2019**, *40*, 4130–4145. [CrossRef]
35. Schafer, R.; Moore, T. Selective Attention from Voluntary Control of Neurons in Prefrontal Cortex. *Science* **2011**, *332*, 1568–1571. [CrossRef] [PubMed]
36. Hopfinger, J.; Luck, S.; Hillyard, S. Selective attention: Electrophysiological and neuromagnetic studies. In *The Cognitive Neurosciences III*; Gazzaniga, M., Ed.; MIT Press: Cambridge, MA, USA, 2004; pp. 561–574.
37. Casteau, S.; Smith, D. Associations and Dissociations between Oculomotor Readiness and Covert Attention. *Vision* **2019**, *3*, 17. [CrossRef] [PubMed]
38. Akshoomoff, N.A. Selective Attention and Active Engagement in Young Children. *Dev. Neuropsychol.* **2002**, *22*, 625–642. [CrossRef] [PubMed]
39. D'Angiulli, A.; Warburton, W.; Dahinten, V.S.; Hertzman, C. Population-Level Associations between Preschool Vulnerability and Grade-Four Basic Skills. *PLoS ONE* **2009**, *4*, e7692. [CrossRef]
40. D'Angiulli, A.; Griffiths, G.; Marmolejo-Ramos, F. Neural correlates of visualizations of concrete and abstract words in preschool children: A developmental embodied approach. *Front. Psychol.* **2015**, *6*, 1–17. [CrossRef]
41. Gioia, G.A.; Espy, K.A.; Isquith, P.K. *Behavior Rating Inventory of Executive Function®–Preschool Version (BRIEF®–P)*; Psychological Assessment Resources: Odessa, FL, USA, 2003.
42. Achenbach, T.M. *Achenbach System of Empirically Based Assessment (ASEBA): Development, Findings, Theory, and Applications*; University of Vermont, Research Center of Children, Youth & Families: Burlington, VT, USA, 2009.
43. D'Angiulli, A.; Devenyi, P. Retooling computational techniques for EEG-based neurocognitive modeling of children's data, validity and prospects for learning and education. *Front. Comput. Neurosci.* **2019**, *13*, 4. [CrossRef]

44. Griffiths, G.; West, R.; D'Angiulli, A. Cognitive modeling of Event-Related Potentials. In Proceedings of the 33th Cognitive Science Society Annual Meeting, Boston, MA, USA, 20–23 July 2011.
45. D'Angiulli, A.; Yeh, W.-H.; Griffiths, G. Correlation between parent-reported executive functions and EEG response during selective-attention and language tasks in preschool children: An event-related and spectral measurement study. *Front. Hum. Neurosci.* **2010**, *82*. [CrossRef]
46. Yeh, W.-H.; D'Angiulli, A. Compensatory Mechanism and Circadian Preference Related Frontal Cortex Activation in Adolescent: The Relationship to Sleep Pattern and Testing Time. *Front. Hum. Neurosci.* **2010**, *4*. [CrossRef]
47. Van Roon, P.; D'Angiulli, A. Preschooler's ERPs of online/offline visualizations and embodiment theory. In Proceedings of the 36th Annual Conference of the Cognitive Science Society, Quebec City, QC, Canada, 23–26 July 2014.
48. Ille, N.; Berg, P.; Scherg, M. Artifact correction of the ongoing EEG using spatial filters based on artifact and brain signal topographies. *J. Clin. Neurophysiol.* **2002**, *19*, 113–124. [CrossRef]
49. Berg, P.; Scherg, M. A multiple source approach to the correction of eye artifacts. *Electroencephalogr. Clin. Neurophysiol.* **1994**, *90*, 229–241. [CrossRef]
50. Luck, S. *An Introduction to the Event-Related Potential Technique*; MIT Press: Cambridge, MA, USA, 2005.
51. Filipović, S.; Andreassi, J.L. Psychophysiology: Human Behavior and Physiological Response. *Psychophysiology* **2001**, *15*, 210–212. [CrossRef]
52. Berman, S.; Friedman, D. The Development of Selective Attention as Reflected by Event-Related Brain Potentials. *J. Exp. Child. Psychol.* **1995**, *59*, 1–31. [CrossRef] [PubMed]
53. Hedayati, N.; Schibli, K.; D'Angiulli, A. El Sistema-inspired ensemble music training is associated with changes in children's neurocognitive functional integration: Preliminary ERP evidence. *Neurocase* **2016**, *22*, 1–10. [CrossRef] [PubMed]
54. Delorme, A.; Makeig, S. EEGLAB: An open source toolbox for analysis of single-trial EEG dynamics including independent component analysis. *J. Neurosci. Methods* **2004**, *134*, 9–21. [CrossRef]
55. Vincent, S.B. *The Functions of the Vibrissae in the Behavior of the White Rat. Behavior Monographs, 1*; University of Chicago: Chicago, IL, USA, 1912.
56. Hilgard, E.R. Methods and procedures in the study of learning. In *Handbook of Experimental Psychology*; Stevens, S.S., Ed.; Wiley: New York, NY, USA, 1951; pp. 517–567.
57. Genest, C. Vincentization Revisited. *Ann. Stat.* **1992**, *20*, 1137–1142. [CrossRef]
58. Rosenthal, R.; Rosnow, R.L.; Rubin, D.B. *Contrasts and Effect Sizes in Behavioral Research: A Correlational Approach*; Cambridge University Press: New York, NY, USA, 2000.
59. Cherniak, C. Neural wiring optimization. *Prog. Brain Res.* **2012**, *195*, 361–371.
60. Jung, T.-P.; Makeig, S.; Westerfield, M.; Townsend, J.; Courchesne, E.; Sejnowski, T.J. Analysis and visualization of single-trial event-related potentials. *Hum. Brain Mapp.* **2001**, *14*, 166–185. [CrossRef]
61. Hyvärinen, A.; Oja, E. A Fast Fixed-Point Algorithm for Independent Component Analysis. *Neural Comput.* **1997**, *9*, 1483–1492. [CrossRef]
62. Lancaster, J.; Fox, P. *Talairach Client Version 2.4.3*; Research Imaging Institute, University of Texas Health Science Center: San Antonio, TX, USA, 2015.
63. Papademetris, X.; Scheinost, D. Yale Bioimage Suite Web. Dept. of Radiology and Biomedical Imaging, Yale School of Medicine. Available online: https://bioimagesuiteweb.github.io/webapp/ (accessed on 22 February 2020).
64. Anderson, J.R.; Lebiere, C. *The Atomic Components of Thought*; Psychology Press: New York, NY, USA, 2012.
65. Stewart, T.C.; Eliasmith, C. Neural Symbolic Decision Making: A Scalable and Realistic Foundation for Cognitive Architectures. In *Biologically Inspired Cognitive Architectures*; Series in Frontiers in Artificial Intelligence and Applications, volume 221; Samsonovich, A.V., Jóhannsdóttir, K.R., Chella, A., Goertzel, B., Eds.; IOS Press: Clifton, VA, USA, 2010; pp. 147–152.
66. Stewart, T.C.; Eliasmith, C. Spiking neurons and central executive control: The origin of the 50-millisecond cognitive cycle. In *Proceedings of the 9th International Conference on Cognitive Modelling 2009*; University of Manchester: Manchester, UK, 2009; Volume 122, pp. 130–131.
67. Brasoveanu, A. Introduction to (Python) ACT-R; semantics seminar: Computing dynamic meanings. 2015. Available online: https://people.ucsc.edu/~{}abrsvn/Intro_to_Python_ACT-R.pdf (accessed on 20 February 2020).

68. Liu, Q.; Zhu, X.; Ziegler, A.; Shi, J. The effects of inhibitory control training for preschoolers on reasoning ability and neural activity. *Sci. Rep.* **2015**, *5*, 14300. [CrossRef]
69. Kim, H. Involvement of the dorsal and ventral attention networks in oddball stimulus processing: A meta-analysis. *Hum. Brain Mapp.* **2013**, *35*, 2265–2284. [CrossRef]
70. Corbetta, M.; Shulman, G.L. Control of goal-directed and stimulus-driven attention in the brain. *Nat. Rev. Neurosci.* **2002**, *3*, 201–215. [CrossRef] [PubMed]
71. Vossel, S.; Geng, J.J.; Fink, G.R. Dorsal and ventral attention systems: Distinct neural circuits but collaborative roles. *Neuroscience* **2014**, *20*, 150–159. [CrossRef] [PubMed]
72. Rossi, A.F.; Pessoa, L.; DeSimone, R.; Ungerleider, L. The prefrontal cortex and the executive control of attention. *Exp. Brain Res.* **2008**, *192*, 489–497. [CrossRef] [PubMed]
73. Sridharan, D.; Levitin, D.J.; Menon, V. A critical role for the right fronto-insular cortex in switching between central-executive and default-mode networks. *Proc. Natl. Acad. Sci. USA* **2008**, *105*, 12569–12574. [CrossRef] [PubMed]
74. Cai, W.; Chen, T.; Ryali, S.; Kochalka, J.; Li, C.-S.R.; Menon, V. Causal Interactions Within a Frontal-Cingulate-Parietal Network During Cognitive Control: Convergent Evidence from a Multisite-Multitask Investigation. *Cereb. Cortex* **2015**, *26*, 2140–2153. [CrossRef] [PubMed]
75. Pergola, G.; Danet, L.; Pitel, A.-L.; Carlesimo, G.A.; Segobin, S.; Pariente, J.; Suchan, B.; Mitchell, A.S.; Barbeau, E.J. The Regulatory Role of the Human Mediodorsal Thalamus. *Trends Cogn. Sci.* **2018**, *22*, 1011–1025. [CrossRef]
76. Robinson, J.L.; Laird, A.R.; Glahn, D.C.; Blangero, J.; Sanghera, M.K.; Pessoa, L.; Uecker, A.; Friehs, G.; Young, K.; Griffin, J.L.; et al. The functional connectivity of the human caudate: An application of meta-analytic connectivity modeling with behavioral filtering. *NeuroImage* **2011**, *60*, 117–129. [CrossRef]
77. Grahn, J.A.; Parkinson, J.A.; Owen, A.M. The cognitive functions of the caudate nucleus. *Prog. Neurobiol.* **2008**, *86*, 141–155. [CrossRef]
78. Hedden, T.; Gabrieli, J.D.E. Shared and selective neural correlates of inhibition, facilitation, and shifting processes during executive control. *NeuroImage* **2010**, *51*, 421–431. [CrossRef]
79. Ardila, A.; Bernal, B.; Rosselli, M. Language and Visual Perception Associations: Meta-Analytic Connectivity Modeling of Brodmann Area 37. *Behav. Neurol.* **2015**, *2015*, 1–14. [CrossRef]
80. Brown, S.P.; Mathur, B.; Olsen, S.R.; Luppi, P.-H.; Bickford, M.E.; Citri, A. New Breakthroughs in Understanding the Role of Functional Interactions between the Neocortex and the Claustrum. *J. Neurosci.* **2017**, *37*, 10877–10881. [CrossRef] [PubMed]
81. Leisman, G.; Melillo, R. The basal ganglia: Motor and cognitive relationships in a clinical neurobehavioral context. *Rev. Neurosci.* **2013**, *24*. [CrossRef] [PubMed]
82. Tipper, S.P.; Weaver, B.; Houghton, G. Behavioural Goals Determine Inhibitory Mechanisms of Selective Attention. *Q. J. Exp. Psychol. Sect. A* **1994**, *47*, 809–840. [CrossRef]
83. Gevins, A. The future of electroencephalography in assessing neurocognitive functioning. *Electroencephalogr. Clin. Neurophysiol.* **1998**, *106*, 165–172. [CrossRef]
84. Cassenti, D.N. ACT-R Model of EEG Latency Data. In Proceedings of the Human Factors and Ergonomics Society Annual Meeting, Belfast, UK, 3–5 September 2007; Volume 51, pp. 812–816.
85. Cassenti, D.N.; Kerick, S.; McDowell, K. Observing and modeling cognitive events through event-related potentials and ACT-R. *Cogn. Syst. Res.* **2011**, *12*, 56–65. [CrossRef]

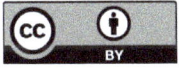

© 2020 by the authors. Licensee MDPI, Basel, Switzerland. This article is an open access article distributed under the terms and conditions of the Creative Commons Attribution (CC BY) license (http://creativecommons.org/licenses/by/4.0/).

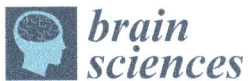

Article

Left-Hemispheric Asymmetry for Object-Based Attention: an ERP Study

Andrea Orlandi * and Alice Mado Proverbio

Neuro-MI, Milan Center for Neuroscience, Dept. of Psychology, University of Milano - Bicocca, Milan 20126, Italy; mado.proverbio@unimib.it
* Correspondence: a.orlandi5@campus.unimib.it; Tel.: +39-02-64483866

Received: 26 September 2019; Accepted: 6 November 2019; Published: 8 November 2019

Abstract: It has been shown that selective attention enhances the activity in visual regions associated with stimulus processing. The left hemisphere seems to have a prominent role when non-spatial attention is directed towards specific stimulus features (e.g., color, spatial frequency). The present electrophysiological study investigated the time course and neural correlates of object-based attention, under the assumption of left-hemispheric asymmetry. Twenty-nine right-handed participants were presented with 3D graphic images representing the shapes of different object categories (wooden dummies, chairs, structures of cubes) which lacked detail. They were instructed to press a button in response to a target stimulus indicated at the beginning of each run. The perception of non-target stimuli elicited a larger anterior N2 component, which was likely associated with motor inhibition. Conversely, target selection resulted in an enhanced selection negativity (SN) response lateralized over the left occipito-temporal regions, followed by a larger centro-parietal P300 response. These potentials were interpreted as indexing attentional selection and categorization processes, respectively. The standardized weighted low-resolution electromagnetic tomography (swLORETA) source reconstruction showed the engagement of a fronto-temporo-limbic network underlying object-based visual attention. Overall, the SN scalp distribution and relative neural generators hinted at a left-hemispheric advantage for non-spatial object-based visual attention.

Keywords: selective attention; object-based attention; hemispheric asymmetry; ERP; selection negativity; swLORETA; anterior cingulate cortex; visual recognition

1. Introduction

It is known that visual attention can be consciously directed towards a selected location in space (spatial attention [1,2]), a stimulus as a whole (object-based attention [3–5]), or specific features of a stimulus (feature-based attention [6–8]). While both behavioral and neural correlates of spatial and feature-related attentional processes have been extensively investigated [9–11], attentive selection for objects requires further consideration. For instance, a processing bias (i.e., increased accuracy and faster response), together with the enhanced engagement of fronto-parietal regions (i.e., frontal eye-field, posterior parietal cortex), was reported for stimuli occurring within a target location [12]. Several studies have also shown that attention directed towards single (or combined) stimulus features (i.e., color, orientation, motion, spatial frequency) leads to increased activity within the visual areas sensitive to the target physical trait (i.e., V4 for color; MT+ (middle temporal) for motion [8,13]).

In the case of attention on an object, a few studies have shown an enhanced engagement of the extrastriate visual cortices for target stimulus processing [3]. At the same time, the neural mechanisms and relative brain regions underlying this top-down modulation of the occipito-temporal regions are not yet entirely clarified [4,14]. In two classic fMRI studies by O'Craven and colleagues [3], the participants were presented with stimuli depicting a transparent face superimposed over a house, with one stimulus moving and the other stationary. They were instructed to press a button when a target attribute (i.e., face, house, or motion) was consecutively repeated. Attention directed towards faces, houses, or visual motion resulted in increased activity in the FFA (fusiform face area), PPA (parahippocampal place area), and MT (middle temporal), respectively [15–17]. This top-down bias signal for the attended attribute also led to enhanced engagement of the areas associated with the processing of the task-irrelevant attribute. This evidence suggests the occurrence of attentive selection processes for the whole object. Similar results were reported in a subsequent study by Serences and colleagues [4], in which two streams of superimposed faces and houses morphed into the next stimuli at a changing rate of 1/s. Target stimuli required the participants to maintain their attention within the current stream or to shift it toward the other stream. Attention directed to faces and houses led to enhanced activity in the right lateral fusiform gyrus and bilateral medial fusiform gyrus, respectively. Additionally, transient shift-related activity was shown in the right superior frontal sulcus/precentral gyrus and the medial superior parietal lobule, suggesting a role of these regions in non-spatial attentional control processes.

More recently, in a MEG (magnetoencephalography) study by Baldauf and Desimone [14], the participants were shown two streams (spatially overlapping) of faces and houses tagged at different presentation frequencies and instructed to attend to one of them (during target detection). Selective attention enhanced the functional connectivity between the stimulus sensitive visual regions (FFA and PPA) and the inferior frontal junction (IFJ, identified using an attention-related fMRI localizer) at the specific tagging frequencies. Increased phase coherence was also visible in the higher gamma range. The phase lag (20 ms) between frontal and temporal areas indicated the IFJ as a potentially key region for top-down modulation of object-based (and feature-based) attention [18,19]. Using a different approach, Valdes-Sosa and colleagues [20] showed evidence for non-spatial, object-based attention selection at an early stage of vision. The authors presented the participants with two superimposed sets of red and green dots. They were instructed to detect coherent motion displacements (in cardinal directions) of one set of dots, ignoring the other one. The two sets could also be stationary or in rigid rotation around the central fixation point in both the same and opposite directions. In the latter baseline condition (perceived as two transparent superimposed surfaces), unattended (rather than attended) stimuli resulted in a suppression of the posterior N1 and P1 components related to the motion onset. This effect was reduced or absent when the two sets were perceived as a single object, while the attended (than unattended) stimuli elicited an increased selection negativity (SN) response.

Another issue that needs more in-depth analysis relates to the roles of the left and right hemispheres in selective attention processes. A right asymmetry has been shown during tasks involving overt and covert attentional shifting to selected spatial locations in healthy and clinical (i.e., neglect syndrome) populations [21–24]. A greater engagement of the right hemisphere has also been shown during tasks requiring sustained attention [25,26]. At the same time, evidence from several studies seems to suggest left-lateralized neural substrates underlying focused attentive selection [27–31]. A case in point is the ERP (event-related potential) study by Proverbio and colleagues [30]. The participants were presented with images of familiar objects and animals that were associated or not associated with the prototypical color. They were instructed to recognize either the shape or color of the stimuli, ignoring the other trait. Target stimuli characterized by the prototypical (vs. unassociated) color/shape combination elicited a larger N2 component (or SN) over posterior sites, during the attention to color condition only. This effect was found over the left but not right hemisphere, as also confirmed by the topographic map of voltage distribution computed on the difference wave (associated minus unassociated targets). These results likely showed specific involvement of the left occipito-temporal cortex for conjoined color and shape processing of real objects.

Moreover, Milham and colleagues [28] showed hemispheric differences in attentional control based on the response (vs. non-response) conflict level. The participants were engaged in a Stroop task during fMRI scanning. The incongruent color words could give rise to either an eligible (color in the response set) or an ineligible (color outside the response set) response. Greater engagement of the right fronto-parietal network (i.e., anterior cingulate cortex (ACC), superior, inferior, and middle frontal gyrus, superior parietal lobule) was reported in response to incongruent-eligible (vs. neutral) stimuli. At the same time, both incongruent types of stimuli (relative to neutral stimuli) elicited greater activity in the left hemisphere (i.e., middle frontal cortex, precuneus, and superior parietal lobule), which was likely associated with attentional control at non-response (semantic and phonological) levels.

These findings also appear to be consistent with the left-lateralized brain network reported for local (vs. global) stimulus processing (i.e., Navon stimuli [32–37]) and perception of high (vs. low) spatial frequencies [38–41]. In this vein, Martínez and colleagues [41] reported a larger SN component in response to target (vs. non-target) spatial frequencies (black and white checkboard patterns). The discrimination of high frequencies (5 cpd, cycles per degree) elicited an enhanced SN over the left (compared to the right) hemisphere, while the opposite result was reported for low frequencies (0.8 cpd). In a previous study by Yamaguchi and colleagues [36], the participants were instructed to recognize a target letter (within compound stimuli) at the hierarchical level, indicated by a pre-stimulus cue. The local and global targets elicited an increased N2 response (250–350 ms) over the left and right hemispheres, respectively. The attentional shift elicited by the local (rather than global) cue also resulted in a larger negative response (starting at 240 ms after the onset) at left (vs. right) scalp sites, and vice versa. These findings are in accordance with attentive-selection-related brain asymmetry reported by Fink and colleagues [37]. In that study, greater engagement of the left inferior occipital cortex was found during attention directed to local stimulus features, while globally directed attention activated the right lingual gyrus. Moreover, the number of attentional switches between hierarchical levels (in a divided attention task) co-variated with the activity in the left posterior aspects of the superior temporal gyrus and in the right temporoparietal–occipital junction. This evidence suggests a role of the temporoparietal regions in attentional control for local/global processing, consistent with previous evidence from unilateral brain-damaged patients [42,43]. Finally, partially conflicting evidence was reported in the ERP study by Johannes and colleagues [44]. The authors presented the participants with images representing hierarchically composed non-linguistic stimuli during a divided attention task (detection of a target stimulus at both local and global levels). Target stimuli elicited a larger posterior negative component (Ne, 250–500 ms) which was larger over the left than the right hemisphere for both local and global targets. Global non-targets (distracters) led to an earlier Ne onset during local target processing, suggesting different mechanisms for local/global analysis. At the same time, the asymmetrical distribution on the Ne possibly indicated a predominant role of the left hemisphere in hierarchical stimulus processing.

The present study aimed to further investigate the neural mechanisms underlying object-based visual attention [3,4], under the assumption of a left-hemispheric advantage [28,44]. The EEG (electroencephalography) technique was used, due to its high temporal resolution. Several subprocesses occurring during a target detection task have been previously revealed, indexed by different ERP components modulated (in amplitude and latency) by selective attention. This includes the frontal N2, occipito-temporal N2 (or SN), and centro-parietal P300 responses. These components are interpreted as an index of response inhibition [45], attention allocation [46], and stimulus categorization [47], respectively. Evidence of an earlier effect of visual attention on stimulus processing has also been reported, opening a debate that remains unresolved. While a few authors have claimed an impact of visual attention starting at the level of the extrastriate cortex (i.e., P1 component at 70–75 ms [48]), other authors have reported evidence of a prior modulation of the striate cortex as well (i.e., C1 component at 40–60 ms [49,50]).

Here, 3D graphics were used to create images of three visually comparable (by percentage of non-empty pixels, spatial distribution, etc.) categories of stimuli (wooden dummies, chairs, structures of cubes), which lacked detail. The participants were presented with the stimuli individually displayed at the center of the screen during EEG recordings. At the beginning of each run, they were told which target category required a motor response (button press with the index finger) when perceived between non-target stimuli [51]. Modulation of the amplitude of the N2 (decrease) and P300 (increase) components in response to correctly identified targets (relative to non-targets) was expected over frontal and centro-parietal sites, respectively [45,47]. Moreover, a left asymmetric distribution of the occipito-temporal selection negativity (N2 to target minus non-target) would suggest a predominant role of the left hemisphere in selective visual attention towards objects [30,51]. This hypothesis was also further investigated by applying the standardized weighted low-resolution electromagnetic tomography (swLORETA) inverse solution to estimate the neural sources in the SN time window.

2. Materials and Methods

2.1. Participants

Twenty-nine healthy, right-handed volunteers took part in the present investigation (13 males and 16 females). They were students at the University of Milano-Bicocca (mean schooling: 16.62 years, SD = 2.03) with an average age of 25 years (mean age: 25.10, SD = 4.96). Each volunteer reported no history of drug abuse or neurological illness, and had normal or corrected-to-normal vision. The right-handedness was assessed using the Italian version of the Edinburgh Handedness Inventory (mean index score: 0.79, SD = 0.17). The experiments were conducted with the understanding and the written consent of each volunteer. The study was conducted in accordance with the Declaration of Helsinki, and the protocol was approved by the Ethics Committee of the University of Milano-Bicocca (protocol number 0000273/14).

2.2. Stimuli

The stimulus set consisted of 240 different color images created as 3D graphics using Blender software v 2.79. The images depicted wooden dummies (80 stimuli), structures of cubes (80 stimuli), and chairs (80 stimuli) on white backgrounds (see Figure 1). The stimuli were composed of modular structures (cylindrical for the dummies, cubical for the cubes, and rectangular for the chair) which lacked detail (i.e., face, hair, hands/feet in the case of the wooden dummies) and were characterized by a light wood-like texture. This method was illustrated in a previous study by our research group [51]. Presently, 16 models were designed for each of the three stimulus categories (i.e., a mannequin with: both arms at side, left arm extended forwards) and then rotated around the vertical/longitudinal z-axis (0°, ±20°, ±40°). For each model, five points of view were obtained. This increased the visual variety and reduced eventual habituation effects due to stimulus repetition (3 types × 16 models × 5 rotations = 240 stimuli). The stimulus categories were balanced for stimulus distribution in the four quadrants of the visual field. The maximum size of the stimuli was 3.75 × 3.95 cm, subtending visual angles of 1° 53' × 1° 59'. No difference in stimulus luminance ($\approx$15.9 cd/m^2, $p = 0.29$) and volume occupation (non-empty pixels: $\approx$10.86%, $p = 0.39$) was revealed by the ANOVAs as a function of stimulus category. Moreover, since each stimulus served as both target and non-target in non-consecutive experimental runs (as illustrated in the following paragraph), there was no difference in mean luminance due to variation in directed attention (target vs. non-target).

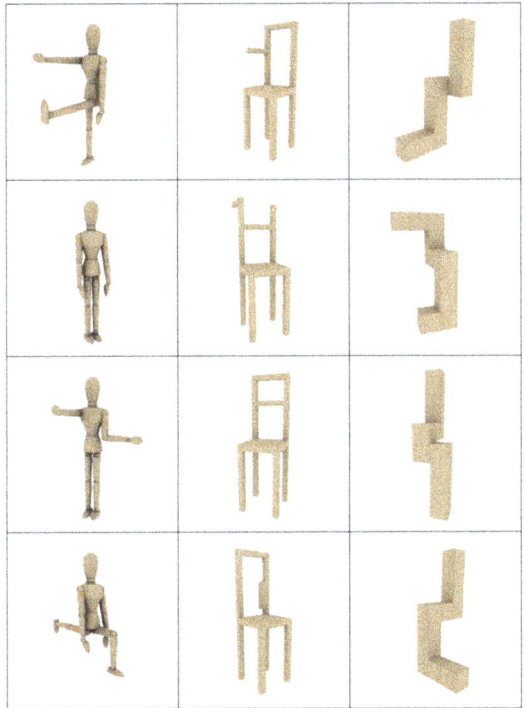

Figure 1. Example of stimuli. The figure shows a few examples of the stimuli used in the present study. Bodies (wooden dummies), objects (chairs), and cube structures were created as 3D graphics. The stimuli set included 240 different images: 16 models for each of the three categories of stimuli, presented from five different points of view obtained by rotating each model along its vertical axis ($-40°$, $-20°$, $0°$, $+20°$, $+40°$).

2.3. Task and Procedure

Once the EEG cap was placed, participants were invited to seat in an acoustically and electrically shielded cabin, facing a high-resolution VGA (video graphics array) computer screen 114 cm away from their eyes. A fixation dot remained at the center of the screen for the entire duration of the experiment. The participants were invited to fixate upon it in order to minimize motion artifacts (i.e., eye gazes, blinks, and body movements) during EEG recording. The stimulus presentation was performed using Eevoke v2.2 (ANT Nneuro, Hengelo, The Netherlands). Each trial consisted of an image centrally displayed for 500 ms and followed by an empty, isoluminant white background for 900 ms ± 100 ms (inter-stimulus interval, ISI). Each of the 240 images was repeated twice during the experiment (in non-consecutive runs) and presented in both upright and upside-down orientations, for a total of 960 stimuli. An experimental run included 80 trials in a pseudo-randomized order, counterbalanced for the type of stimulus (bodies, cubes, chair) and orientation (upright, upside-down). Twelve different runs were created and presented in pseudo-randomized and counterbalanced order to the participants. Before the beginning of the EEG recording, the participants were provided with the experimental instructions (printed and standardized) and engaged in practical training (using two additional runs) to familiarize them with both the task and setting. The participants were asked to identify a specific target stimulus, regardless of the orientation, with a button press on a joypad using the index finger (see Figure 2). The target was verbally indicated by the experimenter at the beginning of each run and represented one-third of the total images displayed in that run. The left and right hand were used alternatively between runs, and the order was counterbalanced across volunteers. All the participants were blinded to the goal of the study and the stimulus proprieties.

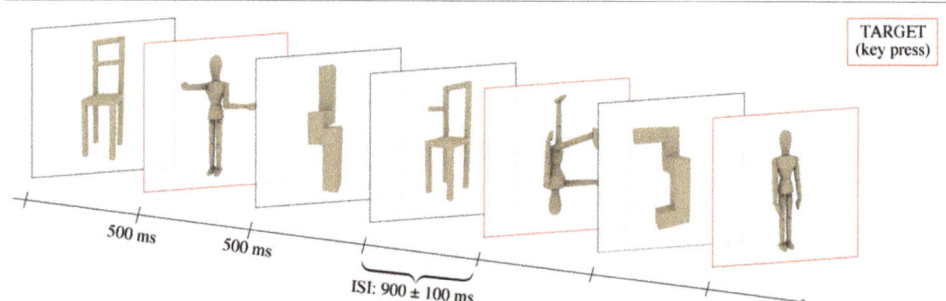

Figure 2. Timescale of the experimental design. The stimuli were presented for 500 ms at the center of the screen, separated by an ISI (inter-stimulus interval) of 900 ± 100 ms. The participants were instructed to recognize a specific target category (i.e., bodies, as illustrated by the red squares in the present figure), indicated at the beginning of each run, by button press.

2.4. EEG Recording and Data Analysis

EEG data were recorded using a standard EEG cap with 128 electrodes located according to the 10–5 International System [52] using EEProbe v2.2 software (ANT Nneuro, Hengelo, The Netherlands). The sampling rate was 512 Hz, and averaged mastoids represented the reference electrode. Electrooculograms (EOG) were also collected. The impedance of the electrodes was maintained below 5 kΩ. The EEGs and EOGs were amplified and subjected to a half-amplitude band-pass filter (0.16–70 Hz, 50 Hz notch). An automated artefact rejection procedure was used to remove EEG segments marked by eye movements (saccades and blinks), muscle-related potentials, or amplifier blockages. Peak-to-peak amplitudes superior to 50 µV were considered artefacts. Trials containing errors (non-targets wrongly indicated as targets) and omissions (wrongly unrecognized targets) were also manually discharged. EEG epochs were synchronized with the stimulus onset. ERPs were averaged, considering −100 ms before the stimulus onset and 1000 ms after the onset. They were subjected to a band-pass filter of 0.16–30 Hz. ERPs were identified and measured with reference to the average baseline voltage, computed as the 100 ms before the stimulus onset. The electrode sites and ERPs' latency were chosen based on the maximum amplitude reached by the components of interest [53] and in accordance with previous literature [45–47]. For the purposes of the present manuscript, only the stimuli presented in the upright orientation were considered (50% of all trials). This avoided any possible confounding effect lead by the inversion of stimuli depicting bodies but not objects [51,54,55]. ERP averages were computed as a function of attention, electrodes, and hemisphere factors. The two levels of the attention factor (target, non-target) were obtained by collapsing all the target and non-target images, respectively, regardless of the content (to increase the EEG signal-noise ratio).

The mean area voltage of the N2 component was measured at AFp3h, AFp4h, AFF1, AFF2, F1, and F2 electrode sites during the 225–265 ms time window (see Figure 3). The mean area voltage of the selection negativity (SN) component was measured at P9, P10, PPO9h, PPO10h, PO7, and PO8 electrode sites during the 240–280 ms time window. The mean area voltage of the P300 component was measured at CPz, Pz, and POz electrode sites during the 350–450 ms time window. The N2 and SN data were subjected to multifactorial repeated measures ANOVA with three within-group factors, including: attention (non-target, target), electrode (three levels depending on the ERP component of interest), and hemisphere (left, right). The P300 data were subjected to multifactorial repeated measures ANOVA with two within-group factors, including attention (non-target, target), and electrode (CPz, Pz, POz) factors. Multiple comparisons were computed using Tukey's post-hoc tests; all the ANOVAs were performed using Statistica software (version 10, Tulsa, OK, USA) by StatSoft.

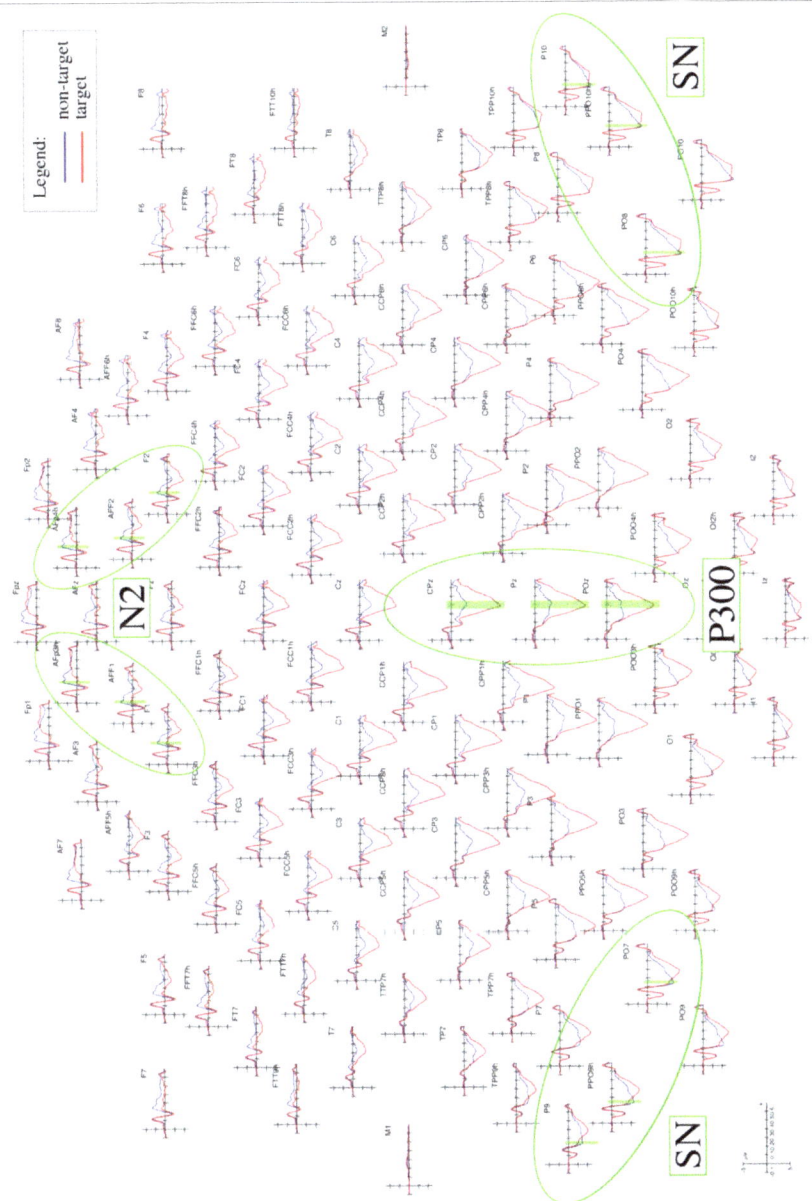

Figure 3. Grand average event-related potential (ERP) waveforms recorded over the scalp. Grand average waveforms (ERPs) recorded over the entire scalp (128 electrodes). The red lines represent the evoked response to target stimuli, while the blue lines represent the evoked response to non-target stimuli. The electrode sites where the three components of interest (N2, SN, and P300) reached the maximum peak are shown by the green circles. The time windows in which the N2 (225–265 ms), SN (240–280 ms), and P300 (350–450 ms) were analyzed are highlighted by the green areas.

Standardized weighted low-resolution electromagnetic tomography (swLORETA) was applied to the difference waves obtained by subtracting the ERPs for the non-target stimuli from those elicited by target stimuli in the SN time window (240–280 ms). LORETA, which is a discrete linear solution to the inverse EEG problem, corresponds to the 3D distribution of neuronal electric activity that yields maximum similarity (i.e., maximum synchronization) in terms of orientation and strength between neighboring neuronal populations (represented by adjacent voxels). In this study, an improved version of the sLORETA (standardized low-resolution electromagnetic tomography) was used, which incorporates a singular value decomposition-based lead field weighting (swLORETA) [56]. The following characteristics for source space were included: five points of grid spacing (the distance between two calculation points) and estimated SNR (Signal-to-Noise Ratio defines the regularization; a higher SNR value leads to less regularization and less blurred results) equal to three. The source reconstruction was performed on group data to identify statistically significant active electromagnetic dipoles ($p < 0.05$).

The accuracy (percentage of hits), reaction times (RTs), and errors (percentage of wrong responses to non-targets) were also recorded and measured. Repeated measures ANOVAs were performed on the mean RTs, and percentages of hits and errors with one within-group factor: hand (left, right).

3. Results

3.1. Behavioral Results

3.1.1. Accuracy

The mean accuracy (HITs) reached the 99.5% level and no difference as a function of handedness was shown ($p = 0.41$). The error rate, intended as the number of non-target stimuli wrongly identified as targets, reached 0.9%, with no difference between the right and left hand ($p = 0.62$).

3.1.2. Reaction Times

The ANOVA performed on the reaction times (RTs) showed an almost significant trend ($F(1,28) = 3.697$, $p = 0.06$, $\eta_p^2 = 0.12$) towards a faster response with the right hand (420 ms, SE: 5.96) relative to the left hand (429 ms, SE: 8.15).

3.2. Electrophysiological Results

3.2.1. Anterior N2 (225–265 ms)

The ANOVA performed on the amplitude values of the N2 component revealed a significant main effect of attention ($F(1,28) = 59.864$, $p < 0.0001$, $\eta_p^2 = 0.68$). The negativity was larger in response to non-target stimuli (−2.24 µV, SE: 0.63) relative to the target stimuli (−0.18 µV, SE: 0.72).

Furthermore, a significant interaction between attention and electrode factors ($F(2,56) = 49.215$, $p < 0.0001$, $\eta_p^2 = 0.64$) was confirmed, with a larger frontal N2 elicited by non-target (compared with target) stimuli at all the electrode site considered ($p < 0.001$). Moreover, the N2 measured at AFp3h–AFp4h was significantly different from those measured at AFF1–AFF2 and F1–F2 in response to both target and non-target ($p < 0.001$) stimuli. At the same time, no difference in the N2 amplitude was found between AFF1–AFF2 and F1–F2 ($p = 0.99$) electrode sites. In addition, the N2 recorded at the AFp3h–AFp4h prefrontal sites (non-target minus target: −2.73 µV was more sensitive to the attentive modulation compared with the N2 at AFF1–AFF2 (non-target minus target: −1.85 µV) and F1–F2 (non-target minus target: −1.59 µV) frontal sites (see Figure 4).

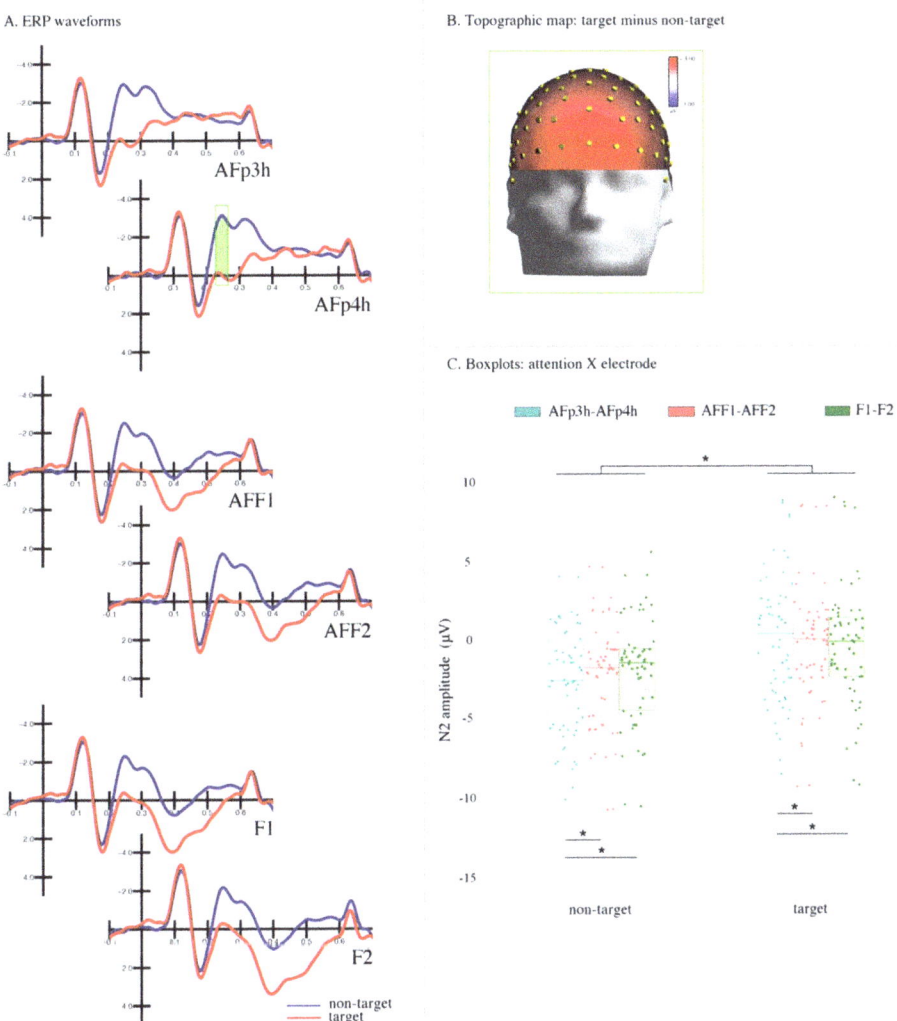

Figure 4. N2 component. (**A**) The grand average ERP waveforms recorded at frontal sites. The correctly recognized targets (in red) relative to non-target stimuli (in blue) led to a reduction of the amplitude of the N2 response between 225–265 ms (area highlighted in green). (**B**) The topographic map (front view) of voltage distribution in the P300 time window (350–450 ms) computed as the difference wave target minus non-target. The positive values are represented in red, while the negative values are represented in blue. (**C**) The boxplots relative to the significant attention X electrode interaction. The N2 response to target (compared with no-target) stimuli was smaller at all electrode sites.

3.2.2. Selection Negativity (240–280 ms)

The ANOVA performed on the amplitude values of the occipito-temporal selection negativity (SN) potential showed a significant main effect of the attention factor ($F(1,28) = 8.512$, $p < 0.007$, $\eta_p^2 = 0.23$).

The SN was more negative in response to target (4.32 µV, SE: 0.51) relative to non-target (4.85 µV, SE: 0.49) stimuli (see Figure 5).

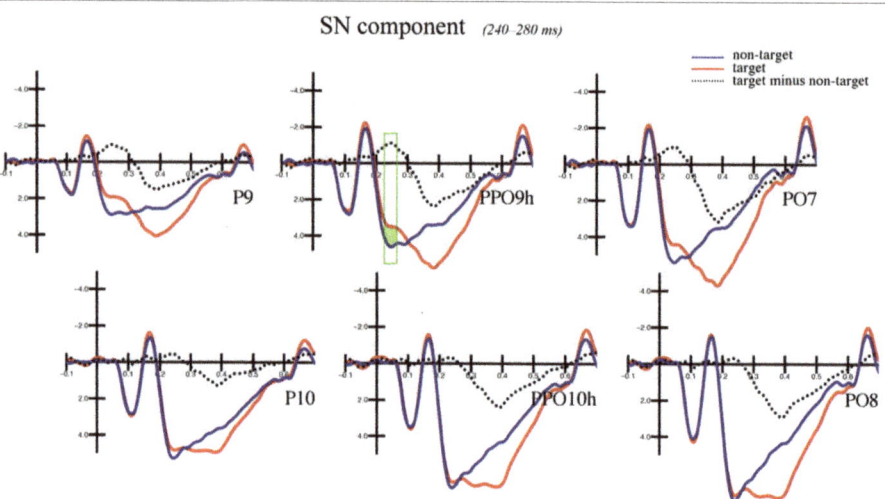

Figure 5. Selection negativity (SN) component: grand average ERP waveforms. The figure illustrates the grand average ERP waveforms recorded at occipito-temporal sites. The correctly recognized targets (in red) relative to non-target stimuli (in blue) led to more negative values of the SN (selection negativity) response between 240–280 ms (area highlighted in green, which also corresponds to the area under the dotted curve). The top row shows electrode sites over the left hemisphere (P9, PPO9h, and PO7), while the bottom row shows those over the right hemisphere (P10, PPO10h, and PO8).

The SN was also larger over the left hemisphere (3.47 µV, SE: 0.46) compared with the right hemisphere (5.70 µV, SE: 0.57), as shown by the significant effect of hemisphere factor on the SN amplitude ($F(1,28) = 46.414$, $p < 0.0001$, $\eta_p^2 = 0.62$).

Moreover, the significant attention by hemisphere interaction ($F(1,28) = 16.756$, $p < 0.001$, $\eta_p^2 = 0.37$) revealed a more negative SN response to target (relative to non-target) stimuli over the left hemisphere (non-target: 3.92 µV, SE: 0.48; target: 3.02 µV, SE: 0.45; $p < 0.0002$), but not the right hemisphere (non-target: 5.78 µV, SE: 0.55; target: 5.62 µV, SE: 0.61; $p = 0.64$) (see Figures 6 and 7).

Finally, the main effect of the electrode factor ($F(2,56) = 67.7041$, $p < 0.0001$, $\eta_p^2 = 0.71$) showed that the SN amplitude maximally peaked at P9–P10 electrode sites (3.38 µV, SE: 0.49) and gradually reduced at PPO9h–PPO10h (4.86 µV, SE: 0.50) and PO7–PO8 (5.52 µV, SE: 0.52), respectively.

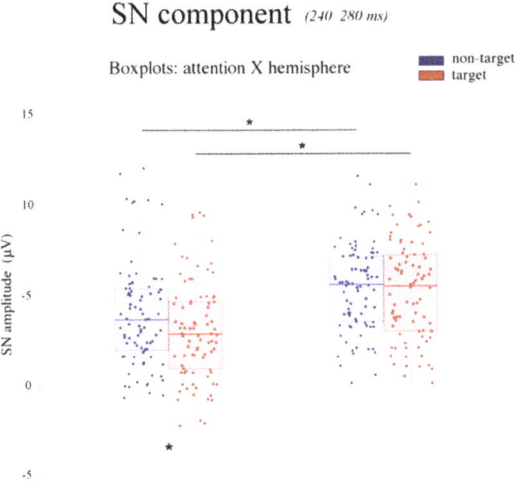

Figure 6. SN component: boxplots. The figure illustrates the boxplots relative to the significant attention by hemisphere interaction for the SN component. The SN was larger over the left than the right hemisphere. Moreover, the SN was more negative in response to the target (in red) compared with non-target (in blue) stimuli over the left, but not the right hemisphere. This evidence suggests that selective attention processes for visual object recognition are left-lateralized.

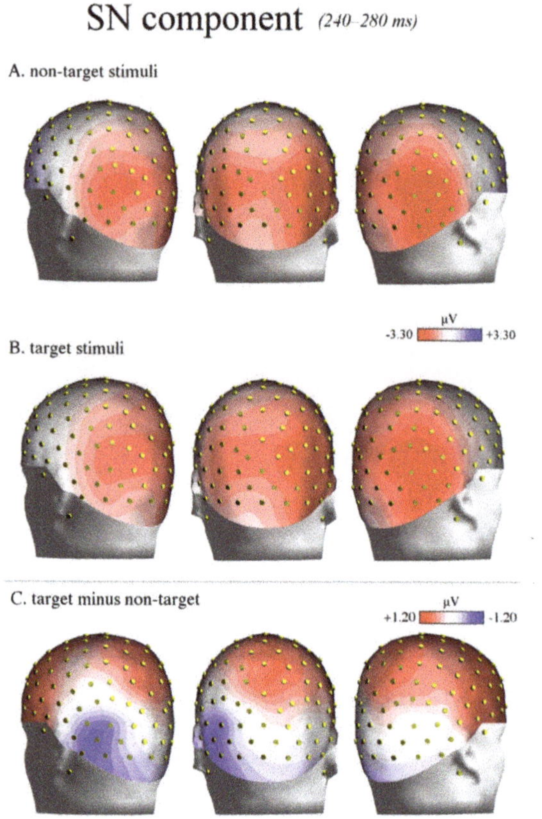

Figure 7. SN component: topographic maps. The figure illustrates the back view of the topographic maps of voltage distribution in the SN time window (240–280 ms) relative to non-target stimuli (**A**), target stimuli (**B**), and the difference wave target minus non-target (**C**). The positive values are represented in red, while the negative values are represented in blue. A strong left-lateralized negative peak is visible at occipito-temporal sites (**C**).

3.2.3. P300 (350–450 ms)

The ANOVA performed on the amplitude values of the P300 component showed a significant main effect of the attention factor ($F(1,28) = 97.756$, $p < 0.0001$, $\eta_p^2 = 0.78$). The positivity evoked by the target stimuli (8.95 µV, SE: 0.77) was larger than that evoked by non-target stimuli (2.78 µV, SE: 0.46), as can be seen in Figure 8.

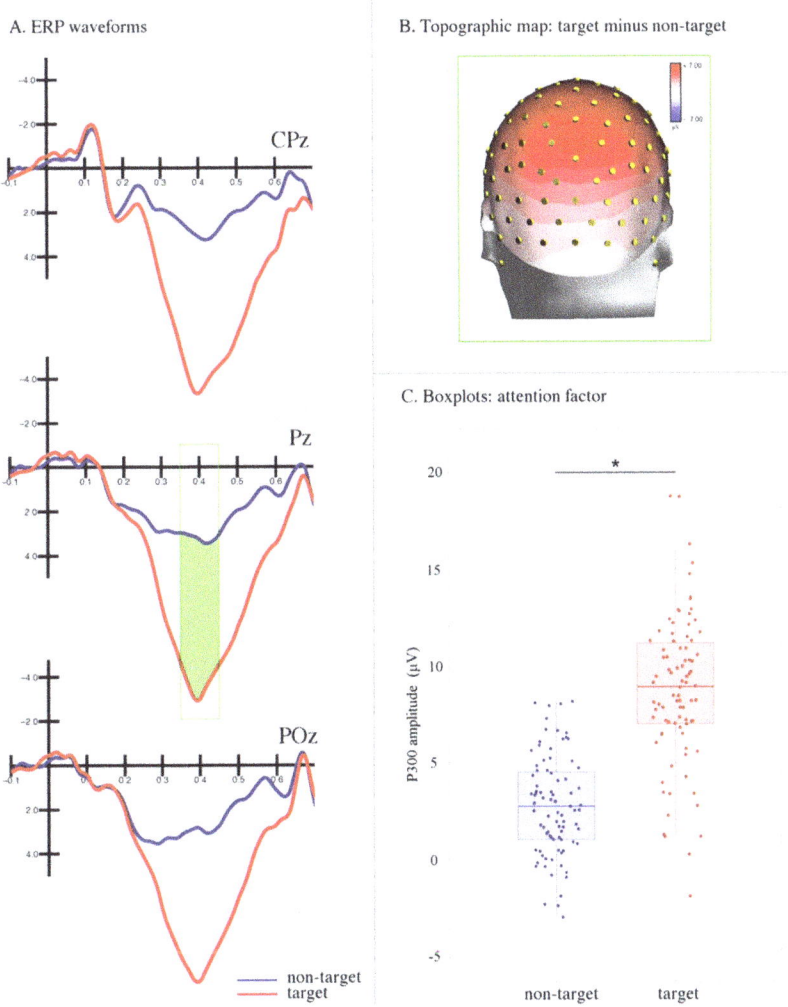

Figure 8. P300 component. (**A**) The grand average ERP waveforms recorded at centro-parietal midline sites. The correctly recognized targets (in red) relative to non-target stimuli (in blue) elicited a larger P300 response between 350–450 ms (area highlighted in green). (**B**) The topographic map (back view) of voltage distribution in the P300 time window (350–450 ms) computed as the difference wave target minus non-target. The positive values are represented in red, while the negative values are represented in blue. (**C**) The boxplots relative to the significant main effect of the attention factor.

3.2.4. swLORETA Source Reconstruction (240–280 ms)

The swLORETA inverse solution investigated the cortical sources of the bioelectrical activity recorded over the scalp underlying selective attention processes for object recognition. For this purpose, the source reconstruction was applied to the difference wave obtained by subtracting the ERP evoked by non-target stimuli from those elicited by target stimuli in the SN time window (240–280 ms). A list of the estimated active electromagnetic dipoles can be found in Table 1. The main dipoles were located in the medial frontal gyrus (BA 11) and right anterior cingulate cortex (BA 24). The uncus (BA 28/36) was also bilaterally engaged, together with the left middle/superior temporal (BA 22) and inferior frontal/precentral (BA 6/9) gyri (see Figure 9).

Table 1. List of estimated electromagnetic dipoles.

Magnitude	T-x (mm)	T-y (mm)	T-z (mm)	Hem	Lobe	Gyrus	BA	Function
18.2	1.5	38.2	−17.9	R	F	MedFG	11	Attentive selection
15.3	1.5	35.3	5.3	R	Lim	ACC	24	
5.5	−38.5	2.4	29.4	L	F	IFG/PrecGyrus	6/9	
16.0	−28.5	−8	−28.9	L	Lim	Uncus	28	Affective response
15.8	21.2	−0.6	−28.2	R	Lim	Uncus	36	
12.8	−48.5	−36.6	−1.3	L	T	MTG/STG	22	

List of the electromagnetic dipoles estimated in response to target minus non-target stimuli in the SN time window (240–280 ms) according to swLORETA, with the relative Talairach coordinates. (Legend: Hem—hemisphere, MedFG—medial frontal gyrus, ACC—anterior cingulate cortex, IFG—inferior frontal/precentral gyrus, MTG/STG—middle/superior temporal gyrus, T—temporal lobe, F—frontal lobe, Lim—limbic system, BA—Brodmann's area, R—right, L—left).

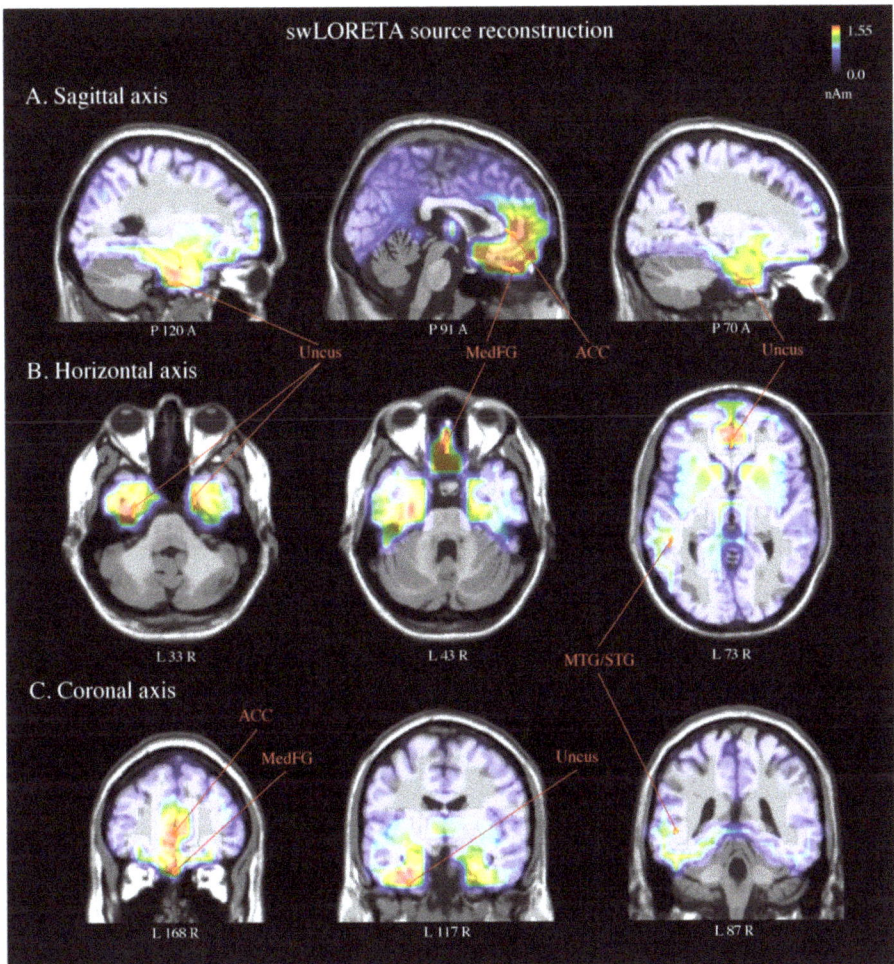

Figure 9. Standardized weighted low-resolution electromagnetic tomography (swLORETA) source reconstruction of surface potentials in the SN time windows. SwLORETA performed on the grand-average waveforms of the difference wave (target minus non-target) in the time window of the SN component (240–280 ms). The sagittal (**A**), horizontal (**B**), and coronal (**C**) anatomical planes of the brain are shown. The engagement of limbic regions is visible, which includes the right anterior cingulate cortex (ACC, BA 24), medial frontal gyrus (MedFG, BA 11), and uncus, bilaterally (BA 28/36). Active dipoles in the left middle/superior temporal gyrus (MTG/STG, BA 22) and inferior frontal/precentral gyrus (IFG, BA 9/6) are also shown. The strongest magnitude values of the signal (nAm) are presented in red.

4. Discussion

The present ERP study investigated the time course and neural correlates of object-based attention, under the assumption of left-hemispheric dominance. For this purpose, healthy, right-handed participants were presented with 3D graphic images depicting the shapes of different categories of stimuli (wooden dummies, chairs, structures of cubes) which lacked detail. They were instructed to pay attention to and detect one given target category (singularly and centrally presented) among non-targets by emitting a motor response (button press). As visible in Figure 3, three main ERP components

(N2, SN, and P300) were shown to be sensitive to selective attention in different time windows, likely highlighting different the cognitive processes involved in recognition of the target objects.

The anterior N2 was the first potential that was modulated by the attentive selection (225–265 ms). The amplitude of this negativity was reduced in response to the target images when compared with the non-targets. Similar results have been previously reported during go/no-go tasks. A larger N2 has been found for non-target (relative to target) item tasks that require response inhibition (no-go) in terms of both actual [45] and imagined [57] motor acts (i.e., button press). This interpretation is supported by source reconstruction studies that have localized the neural generators of the N2 in the anterior cingulate cortex (ACC [58]). The ACC has been associated with cognitive control, as shown by several imaging investigations in both healthy and clinical (i.e., Huntington's disease) individuals [59,60]. The N2 has also been proposed as an index of conflict monitoring [61] and is modulated by stimulus novelty [62], category [63,64], and mismatch [65]. In the present study, the identification of non-target images, which represented two-thirds of the stimuli, required no actual finger movements. Hence, the relative decrease in the N2 amplitude can be considered a correlate of motor inhibition [66]. For instance, in the study by Proverbio and colleagues [66], the participants were presented with four gratings of different spatial frequencies briefly displayed in the four quadrants of the visual field. They were instructed to respond to a target combination of spatial frequency and space location. When compared with the non-targets, the pseudo-targets (stimuli close in spatial frequency to the target and falling within the attended quadrant) elicited both a larger frontal motor N2 and a larger negative prefrontal potential (370–430 ms). This evidence was interpreted as an index of the response inhibition and top-down cognitive control required for irrelevant information suppression. Finally, no hemispheric difference was found here at this stage of stimulus processing (N2 time window). This result is consistent with the increased power in the theta frequency band that has been previously reported at midline frontal scalp sites during target detection tasks [67]. The medial prefrontal cortex has been proposed as a possible neural generator of this effect (i.e., ACC [68]).

Moving forward at the temporal level, the analyses of selection negativity (or posterior N2) response (240–280 ms) revealed an increased amplitude over occipito-temporal areas elicited by target relative to non-target stimuli. This effect is illustrated in Figure 5, which reports the grand average ERP waveforms recorded over posterior sites. The SN was typically obtained subtracting the posterior N2 elicited by non-target stimuli from that evoked by target stimuli. It is considered an index of visual attentive selection processes [46], as it shows sensitivity to several target stimulus features (or a combination of them), including color [69,70], orientation [71], spatial frequency [41,72], and shape [73]. Thus, in the present study, the modulation of the SN may have indicated non-spatial attention allocation towards the specific stimulus shape required for object recognition, consistent with previous evidence [74]. Furthermore, the maximum amplitude of the SN was reached over occipito-temporal scalp sites. The location was compatible with the modulation of associative visual cortex previously reported in several imaging studies on non-spatial attention [3,4].

More importantly, the modulation of the SN was specifically visible over the left but not the right hemisphere, as shown by the topographic maps of voltage distribution depicted in Figure 7 (see also Figure 6). This evidence is consistent with previous ERP studies on shape [51] and color detection [30], as well as local (vs. global) stimulus information processing [32,41] and illusory contour perception [31]. For instance, in a previous study by our research group [51], the participants were presented with images representing upright and inverted bodies (wooden dummies) and structures of cubes. They were instructed to attend to one of the two categories of stimuli (by button press), regardless of the orientation. The occipito-temporal SN was shown to be sensitive to the orientation of the human body shape, being larger in response to the inverted (than upright) body targets. This result likely indicated increased attentive processes for body recognition when presented in non-standard orientations. The negative response was also overall larger over the left than the right hemisphere. This evidence possibly suggests a predominant role of the left hemisphere in shape-related attentive selection processes. It also extends previous findings [30] on conjoined color and shape processing.

These results are also consistent with those reported by Zani and Proverbio [72] in their attentional task (relative to spatial frequency). In that study, the relevant/target (relative to the irrelevant) stimuli elicited larger ERP components at both occipital (N165 and P3b) and frontal (LP, long latency positivity) scalp sites over the left but not the right hemisphere. In another study, larger negativity (N2) was elicited by the perception of illusory contours of a Kanizsa square over the left occipital regions [31], consistent with the idea of left-sided non-spatial feature selection and local (vs. global) stimulus processing [36,37].

Furthermore, the swLORETA inverse solution was applied in this study to the difference wave target minus non-target to estimate the neural sources of the EEG signals in the SN time window (240–280 ms). Several active dipoles underpinned the left-sided SN within a fronto-temporo-limbic network, associated with attentive selection processes. This included the ACC (BA 24), the right medial prefrontal cortex (mPFC, BA 11), and uncus, bilaterally (BA 28/36). Several pieces of evidence have linked the ACC and mPFC to cognitive control [75], with the former region specifically involved in performance and conflict monitoring [60,76]. Both the mPFC and uncus (included in the parahippocampal cortices) are part of the affective system of the human brain [77]. Thus, their engagement may also suggest an affective response [78,79] to target stimuli that were correctly identified. More importantly, the swLORETA showed a selective engagement of the superior/middle temporal (STG/MTG, BA 22) and inferior frontal/precentral gyrus (aka IFJ, BA 6/9) in the left hemisphere. A negative correlation between activity in the left STS and response variability has been reported during the perception of oddball (vs. standard) stimuli in healthy (vs. ADHD) volunteers [80]. At the same time, participants with attentional disorders have shown reduced response to oddball (vs. standard) stimuli in the superior and medial temporal lobe (along with the insula and basal ganglia). The STG/MTG is also considered a key node of an amodal semantic hub, together with the temporal poles [81]. Its involvement may be explained in terms of accessing the knowledge (i.e., name [82]) of the target stimulus category (i.e., bodies, chairs). Finally, previous evidence indicated a role of the IFJ (inferior frontal junction) in the top-down modulation of the inferior temporal cortices when a target object was attended [14,19]. The engagement of left frontal regions (i.e., BA 6) has also been reported during executive (conflict) control, together with the ACC [83]. Overall, these findings seem to support the hypothesis of effective engagement of the left hemisphere in selective attentional processes required by feature recognition (i.e., shape) for objects centrally presented in the visual field [4,27,64,84].

Lastly, the effects of attention were also visible at later latencies (350–450 ms) over centro-parietal sites. An increased positive (P300) response to target stimuli was found when compared with non-target stimuli, which likely suggests the recognition of the target object. The P300 response is generally interpreted as an index of item categorization, updating of the mental representation of stimulus context, and visual awareness [47,85–87]. The P300 is typically maximal in response to stimuli that are identical to a target. Its neural generators have been estimated within the parietal (i.e., inferior parietal lobule, posterior parietal cortex) and inferior temporal regions [85]. At the same time, non-target stimuli that share some visual features with the target stimulus elicit a gradient of increasing P300s as a function of enhanced similarity [88]. Moreover, the maximum peak of this ERP component is concurrent with the RTs when an accurate but fast response is required. In our study, the average RT to targets was 425 ms, included within the P300 time window considered (350–450 ms). A strong tendency towards a faster response with the right (compared with the left) hand was also found. Previous evidence has shown that simple RTs are not often affected by the hand dominance [89]. This result is also consistent with the hypothesis of left-hemispheric dominance for action selection [90,91]. Hence, the right-handedness of the participants can only partially account for the right-hand advantage reported here. It is important to report the case of target detection during spatial attention modulation. Faster RTs have been found for stimuli occurring in the visual field ipsilateral (relative to the contralateral) to the response hand [92–94]. This difference in RTs has been ascribed to the interhemispheric transfer time through the corpus callosum. In the present study, the faster button press obtained with the right hand may have suggested a faster intrahemispheric (vs. interhemispheric) transfer between the contralateral (left) motor cortex and attention-related areas within the left hemisphere. This interpretation, which certainly requires further investigation, is consistent with the assumption of a left-hemispheric dominance in attentive processes for object selection.

A few aspects need further consideration and suggest circumspection in the interpretation of the present results. Firstly, our experimental design likely prevented overt spatial attentional shifting (i.e., central stimuli presentation, stimuli with equal dimensions and number of non-empty pixels, and comparable distribution in the four hemi-quadrants of the visual field), and EEG epochs reporting eye movement were discharged. However, it is also true that covert attentional shifting may have occurred. The introduction of a secondary task would be useful in order to entirely disentangle the contribution of spatial and non-spatial attention [95,96]. This would also strengthen our object-based interpretation of the attention-related results. Secondly, despite a clear left-lateralization of the SN component in our experimental group, individual differences between participants may exist. It is, therefore, desirable for future investigations to account for such variability. Finally, it is necessary to point out that the EEG technique is characterized by a non-ideal spatial resolution [97] compared to functional neuroimaging (i.e., fMRI). This issue can be partially overcome using by high-density caps and state-of-the-art source reconstruction algorithms [98]. Many studies have shown good reliability of swLORETA, since the estimated dipoles were consistent with brain activity found in previous fMRI investigations [99,100]. Caution is still advised when reconstructed neural sources are considered, even when they are in support of main ERP findings, as was the case for the present study.

5. Conclusions

In conclusion, these pieces of evidence seem to support the models of selective attention focused on objects as a whole. In our study, the recognition of the shape of a target object that lacked detail modulated several ERP components associated with motor inhibition (N2), attentive selection (SN), and item categorization (P300) processes at different time latencies and scalp distribution. A fronto-temporo-limbic network seems to underlie such object-based attentive processes. The scalp distribution of the SN component and related neural sources (i.e., left MTG/STG and IFJ) were consistent with the hypothesis of a left-hemispheric advantage for non-spatial visual attention. The present results integrate the previous literature on brain asymmetries relative to attentional control for local and global levels of stimulus processing. They seem to suggest a specific role of the left hemisphere in attentive selection and, thus, recognition of objects and relative features.

Author Contributions: Conceptualization and Methodology, A.O. and A.M.P.; Investigation, A.O.; Formal Analysis, A.O.; Writing – Original Draft Preparation, A.O.; Writing – Review & Editing, A.M.P.; Supervision, A.M.P.

Funding: The authors received no specific funding for this study.

Conflicts of Interest: Authors declare no conflict of interest.

References

1. Mangun, G.R. Neural mechanisms of visual selective attention. *Psychophysiology* **1995**, *32*, 4–18. [CrossRef]
2. Posner, M.I. Orienting of attention. *Q. J. Exp. Psychol.* **1980**, *32*, 3–25. [CrossRef]
3. O'Craven, K.M.; Downing, P.E.; Kanwisher, N. fMRI evidence for objects as the units of attentional selection. *Nature* **1999**, *401*, 584. [CrossRef] [PubMed]
4. Serences, J.T.; Schwarzbach, J.; Courtney, S.M.; Golay, X.; Yantis, S. Control of object-based attention in human cortex. *Cereb. Cortex* **2004**, *14*, 1346–1357. [CrossRef] [PubMed]
5. Blaser, E.; Pylyshyn, Z.W.; Holcombe, A.O. Tracking an object through feature space. *Nature* **2000**, *408*, 196. [CrossRef] [PubMed]
6. Corbetta, M.; Miezin, F.M.; Dobmeyer, S.; Shulman, G.L.; Petersen, S.E. Attentional modulation of neural processing of shape, color, and velocity in humans. *Science* **1990**, *248*, 1556–1559. [CrossRef] [PubMed]
7. Desimone, R.; Duncan, J. Neural mechanisms of selective visual attention. *Annu. Rev. Neurosci.* **1995**, *18*, 193–222. [CrossRef]

8. Schoenfeld, M.A.; Hopf, J.M.; Martinez, A.; Mai, H.M.; Sattler, C.; Gasde, A.; Heinze, H.-J.; Hillyard, S.A. Spatio-temporal analysis of feature-based attention. *Cereb. Cortex* **2007**, *17*, 2468–2477. [CrossRef] [PubMed]
9. Corbetta, M.; Shulman, G.L. Control of goal-directed and stimulus-driven attention in the brain. *Nat. Rev. Neurosci.* **2002**, *3*, 201. [CrossRef]
10. Hopfinger, J.B.; Buonocore, M.H.; Mangun, G.R. The neural mechanisms of top-down attentional control. *Nat. Neurosci.* **2000**, *3*, 284. [CrossRef]
11. Stoppel, C.M.; Boehler, C.N.; Sabelhaus, C.; Heinze, H.J.; Hopf, J.M.; Schoenfeld, M.A. Neural mechanisms of spatial-and feature-based attention: A quantitative analysis. *Brain Res.* **2007**, *1181*, 51–60. [CrossRef] [PubMed]
12. Gitelman, D.R.; Nobre, A.C.; Parrish, T.B.; LaBar, K.S.; Kim, Y.H.; Meyer, J.R.; Mesulam, M.M. A large-scale distributed network for covert spatial attention: Further anatomical delineation based on stringent behavioural and cognitive controls. *Brain* **1999**, *122*, 1093–1106. [CrossRef] [PubMed]
13. Giesbrecht, B.; Woldorff, M.G.; Song, A.W.; Mangun, G.R. Neural mechanisms of top-down control during spatial and feature attention. *Neuroimage* **2003**, *19*, 496–512. [CrossRef]
14. Baldauf, D.; Desimone, R. Neural mechanisms of object-based attention. *Science* **2014**, *344*, 424–427. [CrossRef]
15. Kanwisher, N.; McDermott, J.; Chun, M.M. The fusiform face area: A module in human extrastriate cortex specialized for face perception. *J. Neurosci.* **1997**, *17*, 4302–4311. [CrossRef]
16. Epstein, R.; Harris, A.; Stanley, D.; Kanwisher, N. The parahippocampal place area: Recognition, navigation, or encoding? *Neuron* **1999**, *23*, 115–125. [CrossRef]
17. Grossman, E.; Donnelly, M.; Price, R.; Pickens, D.; Morgan, V.; Neighbor, G.; Blake, R. Brain areas involved in perception of biological motion. *J. Cognit. Neurosci.* **2000**, *12*, 711–720. [CrossRef]
18. Corradi-Dell'Acqua, C.; Fink, G.R.; Weidner, R. Selecting category specific visual information: Top-down and bottom-up control of object based attention. *Conscious. Cogn.* **2015**, *35*, 330–341. [CrossRef]
19. Liu, T. Neural representation of object-specific attentional priority. *Neuroimage* **2016**, *129*, 15–24. [CrossRef]
20. Valdes-Sosa, M.; Bobes, M.A.; Rodriguez, V.; Pinilla, T. Switching attention without shifting the spotlight: Object-based attentional modulation of brain potentials. *J. Cognit. Neurosci.* **1998**, *10*, 137–151. [CrossRef]
21. Corbetta, M.; Kincade, M.J.; Lewis, C.; Snyder, A.Z.; Sapir, A. Neural basis and recovery of spatial attention deficits in spatial neglect. *Nat. Neurosci.* **2005**, *8*, 1603. [CrossRef] [PubMed]
22. Corbetta, M.; Shulman, G.L. Spatial neglect and attention networks. *Annu. Rev. Neurosci.* **2011**, *34*, 569–599. [CrossRef] [PubMed]
23. De Schotten, M.T.; Dell'Acqua, F.; Forkel, S.J.; Simmons, A.; Vergani, F.; Murphy, D.G.; Catani, M. A lateralized brain network for visuospatial attention. *Nat. Neurosci.* **2011**, *14*, 1245. [CrossRef] [PubMed]
24. Shulman, G.L.; Pope, D.L.; Astafiev, S.V.; McAvoy, M.P.; Snyder, A.Z.; Corbetta, M. Right hemisphere dominance during spatial selective attention and target detection occurs outside the dorsal frontoparietal network. *J. Neurosci.* **2010**, *30*, 3640–3651. [CrossRef]
25. Pardo, J.V.; Fox, P.T.; Raichle, M.E. Localization of a human system for sustained attention by positron emission tomography. *Nature* **1991**, *349*, 61. [CrossRef]
26. Whitehead, R. Right hemisphere processing superiority during sustained visual attention. *J. Cognit. Neurosci.* **1991**, *3*, 329–334. [CrossRef]
27. Georgopoulos, A.P.; Whang, K.; Georgopoulos, M.A.; Tagaris, G.A.; Amirikian, B.; Richter, W.; Kim, S.; Uğurbil, K. Functional magnetic resonance imaging of visual object construction and shape discrimination: Relations among task, hemispheric lateralization, and gender. *J. Cognit. Neurosci.* **2001**, *13*, 72–89. [CrossRef]
28. Milham, M.P.; Banich, M.T.; Webb, A.; Barad, V.; Cohen, N.J.; Wszalek, T.; Kramer, A.F. The relative involvement of anterior cingulate and prefrontal cortex in attentional control depends on nature of conflict. *Cognit. Brain Res.* **2001**, *12*, 467–473. [CrossRef]
29. Proverbio, A.M. Left and Right Hemisphere Role for Selective and Sustained Attention: An Electrophysiological Approach. Ph.D. Thesis, University of Padua, Padua, India, 1993.
30. Proverbio, A.M.; Burco, F.; del Zotto, M.; Zani, A. Blue piglets? Electrophysiological evidence for the primacy of shape over color in object recognition. *Cognit. Brain Res.* **2004**, *18*, 288–300. [CrossRef]
31. Proverbio, A.M.; Zani, A. Electrophysiological indexes of illusory contours perception in humans. *Neuropsychologia* **2002**, *40*, 479–491. [CrossRef]
32. Gable, P.A.; Poole, B.D.; Cook, M.S. Asymmetrical hemisphere activation enhances global-local processing. *Brain Cognit.* **2013**, *83*, 337–341. [CrossRef] [PubMed]

33. Navon, D. Forest before trees: The precedence of global features in visual perception. *Cognit. Psychol.* **1977**, *9*, 353–383. [CrossRef]
34. Proverbio, A.M.; Minniti, A.; Zani, A. Electrophysiological evidence of a perceptual precedence of global vs. local visual information. *Cognit. Brain Res.* **1998**, *6*, 321–334. [CrossRef]
35. Van Kleeck, M.H. Hemispheric differences in global versus local processing of hierarchical visual stimuli by normal subjects: New data and a meta-analysis of previous studies. *Neuropsychologia* **1989**, *27*, 1165–1178. [CrossRef]
36. Yamaguchi, S.; Yamagata, S.; Kobayashi, S. Cerebral asymmetry of the "top-down" allocation of attention to global and local features. *J. Neurosci.* **2000**, *20*, RC72. [CrossRef]
37. Fink, G.R.; Halligan, P.W.; Marshall, J.C.; Frith, C.D.; Frackowiak, R.S.J.; Dolan, R.J. Where in the brain does visual attention select the forest and the trees? *Nature* **1996**, *382*, 626. [CrossRef]
38. Baas, J.M.; Kenemans, J.L.; Mangun, G.R. Selective attention to spatial frequency: An ERP and source localization analysis. *Clin. Neurophysiol.* **2002**, *113*, 1840–1854. [CrossRef]
39. Proverbio, A.M.; Zani, A.; Avella, C. Differential activation of multiple current sources of foveal VEPs as a function of spatial frequency. *Brain Topogr.* **1996**, *9*, 59–68. [CrossRef]
40. Proverbio, A.M.; Zani, A.; Avella, C. Hemispheric asymmetries for spatial frequency discrimination in a selective attention task. *Brain Cognit.* **1997**, *34*, 311–320. [CrossRef]
41. Martınez, A.; Di Russo, F.; Anllo-Vento, L.; Hillyard, S.A. Electrophysiological analysis of cortical mechanisms of selective attention to high and low spatial frequencies. *Clin. Neurophysiol.* **2001**, *112*, 1980–1998. [CrossRef]
42. Robertson, L.C.; Lamb, M.R. Neuropsychological contributions to theories of part/whole organization. *Cognit. Psychol.* **1991**, *23*, 299–330. [CrossRef]
43. Robertson, L.C.; Lamb, M.R.; Knight, R.T. Effects of lesions of temporal-parietal junction on perceptual and attentional processing in humans. *J. Neurosci.* **1988**, *8*, 3757–3769. [CrossRef] [PubMed]
44. Johannes, S.; Wieringa, B.M.; Matzke, M.; Münte, T.F. Hierarchical visual stimuli: Electrophysiological evidence for separate left hemispheric global and local processing mechanisms in humans. *Neurosci. Lett.* **1996**, *210*, 111–114. [CrossRef]
45. Patel, S.H.; Azzam, P.N. Characterization of N200 and P300: Selected studies of the event-related potential. *Int. J. Med. Sci.* **2005**, *2*, 147. [CrossRef] [PubMed]
46. Hillyard, S.A.; Anllo-Vento, L. Event-related brain potentials in the study of visual selective attention. *Proc. Natl. Acad. Sci. USA* **1998**, *95*, 781–787. [CrossRef]
47. Polich, J. Updating P300: An integrative theory of P3a and P3b. *Clin. Neurophysiol.* **2007**, *118*, 2128–2148. [CrossRef]
48. Martinez, A.; Anllo-Vento, L.; Sereno, M.I.; Frank, L.R.; Buxton, R.B.; Dubowitz, D.J.; Wong, E.C.; Hinrichs, H.; Heinze, H.J.; Hillyard, S.A. Involvement of striate and extrastriate visual cortical areas in spatial attention. *Nat. Neurosci.* **1999**, *2*, 364. [CrossRef]
49. Proverbio, A.M.; Del Zotto, M.; Zani, A. Electrical neuroimaging evidence that spatial frequency-based selective attention affects V1 activity as early as 40–60 ms in humans. *BMC Neurosci.* **2010**, *11*, 59. [CrossRef]
50. Zani, A.; Proverbio, A.M. Selective attention to spatial frequency gratings affects visual processing as early as 60 msec. poststimulus. *Percept. Motor Skill.* **2009**, *109*, 140–158. [CrossRef]
51. Orlandi, A.; Proverbio, A.M. ERP indices of an orientation-dependent recognition of the human body schema. *Neuropsychologia*. under review.
52. Oostenveld, R.; Praamstra, P. The five percent electrode system for high-resolution EEG and ERP measurements. *Clin. Neurophysiol.* **2001**, *112*, 713–719. [CrossRef]
53. Picton, T.W.; Bentin, S.; Berg, P.; Donchin, E.; Hillyard, S.A.; Johnson, R.; Miller, G.A.; Ritter, W.; Ruchkin, D.S.; Rugg, M.D.; et al. Guidelines for using human event-related potentials to study cognition: Recording standards and publication criteria. *Psychophysiology* **2000**, *37*, 127–152. [CrossRef] [PubMed]
54. Reed, C.L.; Stone, V.E.; Bozova, S.; Tanaka, J. The body-inversion effect. *Psychol. Sci.* **2003**, *14*, 302–308. [CrossRef] [PubMed]
55. Reed, C.L.; Stone, V.E.; Grubb, J.D.; McGoldrick, J.E. Turning configural processing upside down: Part and whole body postures. *J. Exp. Psychol. Hum. Percept. Perform.* **2006**, *32*, 73. [CrossRef] [PubMed]
56. Palmero-Soler, E.; Dolan, K.; Hadamschek, V.; Tass, P.A. swLORETA: A novel approach to robust source localization and synchronization tomography. *Phys. Med. Biol.* **2007**, *52*, 1783–1800. [CrossRef]

57. Angelini, M.; Calbi, M.; Ferrari, A.; Sbriscia-Fioretti, B.; Franca, M.; Gallese, V.; Umiltà, M.A. Motor inhibition during overt and covert actions: An electrical neuroimaging study. *PLoS ONE* **2015**, *10*, e0126800. [CrossRef]
58. Bekker, E.M.; Kenemans, J.L.; Verbaten, M.N. Source analysis of the N2 in a cued Go/NoGo task. *Cognit. Brain Res.* **2005**, *22*, 221–231. [CrossRef]
59. Beste, C.; Saft, C.; Andrich, J.; Gold, R.; Falkenstein, M. Response inhibition in Huntington's disease—A study using ERPs and sLORETA. *Neuropsychologia* **2008**, *46*, 1290–1297. [CrossRef]
60. MacDonald, A.W.; Cohen, J.D.; Stenger, V.A.; Carter, C.S. Dissociating the role of the dorsolateral prefrontal and anterior cingulate cortex in cognitive control. *Science* **2000**, *288*, 1835–1838. [CrossRef]
61. Donkers, F.C.; Van Boxtel, G.J. The N2 in go/no-go tasks reflects conflict monitoring not response inhibition. *Brain Cognit.* **2004**, *56*, 165–176. [CrossRef]
62. Folstein, J.R.; Van Petten, C.; Rose, S.A. Novelty and conflict in the categorization of complex stimuli. *Psychophysiology* **2008**, *45*, 467–479. [CrossRef]
63. Proverbio, A.M.; Del Zotto, M.; Zani, A. The emergence of semantic categorization in early visual processing: ERP indices of animal vs. artifact recognition. *BMC Neurosci.* **2007**, *8*, 24. [CrossRef] [PubMed]
64. Zani, A.; Marsili, G.; Senerchia, A.; Orlandi, A.; Citron, F.M.; Rizzi, E.; Proverbio, A.M. ERP signs of categorical and supra-categorical processing of visual information. *Biol. Psychol.* **2015**, *104*, 90–107. [CrossRef] [PubMed]
65. Folstein, J.R.; Van Petten, C. Influence of cognitive control and mismatch on the N2 component of the ERP: A review. *Psychophysiology* **2008**, *45*, 152–170. [CrossRef] [PubMed]
66. Proverbio, A.M.; Del Zotto, M.; Crotti, N.; Zani, A. A no-go related prefrontal negativity larger to irrelevant stimuli that are difficult to suppress. *Behav. Brain Funct.* **2009**, *5*, 25. [CrossRef]
67. Harper, J.; Malone, S.M.; Bernat, E.M. Theta and delta band activity explain N2 and P3 ERP component activity in a go/no-go task. *Clin. Neurophysiol.* **2014**, *125*, 124–132. [CrossRef]
68. Bokura, H.; Yamaguchi, S.; Kobayashi, S. Electrophysiological correlates for response inhibition in a Go/NoGo task. *Clin. Neurophysiol.* **2001**, *112*, 2224–2232. [CrossRef]
69. Anllo-Vento, L.; Hillyard, S.A. Selective attention to the color and direction of moving stimuli: Electrophysiological correlates of hierarchical feature selection. *Percept. Psychophys.* **1996**, *58*, 191–206. [CrossRef]
70. Müller, M.M.; Keil, A. Neuronal synchronization and selective color processing in the human brain. *J. Cognit. Neurosci.* **2004**, *16*, 503–522. [CrossRef]
71. Proverbio, A.M.; Esposito, P.; Zani, A. Early involvement of the temporal area in attentional selection of grating orientation: An ERP study. *Cognit. Brain Res.* **2002**, *13*, 139–151. [CrossRef]
72. Zani, A.; Proverbio, A.M. ERP signs of early selective attention effects to check size. *Electroen. Clin. Neurophysiol.* **1995**, *95*, 277–292. [CrossRef]
73. Smid, H.G.; Jakob, A.; Heinze, H.J. An event-related brain potential study of visual selective attention to conjunctions of color and shape. *Psychophysiology* **1999**, *36*, 264–279. [CrossRef] [PubMed]
74. Eimer, M. An event-related potential (ERP) study of transient and sustained visual attention to color and form. *Biol. Psychol.* **1997**, *44*, 143–160. [CrossRef]
75. Ridderinkhof, K.R.; Van Den Wildenberg, W.P.; Segalowitz, S.J.; Carter, C.S. Neurocognitive mechanisms of cognitive control: The role of prefrontal cortex in action selection, response inhibition, performance monitoring, and reward-based learning. *Brain Cognit.* **2004**, *56*, 129–140. [CrossRef] [PubMed]
76. Botvinick, M.; Nystrom, L.E.; Fissell, K.; Carter, C.S.; Cohen, J.D. Conflict monitoring versus selection-for-action in anterior cingulate cortex. *Nature* **1999**, *402*, 179. [CrossRef] [PubMed]
77. Patterson, D.W.; Schmidt, L.A. Neuroanatomy of the human affective system. *Brain Cognit.* **2003**, *52*, 24–26. [CrossRef]
78. Proverbio, A.M.; Cozzi, M.; Orlandi, A.; Carminati, M. Error-related negativity in the skilled brain of pianists reveals motor simulation. *Neuroscience* **2017**, *346*, 309–319. [CrossRef]
79. Vocks, S.; Busch, M.; Grönemeyer, D.; Schulte, D.; Herpertz, S.; Suchan, B. Neural correlates of viewing photographs of one's own body and another woman's body in anorexia and bulimia nervosa: An fMRI study. *J. Psychiatr. Neurosci.* **2010**, *35*, 163. [CrossRef]
80. Rubia, K.; Smith, A.B.; Brammer, M.J.; Taylor, E. Temporal lobe dysfunction in medication-naive boys with attention-deficit/hyperactivity disorder during attention allocation and its relation to response variability. *Biol. Psychiatr.* **2007**, *62*, 999–1006. [CrossRef]

81. Visser, M.; Jefferies, E.; Embleton, K.V.; Lambon Ralph, M.A. Both the middle temporal gyrus and the ventral anterior temporal area are crucial for multimodal semantic processing: Distortion-corrected fMRI evidence for a double gradient of information convergence in the temporal lobes. *J. Cognit. Neurosci.* **2012**, *24*, 1766–1778. [CrossRef]
82. Tyler, L.K.; Stamatakis, E.A.; Dick, E.; Bright, P.; Fletcher, P.; Moss, H. Objects and their actions: Evidence for a neurally distributed semantic system. *Neuroimage* **2003**, *18*, 542–557. [CrossRef]
83. Fan, J.; McCandliss, B.D.; Fossella, J.; Flombaum, J.I.; Posner, M.I. The activation of attentional networks. *Neuroimage* **2005**, *26*, 471–479. [CrossRef] [PubMed]
84. Eimer, M. The N2pc component as an indicator of attentional selectivity. *Electroencephalogr. Clin. Neurophysiol.* **1996**, *99*, 225–234. [CrossRef]
85. Bledowski, C.; Prvulovic, D.; Hoechstetter, K.; Scherg, M.; Wibral, M.; Goebel, R.; Linden, D.E. Localizing P300 generators in visual target and distractor processing: A combined event-related potential and functional magnetic resonance imaging study. *J. Neurosci.* **2004**, *24*, 9353–9360. [CrossRef] [PubMed]
86. Orlandi, A.; Proverbio, A.M. Bilateral engagement of the occipito-temporal cortex in response to dance kinematics in experts. *Sci. Rep.* **2019**, *9*, 1000. [CrossRef]
87. Picton, T.W. The P300 wave of the human event-related potential. *J. Clin. Neurophysiol.* **1992**, *9*, 456–479. [CrossRef]
88. Azizian, A.; Freitas, A.L.; Watson, T.D.; Squires, N.K. Electrophysiological correlates of categorization: P300 amplitude as index of target similarity. *Biol. Psychol.* **2006**, *71*, 278–288. [CrossRef]
89. Nisiyama, M.; Ribeiro-do-Valle, L.E. Relative performance of the two hands in simple and choice reaction time tasks. *Braz. J. Med. Biol. Res.* **2014**, *47*, 80–89. [CrossRef]
90. Johnson-Frey, S.H.; Newman-Norlund, R.; Grafton, S.T. A distributed left hemisphere network active during planning of everyday tool use skills. *Cereb. Cortex* **2004**, *15*, 681–695. [CrossRef]
91. Schluter, N.D.; Krams, M.; Rushworth, M.F.S.; Passingham, R.E. Cerebral dominance for action in the human brain: The selection of actions. *Neuropsychologia* **2001**, *39*, 105–113. [CrossRef]
92. Corballis, M.C. Hemispheric interactions in simple reaction time. *Neuropsychologia* **2002**, *40*, 423–434. [CrossRef]
93. Marzi, C.A.; Bisiacchi, P.; Nicoletti, R. Is interhemispheric transfer of visuomotor information asymmetric? Evidence from a meta-analysis. *Neuropsychologia* **1991**, *29*, 1163–1177. [CrossRef]
94. Weber, B.; Treyer, V.; Oberholzer, N.; Jaermann, T.; Boesiger, P.; Brugger, P.; Regard, M.; Buck, A.; Savazzi, S.; Marzi, C.A. Attention and interhemispheric transfer: A behavioral and fMRI study. *J. Cognit. Neurosci.* **2005**, *17*, 113–123. [CrossRef] [PubMed]
95. Soto, D.; Blanco, M.J. Spatial attention and object-based attention: A comparison within a single task. *Vis. Res.* **2004**, *44*, 69–81. [CrossRef] [PubMed]
96. Han, S.; Liu, W.; Yund, E.W.; Woods, D.L. Interactions between spatial attention and global/local feature selection: An ERP study. *Neuroreport* **2000**, *11*, 2753–2758. [CrossRef]
97. Zani, A.; Proverbio, A.M. Cognitive Electrophysiology of Mind and Brain. In *The Cognitive Electrophysiology of Mind and Brain*; Elsevier-Academic Press: Amsterdam, The Netherlands; San Diego, CA, USA, 2003; pp. 3–12.
98. Grech, R.; Cassar, T.; Muscat, J.; Camilleri, K.P.; Fabri, S.G.; Zervakis, M.; Xanthopoulos, P.; Sakkalis, V.; Vanrumste, B. Review on solving the inverse problem in EEG source analysis. *J. Neuroeng. Rehabil.* **2008**, *5*, 25. [CrossRef]
99. Boughariou, J.; Jallouli, N.; Zouch, W.; Slima, M.B.; Hamida, A.B. Spatial resolution improvement of EEG source reconstruction using swLORETA. *IEEE Trans. Nanobiosci.* **2015**, *14*, 734–739. [CrossRef]
100. Cebolla, A.M.; Palmero-Soler, E.; Leroy, A.; Cheron, G. EEG spectral generators involved in motor imagery: A swLORETA Study. *Front. Psychol.* **2017**, *8*, 2133. [CrossRef]

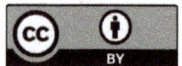

© 2019 by the authors. Licensee MDPI, Basel, Switzerland. This article is an open access article distributed under the terms and conditions of the Creative Commons Attribution (CC BY) license (http://creativecommons.org/licenses/by/4.0/).

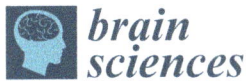

Article

Spatiotemporal Dynamics of Multiple Memory Systems during Category Learning

Kyle K. Morgan [1,2,*], Dagmar Zeithamova [2], Phan Luu [1] and Don Tucker [1,2]

1. Brain Electrophysiology Laboratory Company, Eugene, OR 97403, USA; phan.luu@belco.tech (P.L.); don.tucker@belco.tech (D.T.)
2. Department of Psychology, University of Oregon, Eugene, OR 97403, USA; dasa@uoregon.edu
* Correspondence: kyle.morgan@belco.tech; Tel.: +1-541-525-9798

Received: 6 March 2020; Accepted: 7 April 2020; Published: 9 April 2020

Abstract: The brain utilizes distinct neural mechanisms that ease the transition through different stages of learning. Furthermore, evidence from category learning has shown that dissociable memory systems are engaged, depending on the structure of a task. This can even hold true for tasks that are very similar to each other, which complicates the process of classifying brain activity as relating to changes that are associated with learning or reflecting the engagement of a memory system suited for the task. The primary goals of these studies were to characterize the mechanisms that are associated with category learning and understand the extent to which different memory systems are recruited within a single task. Two studies providing spatial and temporal distinctions between learning-related changes in the brain and category-dependent memory systems are presented. The results from these experiments support the notion that exemplar memorization, rule-based, and perceptual similarity-based categorization are flexibly recruited in order to optimize performance during a single task. We conclude that these three methods, along with the memory systems they rely on, aid in the development of expertise, but their engagement might depend on the level of familiarity with a category.

Keywords: category learning; eeg; machine learning; erp; memory; learning; multiple memory systems; p300

1. Introduction

Category learning has been a productive paradigm for studying learning and memory and it refers to the development of the ability to group objects belonging to the same category and differentiate objects belonging to different categories [1]. There is not a single mechanism of category learning. Research using category learning models have outlined that there are distinct neural mechanisms associated with different learning stages [2]. Furthermore, we know that different tasks engage dissociable memory systems that are optimized for the type of learning involved—even for seemingly similar tasks, such as in categorization [3–7]. This makes it difficult to uniquely attribute the changes in brain activity to either distinct learning systems or representations of the distinct mechanisms that are associated with different task sets. In other words, the two bodies of literature can complicate comparing brain activity across tasks as subjects between those tasks could either be at different stages of learning or be relying on different categorization strategies that are served by dissociable memory systems.

From the skill acquisition perspective, a succinct model of learning has been proposed that describes reliance upon executive functions, depending on the stage of learning: early or late. Under the dual-stage model, the early stage of learning is marked by being heavily reliant on controlled processes, requiring a person to be actively attentive and dependent on limited working memory capacity. In contrast, the late stage is defined by its lack of reliance on controlled processes, reflected as automated performance, and it is not limited by working memory capacity and can be subconsciously carried out under the right context [2].

Modern imaging evidence has delineated distinct brain networks that are involved in the two learning stages [8]. The frontal lobe is responsible for the executive monitoring of unfamiliar stimuli; a process that is integral to the early stages of learning. In contrast, cortical regions of the posterior corticolimbic system are engaged when subjects demonstrate proficient performance in the late stages of learning [8,9]. These posterior corticolimbic structures, which include the hippocampus and posterior cingulate cortex (PCC), consolidate information and, with sufficient practice, enable performance to be more automated, thus removing the need for executive control.

Finer details regarding how the brain changes as a person learns to recognize category structures can be understood from the perspective of the dual stage theory [10]. The dual model of sensory information processing is based on evidence that suggests two separable and parallel systems operate on incoming sensory data. The first is a ventral "what" system that is responsible for the identification of an event or object and it includes the sensory specific cortices (such as visual cortex) and the ventral limbic system, which includes the parahippocampal gyrus, piriform, entorhinal cortex, and the amygdala [11,12]. The second processing stream, as exemplified by dorsal cortical regions of the parietal lobe, is referred to as the dorsal or "where" pathway, and it specializes in spatial analysis of stimuli [11,12]. Information from both streams converge at the hippocampus, which is a structure situated in the medial temporal lobe (MTL) that plays a key role in organizing input to link memories by their contextual representation [13]. This feedback structure allows for the hippocampus to organize memory retrieval based off "what" occurred or "where" something occurred and makes it an essential mechanism for memory retrieval. With further training, the hippocampus is able to perform declarative recall with less need for controlled attention and input from these two sensory pathways; reflecting the early/late transition outlined in the dual stage model. However, a relevant shortcoming to both the dual processing and dual stage models is that as they exist, they do not account for the evidence of other types of memory systems and their possible differential reliance on the brain mechanisms that are described in the models. Another shortcoming is that they do not consider the possibility that different memory systems could be simultaneously engaged during a task, either in competition or working in conjunction, and at different learning stages to optimize learning.

Multiple mechanisms that rely on dissociable memory systems have been implicated in categorization and category learning. One distinction is between strategies that require the application of an explicit rule (rule-based categorization) and those that rely on perceptual similarity (examples: [14,15]). For example, in a family resemblance structure, stimuli that belong to the same category share several common features, with none of them being necessary or sufficient for category membership [16,17]. Categorization relies on the overall similarity rather than an explicit rule. The perceptual similarity system involves posterior visual areas and does not heavily rely on working memory [18–20]. Perceptual similarity allows for making rapid judgements regarding category membership without using much cognitive resources, but falls short in its ability to classify objects when within-category similarity is low or between category similarity is high [21].

In contrast, in rule-based categorization, category membership is dictated by an explicit, verbalizable rule [15]. Rule discovery is commonly achieved through explicit reasoning and hypothesis testing that heavily relies on working memory and selective attention, which are supported by the working memory system in prefrontal cortex and caudate nucleus [22]. The working memory system, within the context of rule-based categorization, allows for participants to focus on individual diagnostic dimensions while ignoring the irrelevant features within the task. This allows for accurate categorization when the within-category variance is high and between-category variance is low. However, rule-based categorization is cognitively expensive and sensitive to distractions when compared to the perceptual similarity system [3,23].

Prior research has focused on creating tasks that exaggerate the preferential recruitment of one system over another to provide compelling evidence for the existence of multiple systems. Evidence from these studies has shown that performance is hindered when the participants fail to engage the memory system optimal for a given category structure. The composition of natural categories contains elements of rule-, *and* perceptual-based systems, suggesting people may be switching between systems within a single task. Identifying signatures of distinct memory systems within single tasks would allow us to better understand how each system contributes to performance and how these systems fit within the expertise development framework.

The main goals of the presented studies were to understand the degree to which distinct learning and memory systems are recruited within the same, real-world task. We implemented a categorization task that was designed to encourage participants to switch between categorization strategies on a trial-by-trial basis and then measured the underlying neural activity in two separate experiments while using functional Magnetic Resonance Imaging (fMRI) and dense-array Electroencephalography (dEEG). The goal of our first experiment, which was a low-sample pilot, was to utilize the spatial resolution of fMRI to establish the overall effectiveness of our task in engaging different memory systems for different trials within the same task. A successful proof-of-concept and spatial distribution in the fMRI pilot then motivated the second, dEEG experiment. In our fully powered dEEG experiment, we studied the time course by which these strategies (and their underlying memory systems) were engaged on a trial-by-trial basis. More specifically, we were interested in understanding when, on a given trial, we can accurately dissociate between verbal and non-verbal rules and the associated memory systems. As the brief involvement of limited attentional and working memory resources may beneficial for the optimization of categorization strategy to the task [24], mapping the timing of the initial convergence and subsequent divergence of distinct categorization processes can provide new insights regarding how distinct systems compete and cooperate to optimize performance. Rough estimates of the anatomical differences between these systems were made while using the EEG data and a novel machine learning approach.

2. fMRI Pilot Experiment

2.1. Materials and Methods

2.1.1. Participants

Eleven right-handed subjects between the ages of 18 and 30 ($M = 24.2$) were recruited from the University of Oregon Human Subjects Pool to participate in our pilot experiment (five males, six females). The subjects had no self-reported neurological or psychiatric conditions, as well as no MRI contraindications. Subjects were compensated $35 for their participation and the Electrical Geodesics, Inc. and University of Oregon IRBs approved the protocol.

2.1.2. Task

The task used was designed to interchangeably recruit a rule-based or similarity-based categorization strategy to categorize three categories of football defensive formations. When between-category similarity is low and within-category similarity is high, visual similarity can guide categorization without the need of limited cognitive resources. However, when between-category similarity is relatively high compared to within-category similarity, successful categorization requires the discovery and an application of an explicit categorization rule, which taxes limited resources, such as working memory and attention. Thus, we chose two formation categories that were visually similar to each other and one category that was visually distinct from the other two. For the two similar categories, the subjects needed to discover an explicit counting rule in order to categorize the members of these two groups reliably: One category of formations displayed three people on the line of scrimmage (and four behind them, 3-4 category), while the other had four people on the line of scrimmage (and three behind them, 4-3 category) (Figure 1). Because of the variable starting positions among players, the formations that fell into one category (e.g., 3-4) could look different from each other (within-category variability). In addition, some of the formations in the 3-4 category were visually very similar to some of the formations in the 4-3 category (high between-category similarity). Thus, the participants could not easily rely on visual similarity and instead needed to discover the rule (number of people on the line of scrimmage) that differentiated the categories. This forced subjects to focus their attention to the line of scrimmage while ignoring irrelevant players positioned elsewhere on the field. We expected that, although these were two categories that participants needed to differentiate between, stimuli from both categories would evoke the same cognitive processes (explicit, rule-based categorization). We collapsed over them in neuroimaging analyses when looking for neural processes associated with these rule-based trials, as subsequent analyses confirmed that participants' performance was comparable for the 3-4 and 4-3 categories on all metrics.

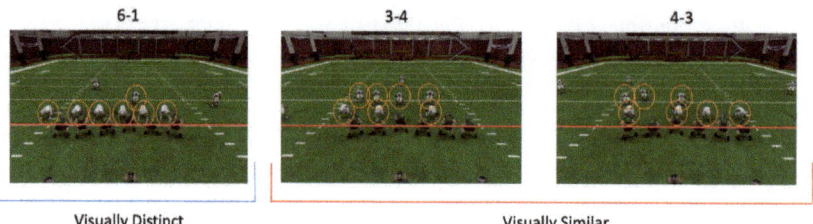

Figure 1. Standard formations used in the experiment. Left (blue underline): A 6-1 formation, which represents the visually distinct category, had six white players on the line of scrimmage (red line) and one player lined up behind them. Middle and Right (red underline): A 3-4 or 4-3 formation, which represent the visually similar categories, had three players (3-4) or 4 players (4-3) on the line of scrimmage (red line) and either four players (3-4) or 3 players (4-3) lined up behind them. The position of the green players did not vary significantly between formations.

For the visually distinct category, there was also an explicit rule, with six people on the line of scrimmage and one person behind (6-1) (Figure 1). However, this category was visually sufficiently distinct from the 3-4 and 4-3 categories, so subjects could rely on visual similarity alone during categorization, rather than having to discover and invoke an explicit rule.

Every category had three separate formations, each sharing the defining number of players on the line of scrimmage for that category, for a total of nine formations used throughout the experiment. On each training trial, the subjects were shown a random formation for 2.5 s and were tasked with pressing a button on a keypad to place the formation into one of the three categories during the 2 s window (Figure 2). Corrective feedback was given to the subject immediately after making their response and it was on the screen for 1.5 s. The inter-trial-interval was optimized for event-related-design while using Optseq2 software and varied between 2 and 8 s [24]. Each formation was shown six times during each training block and there were six total training blocks.

A generalization block was implemented at the end of the experiment in order to test the subject's ability to generalize the strategies that they acquired during training. During this block, the nine old formations were intermixed with nine new formations that belonged to the learned category structures. Each stimulus was randomly shown one at a time and was on the screen for 2 s while the subject used a response pad to categorize the stimulus. No feedback was given during this block, and instead a black fixation screen was shown for 10 s before the next stimulus was presented—resulting in a total fixed trial length of 12 s (Figure 3). Each new and old stimulus was shown only once during the generalization block. The inclusion of a generalization block allowed for us to test whether the participants indeed discovered the category structure rather than memorized labels for individual examples, as rote memorization during training would hinder their categorization performance on the new formations.

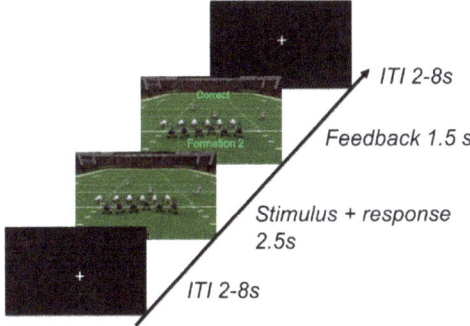

Figure 2. Formations were shown for 2.5 s. Immediately following a response, contingent feedback was shown for 1.5 s. Upon feedback termination, a fixation mark was shown for the duration of the inter-trial interval of 2–8 s before the next formation was presented.

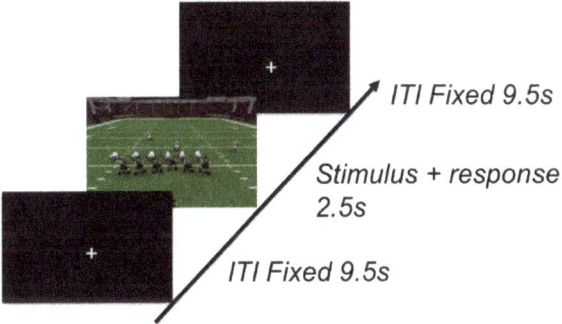

Figure 3. Formations were shown for 2.5 s, regardless of when a subject made a response. No feedback was given. Instead, a fixation cross appeared for a fixed 9.5 s until the next formation was shown.

2.1.3. Procedure

Before coming to the scanning center, the subjects were pre-screened over the telephone to ensure eligibility. Upon arrival at the center, a structural T1 scan was acquired, followed by an exposure block with simultaneous scanning. During this block, the subjects were asked to passively look at the screen and refrain from pressing any buttons. No other context or instructions were given. Each of the nine training formations were shown one at a time for 2 s each before a fixed 10 s ITI. Each formation was shown four times for 36 total trials. Following the exposure block, subjects were read instructions for the experiment. They were told how many formations there would be in the experiment, along with the set number of categories the formations belonged to. Their job was to figure out which formations belong to each category by pressing the buttons on their response pad and utilizing the corrective feedback. A brief practice test (un-scanned) was given, where they learned to categorize unrelated formations. After practice, six training blocks were run with brief breaks in-between and, after training, the subjects sat through another exposure block where they passively viewed each stimulus. To end the experiment, the subjects went through the generalization block, given only the instructions that they were going to go through a final block with no feedback. They were not told whether there would be novel formations in this block. The subjects were asked to write-down their strategies in a debrief questionnaire for categorizing the formations before receiving compensation and leaving the center.

2.1.4. fMRI Acquisition and Pre-Processing

MRI data were acquired with a 3T Siemens Skyra. A high-resolution T1-weighted MPRAGE was acquired for co-registration and normalization before the task was administered (TR = 2.5 s, TE = 3.41 ms, flip angle = 7°, matrix size = 256 × 256, FOV = 256 mm, 1 mm isotropic). Whole-brain fMRI was acquired using a gradient-echo EPI pulse sequence: TR = 2 s, TE = 26 ms, 100 × 100 matrix, FOV = 200 mm, 72 oblique axial slices, no skip, 2 mm isotropic voxels, GRAPA factor 2, multiband factor 3. Preprocessing was carried out in FSL version 5.0.9 (www.fmrib.ox.ac.uk/fsl). The functional images were skull stripped using BET (brain extraction tool), motion corrected, co-registered to the T1 anatomical image, and smoothed with a 4mm FWHM kernel. Two sets of analyses were performed: traditional whole-brain univariate analyses and trial-by-trial multivoxel pattern classification analyses within a set of a priori ROIs. For univariate whole-brain group analyses, functional data were registered to standard MNI space. For multivoxel pattern classification, the data were kept in native space of each participant and trial-specific activation patterns (betaseries) for classification analysis within each participant were extracted using a general linear model with a separate regressor for each trial [25]. A detailed description of each of these analysis approached is provided together with results for better readability.

2.2. Results

2.2.1. Behavioral Results

Data from one participant were excluded due to noise caused by motion during scanning, leaving 10 out of the 11 subjects for analysis. Figure 4 shows the average classification accuracy for each category across the six training runs. Visual inspection indicates that participants learned the visually distinct category faster when compared to the two visually similar categories, but by the end of run 4 they were able to accurately identify members of all categories.

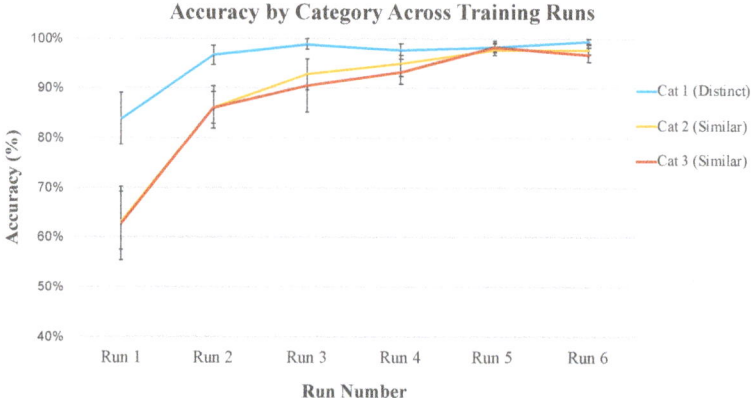

Figure 4. Subjects accurately categorized the visually distinct category quicker than the two visually similar categories. Accuracy for the visually similar categories peaked between runs 4 and 5, which we infer is the time at which subjects discovered the counting rule.

A confusion matrix shows that subjects commonly mixed up the two visually similar categories when making errors, and rarely mixed up the visually distinct category with any other. By block 4, the subjects limited their confusion, which is indexed by the mostly uniformly colored bars in Figure 5. We can infer that this was the point at which most subjects discovered the explicit counting rule that allowed for them to differentiate between members of the two visually similar categories (Figure 5).

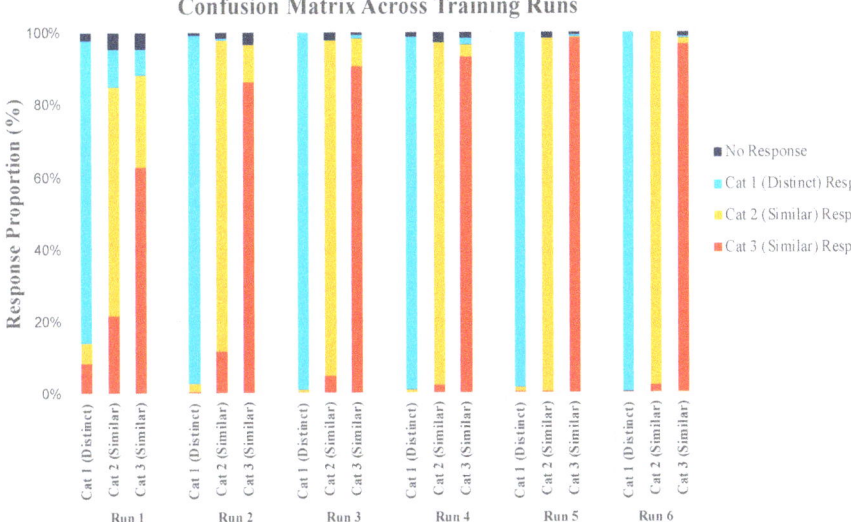

Figure 5. Visualization of the confusion matrix during classification. During the first 3 training blocks, subjects commonly confused the two visually similar categories for one another. By run 4, subjects were able to accurately dissociate between these two categories. Subjects rarely confused any other category when classifying formations in the visually distinct category.

The generalization run was included to test for the hallmark of category knowledge—the ability to generalize category labels to novel category examples. On average, the subjects completed the generalization run with 92% accuracy for the visually distinct category and 88% accuracy for the visually similar categories (Figure 6). Had subjects been relying on the declarative recall of individual stimuli throughout training, their performance in the generalization run would have been closer to chance (33%).

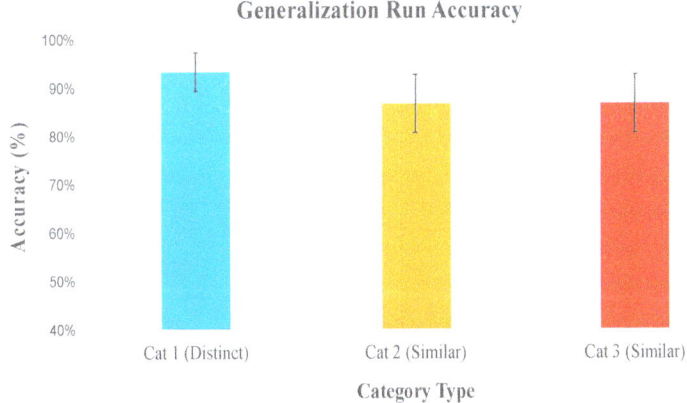

Figure 6. Categorization accuracy in the generalization block.

In the post-test questionnaire, nine out of 10 participants indicated that they used a counting strategy to distinguish between the visually distinct categories, meaning that they accurately identified the defining number of players on the line of scrimmage separating the two categories. The same participants reported relying on perceptual similarity to identify formations in the visually distinct category. This indicates that participants treated the stimuli as expected, using an explicit rule specifically when between-category similarity was high as compared to the within-category similarity. The remaining one participant reported using declarative recall for all stimuli, whereby they memorized each formation individually instead of relying on the intended counting rule. This participant categorized new stimuli in the visually similar categories with an accuracy near chance during the generalization block, which indicated that relying on declarative recall instead of discovering the counting rule was ineffective for generalization in this task.

2.2.2. Univariate fMRI Analysis

Training Analysis

Data from each training run and each participant were separately analyzed at a first level analysis using FSL [26]. Visually distinct and visually similar correct trials were separately modeled as two predictors. Each stimulus onset time was convolved with a hemodynamic response function and entered into a general linear model with their temporal derivatives to estimate beta weights. Contrasts of interests were set that tested for differential activation to the two types of categorization trials. Even after performance becomes equated, we focused on data from runs 4, 5, and 6 to explore whether participants engage distinct processes for visually similar vs. visually distinct categories (the runs after subjects could perform the task with proficiency for all three categories: see Figure 4). Data from the three runs within each subject were combined at a second level while using fixed-effects analysis. Data across participants were then combined at the third level using a random-effects analysis (FLAME 1). Figure 7 depicts regions that were more engaged during visually distinct trials over visually similar categorization trials (blue), and vice-versa (red). Individual voxels were considered to be active when reaching a $Z > 1.8$ and surviving a whole-brain cluster size threshold set at $p < 0.05$ [27]. This threshold was used based on the exploratory nature of our small sample pilot experiment, and the reported results were interpreted for the purposes of motivating Experiment 2.

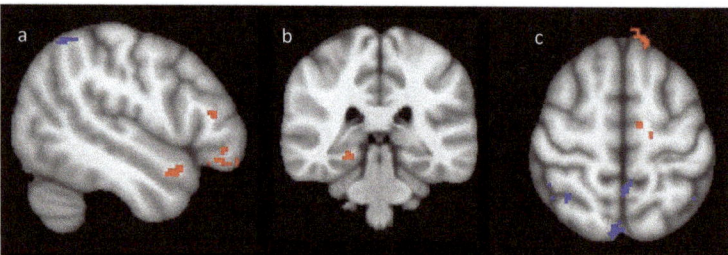

Figure 7. Univariate contrasts of visually similar > visually distinct (Red) and visually distinct > visually similar (Blue) during training displayed in (**a**) sagittal, (**b**) coronal, and (**c**) axial views. Red: dorsal lateral and inferior frontal areas along with hippocampus were engaged significantly more during rule application compared to perceptual similarity analysis. Blue: Fusiform gyrus and lateral occipital cortex were engaged significantly more during perceptual similarity analysis compared to rule application.

The superior and inferior frontal gyri were engaged significantly more on visually similar categories when compared to the visually distinct category (red clusters, Figure 7). The right hippocampus, a region associated with declarative recall, was also engaged during the classification of visual similar categories, which is consistent with prior work indicating the role of hippocampus in rule-based categorization [28]. During classification to the visually distinct category, the lateral occipital cortex and fusiform gyrus were engaged significantly more as compared to visually similar categories (blue clusters, Figure 7), consistent with what might be expected for similarity-based categorization. Tables 1 and 2 illustrate a summary of the top 11 regions associated with each condition.

Table 1. Cluster location and size for similar > distinct contrast in blocks 4, 5, and 6.

Location	Cluster Size	Z-Value	X	Y	Z
L Sup. Fr. Gyrus	58	2.79	−54	44	−10
L. IFG	50	2.95	−50	30	14
L. Sup. Fr. Gyrus	38	2.72	−12	40	56
L. Sup. Fr. Gyrus	34	2.47	−16	56	38
R. Hippocampus	26	2.88	22	−34	−10
L. Sup. Temp. Gyrus	25	2.67	−50	10	−16
R. Fusiform Gyrus	25	3.04	40	−44	−20
R. Lateral Occipital Cortex	24	2.72	−10	−12	56
L. Suppl. Motor Cortex	22	2.42	58	−64	24
Brain Stem	22	2.63	6	−22	−28
R. Mid. Temp. Gyrus	20	2.56	40	−58	2

Table 2. Cluster location and size for distinct > similar contrast in blocks 4, 5, and 6.

Location	Cluster Size	Z-Value	X	Y	Z
R. Lateral Occipital Cortex	519	3.16	6	−74	36
R. Lateral Occipital Cortex	154	2.87	34	−62	62
L. Fusiform Gyrus	106	3.17	−20	−66	−18
L. Lateral Occipital Cortex	98	2.83	−36	−56	38
R. IFG	89	3.25	20	56	−6
L. Post. Cingulate Gyrus	70	2.88	−8	−40	48
R. Lateral Occipital Cortex	55	2.47	20	−88	38
R. Fusiform Gyrus	52	2.62	20	−54	−16
L. Middle Frontal Gyrus	49	2.77	−38	45	18
R. Occipital Pole	41	2.34	20	−104	−10
Brain Stem	40	3.05	22	−32	−42

Generalization

When modeling the generalization block, visually distinct and visually similar trials were further separated, depending on whether they were used during training (old) or whether they were new examples of each category. This resulted in four separate predictors (i.e., Novel-Similar, Novel-Distinct, Old-Similar, Old-Distinct), with the data from each subject being separately analyzed at a first-level analysis. Each stimulus onset time was convolved with a hemodynamic response function and entered into a general linear model with their temporal derivatives to estimate beta weights. Contrast maps were created for each subject, showing areas that were differentially engaged during visually similar vs. visually distinct categories. A group analysis was then run using FLAME 1, combining contrast maps across participants. Figure 8 shows regions that were more engaged during visually distinct trials over visually similar trials (red), and vice-versa (blue). Individual voxels were considered to be active when reaching $Z > 1.8$ and surviving a whole-brain cluster size threshold set at $p < 0.05$ [27].

The results from our univariate analysis show that the left caudate nucleus, left superior frontal gyrus, and left inferior frontal gyrus were significantly more engaged on visually similar trials when compared to visually distinct trials (Figure 8). Caudate nucleus, instead of hippocampus, is one of the only observable differences between the training and generalization contrasts for this condition. Table 3 presents a list of the top 11 clusters from this contrast. In addition, the lateral occipital cortex and right fusiform gyrus were engaged significantly more for distinct trials over visually similar trials during generalization. Table 4 shows a summary of the top 11 clusters.

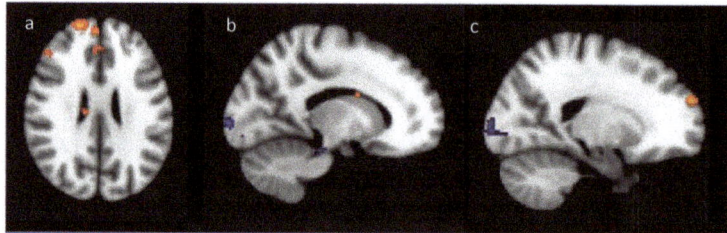

Figure 8. Univariate contrasts of visually similar > visually distinct (Red) and visually distinct > visually similar (Blue) during generalization displayed in (**a**) axial, (**b**) medial sagittal, and (**c**) more lateral sagittal views. Red: Frontal control regions were engaged significantly more during the visually similar trials compared to visually distinct trials during generalization. A cluster over caudate nucleus was also found. Blue: Visually distinct trials relied more heavily on lateral occipital cortex compared to trials separable by a counting rule.

Table 3. Cluster location and size for similar > distinct contrast in generalization block.

Location	Cluster Size	Z-Value	X	Y	Z
L. Caudate Nucleus	290	3.5	−8	−10	24
Cerebellum	129	3.22	16	−72	−28
Cerebellum	125	3.43	32	−80	−22
Cerebellum	90	3.18	4	−50	−10
L. Sup. Frontal Gyrus	88	3.21	−28	6	64
L. Lateral Occipital Cortex	73	3.17	−26	−78	50
R. Lateral Occipital Cortex	71	3.08	40	−74	42
L. Inf. Frontal Gyrus	67	3.22	−42	22	4
Cerebellum	63	3.3	−26	−90	−26
L. Sup. Frontal Gyrus	59	3.17	−42	46	20
Brain Stem	58	2.92	14	−16	−38

Table 4. Cluster location and size for distinct > similar in generalization block.

Location	Cluster Size	Z-Value	X	Y	Z
R. Lateral Occipital Cortex	1922	4	18	−100	6
R. Fusiform Gyrus	335	3.41	12	−72	−2
R. Inf. Frontal Gyrus	213	3.11	62	6	12
Postcentral Gyrus	144	3.35	−40	−26	54
L. Sup. Temporal Gyrus	143	3.49	68	−24	28
Cerebellum	113	3.09	−20	−72	−52
L. Fusiform Gyrus	100	2.88	38	−54	−24
R. Mid. Temporal Gyrus	99	3.13	66	−40	2
R. Mid. Frontal Gyrus	82	3.25	32	18	30
R. Mid Temporal Gyrus	79	3.37	54	−6	−28
R. Angular Gyrus	70	3.7	56	−46	30

2.2.3. Multi-Voxel Pattern Analysis

The univariate analyses provided preliminary evidence that participants may engage distinct neurocognitive processes when categorizing visually distinct vs. visually similar trials, albeit at an exploratory threshold. As a second approach, we employed multi-voxel pattern analysis (MVPA; e.g., [29]), which might provide additional sensitivity. Specifically, we asked whether a machine-learning classifier could distinguish, based on the pattern of activation across voxels, into which condition a current trial belonged. First, cortical parcellation and subcortical segmentation was performed while using Freesurfer software for each participant [30,31]. Given prior work on visual memory and the dissociations between rule-based and similarity-based categorization, we focused on regions within the frontoparietal attentional network and the midline, in addition to the posterior visual cortex [32–34]. Specific Freesurfer-defined ROIs included superior parietal lobe, anterior cingulate cortex (ACC), medial orbitofrontal cortex (MOFC), inferior parietal lobe, inferior frontal gyrus (IFG), and fusiform gyrus.

One participants' data were lost between the time we performed the univariate analysis and MVPA due to a site-wide data loss, which left nine out of 11 subjects for MVPA. We modeled the functional data using a separate regressor for each trial to construct a betaseries representing activation patterns that are associated with each individual trial to obtain trial-specific activation patterns for each participant [35]. Each betaseries was smoothed ($\sigma = 3$) before being co-registered to each participant's high-resolution anatomical image while using Advanced Neuroimaging Tools (ANTs) toolbox [36]. Data were kept in native the space of each participant for the classification. Classification analysis used a linear Support Vector Machine (SVM), as implemented by the LinearCSVMC classifier in PyMVPA (pymvpa.org). Data from all runs were included to obtain enough training samples for the classifier. A leave-one-run-out crossvalidation was chosen, as it would maximize the amount of data in each training fold for our sample size [37,38]. Within each ROI separately, the classifier was trained on data from five out of six training runs and tested on the left-out run. The classification accuracy was then averaged across the six cross-validation folds. Two binary (pairwise) classifications were performed: visually similar category 1 vs. visually distinct category, and visually similar category 2 vs. visually distinct category. We subsequently averaged their results together, as there were no differences in classification accuracy between the two (as expected).

A one-sample t-test was used against a baseline value of 0.5 (50% chance for two equally frequent categories). Figure 9 shows the classification analysis in each ROI, indicating dissociable patterns of activation evoked during categorization of stimuli that presumably required rule application vs. those who could be based on perceptual similarity. The IFG ($M = 0.66$; $t(8) = 4.23$, $p = 0.003$), inferior parietal lobe ($M = 0.70$; $t(8) = 3.65$, $p = 0.007$), superior parietal lobe ($M = 0.76$; $t(8) = 5.8$, $p < 0.001$), MOFC ($M = 0.58$; $t(8) = 3.3$, $p = 0.011$), and fusiform gyrus ($M = 0.62$; $t(8) = 3.75$, $p = 0.006$) all predicted category membership with statistically significant accuracy. The ACC ($M = 0.58$) did not reach significance, $t(8) = 2.02$, $p = 0.078$.

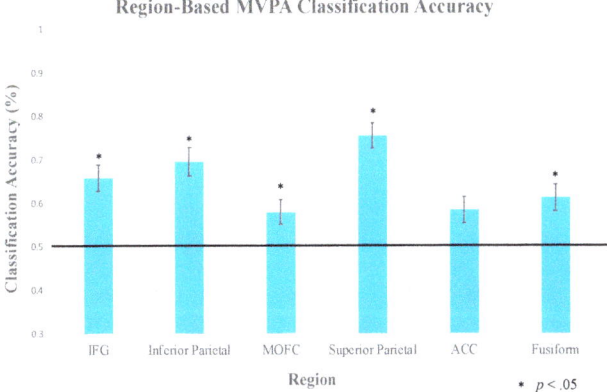

Figure 9. The inferior frontal gyrus (IFG), inferior parietal cortex, medial orbitofrontal cortex (MOFC), superior parietal cortex, and fusiform gyrus were able to classify between our two conditions with significantly above-chance accuracy. Amongst these regions, the superior and inferior parietal cortices provided the most reliable classification. The Anterior Cingulate Cortex (ACC) did not reach statistical significance.

3. dEEG Experiment

3.1. Materials and Methods

3.1.1. Participants

The results from the fMRI pilot motivated the design and interpretation of our fully-powered EEG experiment. Forty-four right-handed participants were recruited from the University of Oregon Human Subjects Pool (22 males, 22 females), with ages ranging between 18 and 39 years old ($M = 19.5$, $SD = 3.2$). All of the participants had normal or corrected-to-normal vision, had no history of head trauma or seizures, and were not consuming medication that could affect their EEG. The participants were pre-screened online for their experience with football to reduce the chance of contextual familiarity confounding differences in skill acquisition rate. Only those subjects that were comfortable recognizing football defensive formations were allowed to participate. The University of Oregon and Brain Electrophysiology Laboratory Company (BELCO) institutional review boards approved the research protocol, and the study took place in the laboratory of BELCO.

3.1.2. Task

The task used in this study was an EEG analogue of the fMRI task used in the pilot. Stimuli in this task consisted of three categories of football defensive formations, with two categories being very visually similar to each other and one category being visually distinct from the other two. For the two similar categories, the subjects needed to discover an explicit counting rule to reliably categorize members of these two groups. For the visually distinct category, subjects could rely on a simple visual similarity analysis to recognize members of this category. Within each category, all of the players were shuffled around the field of view with the exception of the players on the line of scrimmage, as the number of players on the line dictated category membership (Figure 10). This forced subjects to focus their attention to the line of scrimmage over time while ignoring irrelevant players that are positioned elsewhere on the field.

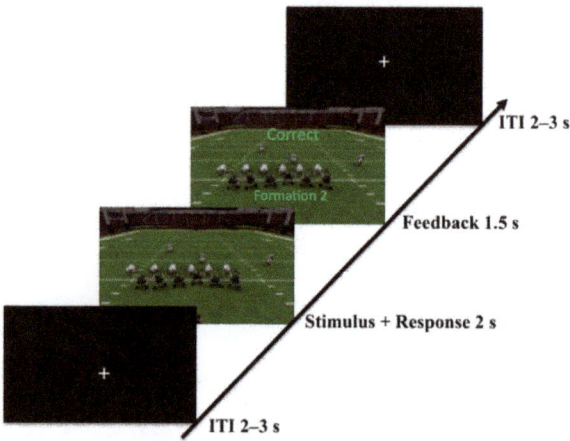

Figure 10. From bottom-left to top right: A fixation cross was shown for 2–3 s. Formations were shown for 2 s while subjects made their response. Immediately following a response, contingent feedback was shown for 1.5 s. Upon feedback termination, a fixation mark was shown for the duration of the inter-trial interval of 2–3 s before the next formation was presented.

Every category had three formations, each sharing the defining number of players on the line of scrimmage for that category, for a total of nine formations used throughout the experiment. On a given trial, the participants were randomly shown one of the nine formations for 2000 ms and they were instructed to place the stimulus into one of the three categories by pressing a button on a response box within the stimulus exposure window. Once they made a response the stimulus disappeared, and the subject was presented with a corrective feedback screen, which indicated whether they were correct along with text describing the correct category for the stimulus (Figure 10). The feedback was on the screen for 1500 ms, after which a fixation cross with a variable inter-stimulus-interval was shown for 2000–3000 ms. The task was divided into eight training blocks that consisted of 90 trials (or 10 exposures per stimulus) per block, which totaled 80 exposures of every stimulus throughout training.

After the final training block, a generalization block was used, which tested each subject's ability to apply any rules they developed during training to novel stimuli similar to the fMRI pilot. During the training block, a mixture of the nine training stimuli and nine novel stimuli belonging to the same categories were used. The subjects were not told that the generalization block would include novel stimuli. No feedback was given to the participants after pressing a button to categorize each formation. Instead, a black screen was shown for 1500 ms after a response was made before the fixation cross appeared to begin the next trial. Each old and novel stimulus (18 total stimuli) was shown five times for a total of 90 trials in the generalization block.

3.1.3. Procedure

Following the informed consent process, the participants were fitted with a 256-channel EEG net and placed 55 cm in front of a computer monitor. A chinrest was used to minimize head movements and keep the distance to the monitor fixed for every participant. The participants were explicitly told that there were nine defensive formations in this study belonging to three categories, and that they must learn which formations go into each category. The response feedback that would help teach the participant to make the correct decision was explained clearly, and the participants were allowed to ask questions before the experiment began.

Once the participant could demonstrate an understanding of the study to the research assistant, a short practice block that consisted of 12 trials followed. The formations used in the practice block resembled different basketball formations to avoid familiarity effects once the real training began. After the practice block, eight training blocks occurred, followed by a final generalization block to test a subject's strategies to novel members of the acquired categories. At the end of the experiment, the participants filled out a debriefing questionnaire, which asked them to describe the strategies that they used to categorize each group of formations. Each session lasted around 2.5 H, and the participants were compensated course credit for their participation.

3.1.4. Learning Criterion

We used the fixed-number of consecutive responses method (FCCR) to simplify the analysis process in order to determine when a participant had sufficiently acquired the response mapping, as we have done in the past [38]. With this method, a subject fulfilled the learning criterion when they could make four correct responses (or non-responses) in a row for each stimulus.

3.1.5. EEG Recording and Pre-Processing

The dEEG was recorded using a 256-channel HydroCel Geodesic Sensor Net (HCGSN) and the data were amplified using a Net Amps 400 Amplifier (Electrical Geodesics, Inc., Eugene, OR). The recordings were referenced to Cz and impedances were maintained below 50 kΩ. dEEG was bandpass filtered (0.1–100 Hz) upon being sampled at 250 s/s with a 16-bit analog-to-digital converter.

After recording, the signals were filtered between 0.1–30 Hz bandpass and segmented into 1200 ms long segments time-locked to the onset of each stimulus (segments extended 200 ms before and 1000 ms after the stimulus onset). Segments containing eyeblinks, muscle tension, major eye movements, or large head movements with 10 or more channels exceeding an absolute voltage threshold of 140 µV were excluded from a participant's average. Segments containing minor eye movements (saccades) were not fully rejected, given the lack of overlap between the latency and distribution of the saccades with the latency and location of the Medial Frontal Negativity (MFN), LIAN, and P300b (P3b). All of the data were re-referenced to the average reference for analysis.

3.2. Results

3.2.1. Behavioral Analysis

Figure 10 shows learning curves for each category. Similar to the behavioral data from our pilot experiment (Figure 4), the participants acquired the visually distinct category first, and there were no performance differences between the two visually similar categories. Based on this, behavioral measures for the two visually distinct categories were averaged together to represent a single visually similar condition in our experiment in order to streamline comparison to the visually distinct category. A paired-samples *t*-test revealed that, on average, across training blocks, the subjects were significantly better at categorizing the visually distinct category (95%) than the visually similar categories (90%), $t(43) = 5.45$, $p < 0.001$. Figure 11 indicates that this difference was driven by early runs, but by Run 5 there were virtually no performance differences across all categories.

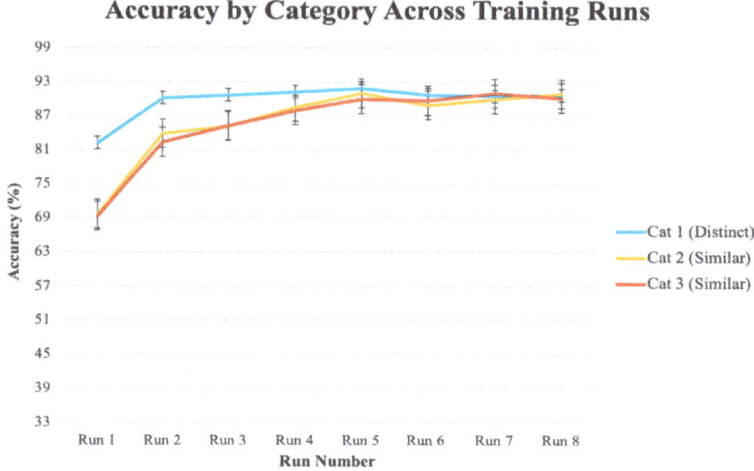

Figure 11. Behavioral performance across training for each category. Participants acquired the visually distinct category first followed by the two visually similar categories. Additionally, there are no behavioral differences between the two visually similar categories. Performance on the two types of categories became equivalent in the second half of training.

Experiment 2 also included a questionnaire that explicitly asked participants to describe the strategies that they used to categorize each formation category. For categorizing visually similar categories, 91% of participants indicated that they used a counting rule when differentiating between the two visually similar categories (e.g., "I counted four players on the line of scrimmage for the first category, and three on for the second category."), 9% of participants relied on declarative memory for these two categories, and no participant reported reliance on similarity. For categorizing visually distinct formations, 21% of participants reported using an explicit counting rule (e.g., "I counted six people on the line of scrimmage"), 68% reported using declarative recall (e.g., "I memorized each formation individually"), and 11% reported using a perceptual similarity strategy (e.g., "There appeared to be a lot of people on the line of scrimmage for formations in this category, such that I did not need to count any players"). Thus, the self-reported strategies differed between the visually-similar vs. visually-distinct trials, although the distinction was less pronounced than in Experiment 1.

3.2.2. Event-Related Potentials (ERPs) Selection Motivation and Analysis

All EEG data were analyzed using Philips Neuro Net Station 5 software. Classic ERP analysis was chosen, as it allows us to evaluate latency and amplitude differences as a function of categorization strategy. The distinct nature of individual ERPs enables us to attribute any observed differences as occurring within the well-studied circuitry that produces each ERP. In the past we utilized two ERPs to track learning-related changes in the brain: The Medial Frontal Negativity (MFN) and P300b (P3b)—for review see [13,39,40]. The MFN is a stimulus-locked medial frontal component with its primary sources in the Anterior Cingulate Cortex (ACC) [13]. The ACC plays a major role in error monitoring and attention during reward-based learning, which makes it an ideal component for indexing effortful control seen in the early stage of category learning [41]. On the other hand, the P300 is elicited under an array of conditions and there is now a well-defined family of different P300 components. Most relevant to learning, the amplitude of the Late Positive Component (referred to as the P3b) mirrors accuracy improvements during categorization tasks [39,40]. The P3b is hypothesized to reflect a constant monitoring and updating of the context under which learning occurred. As context is formed through learning, the maintenance and updating of the context helps to guide a person toward selecting an action quickly and efficiently. Although the sources of the P3b are still being debated, intracranial EEG and animal studies suggest multiple sources, including Posterior Cingulate Cortex (PCC), medial temporal lobe, and superior temporal sulcus—structures that are integral to the late learning stage [42–49]. In the current experiment, we were interested in examining amplitude and latency differences in these two components as a function of the categorization strategy used on a given trial. In theory, the strategies should differ in their reliance on frontal control areas and posterior corticolimbic structures to complete the task, as seen in Experiment 1. Using ERPs allows for us to interpret latency differences between trial types (distinct vs similar) as reflecting the time-course under which the categorization strategies (and their underlying memory systems) are engaged.

The Lateral Inferior Anterior Negativity (LIAN) is a third component that could potentially dissociate between the two categorization strategies. The LIAN is a lesser-known bilateral component that has shown clear dissociations between the recognition of spatial targets and digit targets in a visuomotor association task [39]. Specifically, the amplitude of the right LIAN is anticorrelated with acquiring the ability to recognize spatial configurations and it shows no changes when targets invoke the phonological loop. However, the amplitude of the left LIAN is positively correlated with learning to recognize phonological targets and it is insensitive to acquiring an ability to perform spatial analyses. The Inferior Frontal Gyrus (IFG) is inferred to be the primary source of these components, but it is worth mentioning that the LIAN is rarely discussed in the literature, where it does not receive any mention outside of its role in visuomotor learning. This component was selected, as it might show a dissociation between the two categorization strategies, since they inherently differ in how they engage the phonological loop.

Please see Section 3.1.5 for a review of how all of the signals were pre-processed. For the MFN analysis, a cluster of 12 electrodes that best represent the medial frontal distribution of the component were chosen (see pink electrodes, Figure 12). Consistent with how we have quantified the MFN in the past, an adaptive mean amplitude corresponding to 20 ms before and 20 ms after the maximum negative peak amplitude in a window that extends from approximately 180–300 ms after stimulus onset was computed for the MFN electrode cluster [13,39]. The MFN was referenced to the preceding positive peak (P200) around 150–200 ms after stimulus onset. This method was applied for the post-learning trials for all three formation categories. The trials in the visually distinct category were averaged together to form a single ERP for the similarity-based condition. After analyzing both visually similar categories individually, we determined that there were no amplitude or latency differences in the MFN between these two categories, consistent with the idea that both would require the engagement of explicit, rule-based categorization. In light of this, trials in the two visually similar categories were averaged together to form a single ERP for the visually similar condition. A paired-samples t-test was run to evaluate the differences in MFN amplitude for the visually distinct and visually similar categories. The test revealed a marginally significant effect, such that the MFN was the largest for the visually distinct category ($M = -2.31$ µV) as compared to the visually similar categories ($M = -2.07$ µV), $t(43) = -1.98$, $p = 0.054$ (Figure 13).

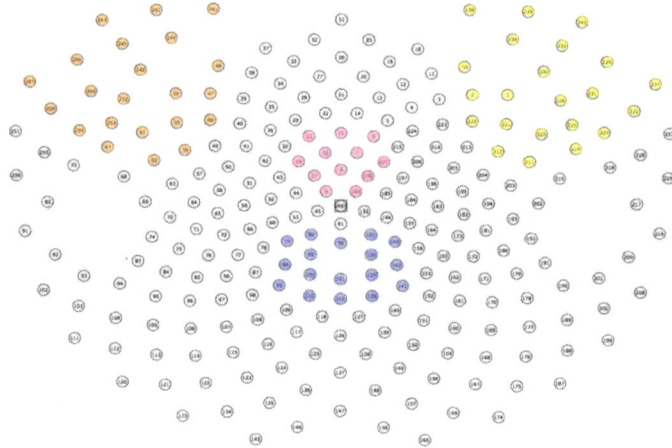

Figure 12. Electrode montages used for the Medial Frontal Negativity (MFN), P300b (P3b), and Lateral Inferior Anterior Negativity Event-Related Potential (LIAN ERP) components. Orange and yellow: Electrodes used for the LIAN analysis. Pink: Electrode cluster used to quantify the MFN. Blue: Electrodes used to quantify the P3b.

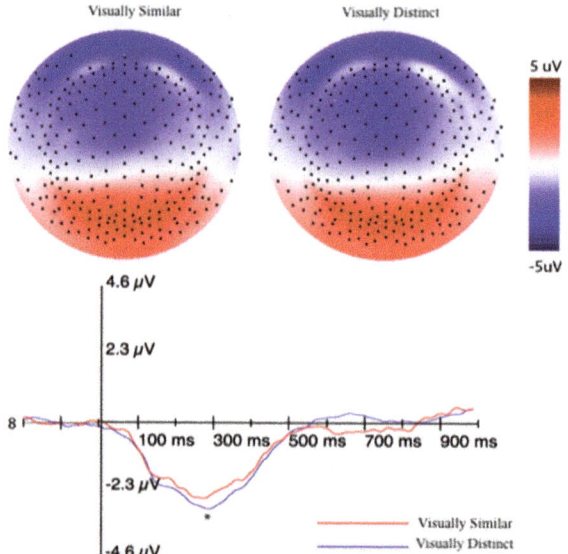

Figure 13. Top: A voltage map displays the voltage across the scalp for the similar and distinct conditions at the peak of the MFN (asterisk in bottom waveform image). A stronger negative voltage is seen over the medial frontal areas for the visually distinct condition. Bottom: Representative waveform (i.e., a single channel over the middle of the negative scalp potential) showing the shape of the MFN for both conditions. This waveform was derived from the grand-average of all the analyzed subjects. The amplitude of the MFN is higher (more negative) for the visually distinct condition.

For the P3b analysis, a set of 17 channels that corresponded to the posterior-parietal distribution of the component were used (see blue electrodes, Figure 12). An adaptive mean amplitude corresponding to 22 ms before and after the peak amplitude window extending from approximately 450–950 ms after stimulus onset was computed for the group of electrodes to quantify the component. This method was applied for the post-learning trials for all three formation categories and is consistent with how we have quantified the P3b in previous experiments [40]. Separate ERPs were computed for the visually similar and distinct categories similar to the method described for the MFN after establishing that there were no differences in amplitude between visually similar categories. A paired samples t-test revealed that the amplitude of the P3b for the distinct category (6.02 µV) was significantly larger than the similar categories (5.34 µV), $t(43) = 4.17$, $p < 0.001$. Figure 14 displays this effect.

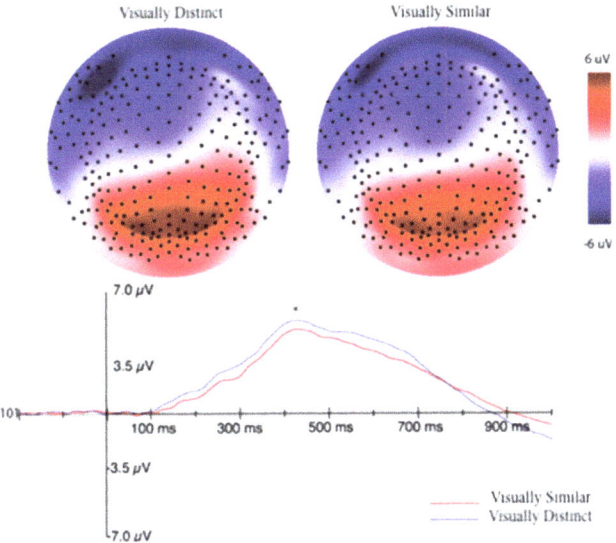

Figure 14. Top: A voltage map displays the voltage across the scalp for the visually similar and distinct conditions at the peak of the P3b (asterisk in bottom waveform image). A stronger positive voltage is seen over the posterior parietal areas for the distinct condition. Bottom: Representative waveform showing the shape of the P3b for both conditions. This waveform was derived from the grand-average of all analyzed subjects. The amplitude of the P3b is higher (more positive) for the visually distinct condition.

The LIAN was quantified by utilizing a cluster of 22 channels in the left or right frontoparietal regions (see orange and yellow electrodes in Figure 12, respectively). An adaptive mean amplitude of these clusters corresponding to 22 ms before and after the peak negative amplitude in a window that extended from 450–950 ms (the same window as the P3b) was used to quantify the component. This method was applied for all post-learning trials for all three categories in each subject. Similar to the P3b and MFN, separate ERPs were computed for the visually similar and distinct categories for both the left and right LIAN after establishing no differences between the visually similar categories. A paired-samples t-test showed that the amplitude of the left LIAN was largest for the distinct category (−7.06 µV) as compared to the amplitude of the visually similar categories (−5.54 µV), $t(43) = -2.98$, $p = 0.004$ (Figure 15). However, no significant amplitude difference for the right LIAN were found between the similar categories (−3.55 µV) and distinct category (−2.92 µV), $t(43) = 1.23$, $p = 0.23$.

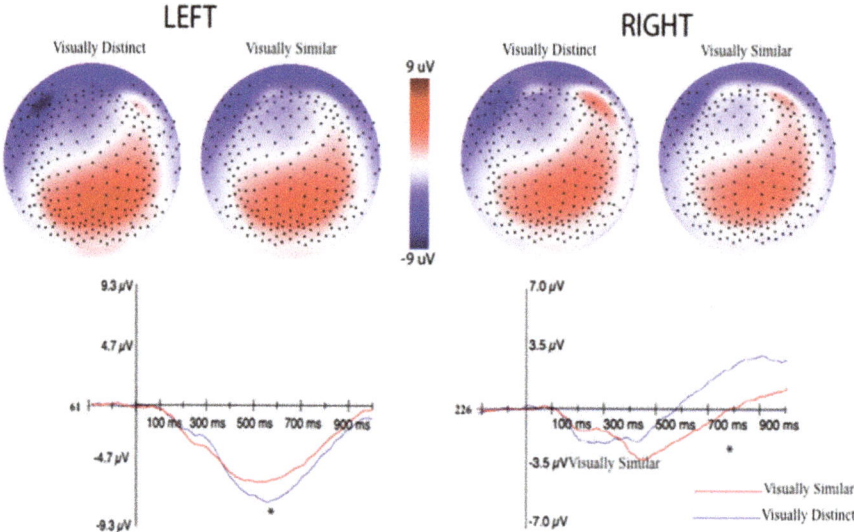

Figure 15. Top: Voltage maps display the voltage across the scalp for the similar and distinct conditions at the peak of the LIAN on the left and right sides (asterisks in bottom waveform images). A stronger negative voltage is seen over the left frontal areas for the visually distinct condition and a stronger negative voltage is seen over the right frontal areas for the visually similar condition. Bottom: Representative waveforms showing the shape of the LIAN for both conditions in the left and right hemispheres. The amplitude of the left LIAN is higher (more negative) for the distinct condition, whereas the right LIAN is higher (more negative) for the similar condition.

3.2.3. EEG Machine Learning Analysis

In addition to traditional ERP analysis, we chose to utilize machine learning, as it provides a more data-driven approach to measuring functional differences. We were interested in tracking the earliest timepoint at which brain responses become distinguishable for visually similar vs visually distinct categories. Group-clusters were used to evaluate the general location of these early temporal dissociations. This novel approach has the advantage of utilizing information in the entire pattern of amplitudes across the whole brain, which can potentially increase the sensitivity to subtle differences or engagement of different networks that may include overlapping regions.

For every subject, post-learning trials were chunked into individual segments extending 200 ms before and 1000 ms after stimulus onset for each category. Segments containing ocular or movement artifacts were rejected from analysis. Each segment was baseline corrected while using a 200 ms pre-stimulus baseline before averaging the segments together to form one averaged waveform for each category of stimuli. Waveforms for the two visually similar categories were averaged together to be compared against the distinct category before re-referencing to an average reference. The waveforms were then broken down into their individual samples, which, at a sampling rate of 250 samples/second, resulted in 300 total samples per waveform (each sample representing 4 ms of recording).

We averaged together the raw voltages of electrodes within 10 regions in order to reduce the number of predicting elements in this analysis: left frontal, right frontal, medial prefrontal, medial frontal, posterior parietal, left temporoparietal, right temporoparietal, left occipital, right occipital, and medial occipital (Figure 16). This process was done for each individual sample for both categories. We then averaged together every five consecutive samples together, resulting in 60 timepoints for each waveform with every timepoint representing 20 ms of data. The first 10 timepoints were used in the baseline correction and, thus, not included in the analysis. In the end, this gave us two matrices (one for visually similar and one for visually distinct) for each subject with dimensions 50 (timepoints) × 10 (electrode groups).

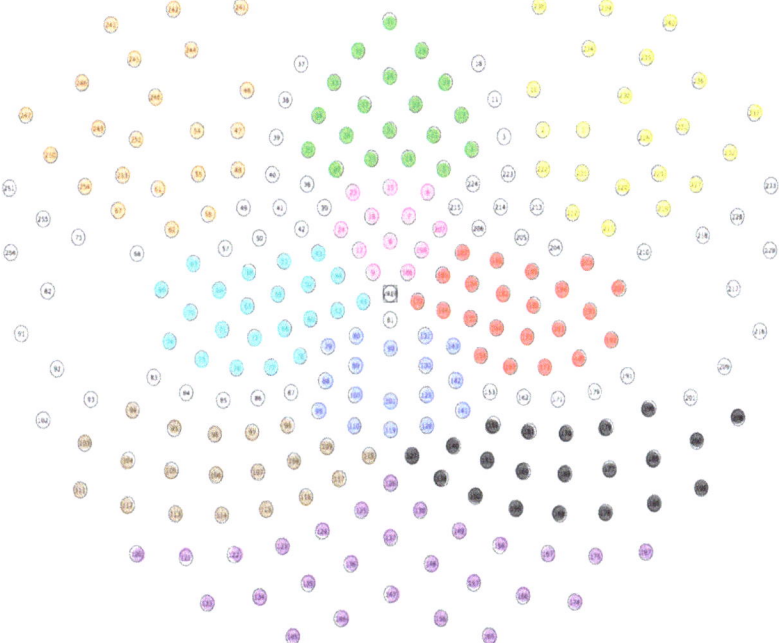

Figure 16. Electrode montages used to define regions during machine-learning analysis. Orange = left frontal, yellow = right frontal, green = medial prefrontal, pink = medial frontal, blue = posterior parietal, cyan = left temporoparietal, red = right temporoparietal, brown = left occipital, purple = medial occipital, and black = right occipital.

For each timepoint, a linear Support Vector Machine (SVM) classifier, as implemented in Matlab, was trained to classify patterns of EEG voltages associated with visually similar vs. visually distinct categories across subjects. The patterns of voltages across all 10 electrode groups associated with each condition for each subject served as the patterns to be classified. Leave-one-subject-out cross validation was carried out, such that patterns from 43 out of the 44 subjects were used to train the classifier, and the subject that was left out of training was used as the test subject. This type of training and test format was iteratively performed until all subjects were used as a test subject. For each iteration and timepoint, the classifier provided an estimate of how likely each of the two test patterns from the left-out subject (one pattern for visually similar trials and one for visually distinct trials) represented the visually similar category. Because there were two categories (distinct vs similar), the classifier-estimated probability that a pattern represents the visually distinct category was always 1 minus visually similar. The test pattern with greater visually similar evidence was labeled as the classifier's guess for which pattern represents the visually similar category. The other test pattern was labeled as the visually distinct guess. When the classifier's guess matched the actual condition, the classification was considered correct for the given test participant and timepoint. The classification accuracies from both pairwise classifications (visually similar 1 vs visually distinct, visually similar 2 vs visually distinct) were averaged together. This was done to provide an overall estimate of how well the classifier could distinguish between each of the two visually similar categories vs. the visually distinct category.

The classification accuracy for each timepoint was averaged across iterations and a one-sample *t*-test was performed against a theoretical chance mean (50%, as we performed pairwise classifications). The cross-validated classification accuracy for each timepoint is chronologically plotted in Figure 17, and timepoints that had a classification accuracy significantly above chance at $p < 0.05$ (uncorrected) are denoted by a blue diamond along the X axis. From this figure, the earliest timepoints at which the classifier was able to reliable differentiate between the two categories was between 260 and 320 ms, which coincides with the onset and peak of the MFN. Another extended period reliably above chance was between 440 and 700 ms, which corresponded to the peak and onset of the LIAN and P3b.

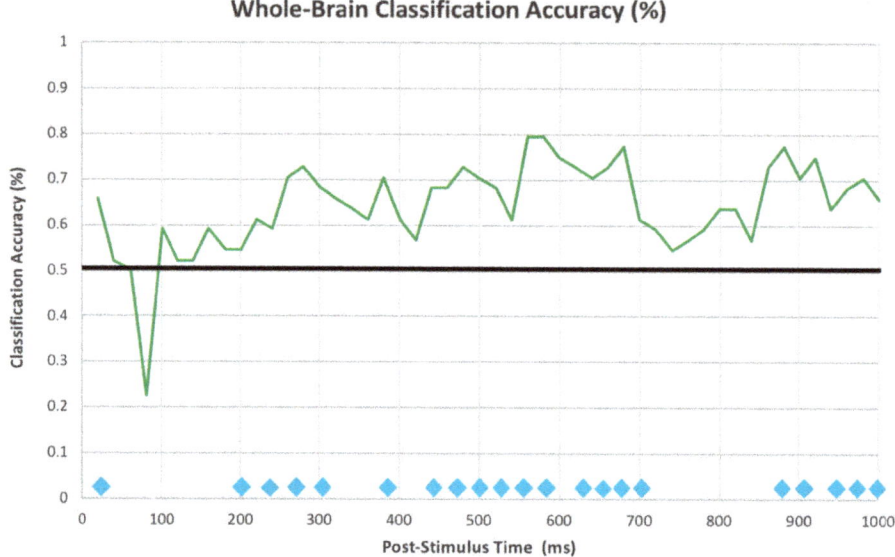

Figure 17. Whole-brain classification accuracy over time on an experimental trial. Blue diamonds along the X-axis represent timepoints where classification accuracy is significantly above chance ($p < 0.05$). The earliest string of above-chance classification accuracies is observable between 200 and 300 ms after stimulus onset, followed by another group between 430–700 ms. A late string of reliable classification occurs around 890–1000 ms.

The same SVM classification was run again using only the voltages in each region individually to determine whether any one particular region was driving the classification accuracy at each timepoint. The overall classification within each region indicated that the medial prefrontal, left frontal, and posterior parietal regions show the earliest reliable (and strongest) classification accuracy amongst all regions, with a maximum classification accuracy of 82% (Figure 18). Within these regions, reliable differentiation between categories occurs around 250 ms and remains stable until around 740 ms. The classification accuracy peaked earlier in the posterior parietal region compared to the medial prefrontal and left frontal regions, even though we can differentiate between the two categories with reliable accuracy using any of these three regions within the entire 500 ms window.

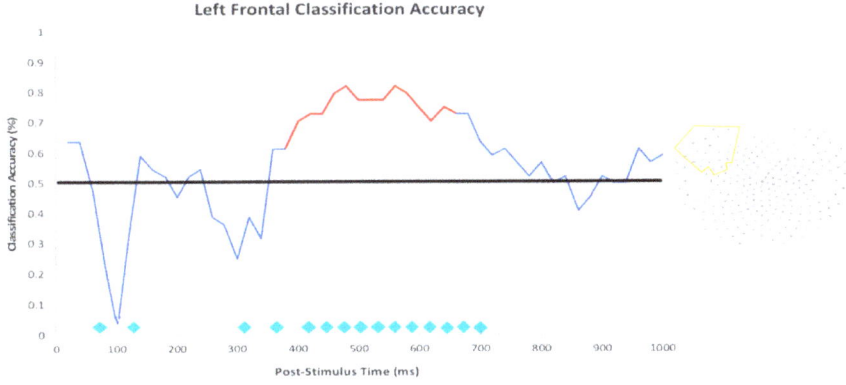

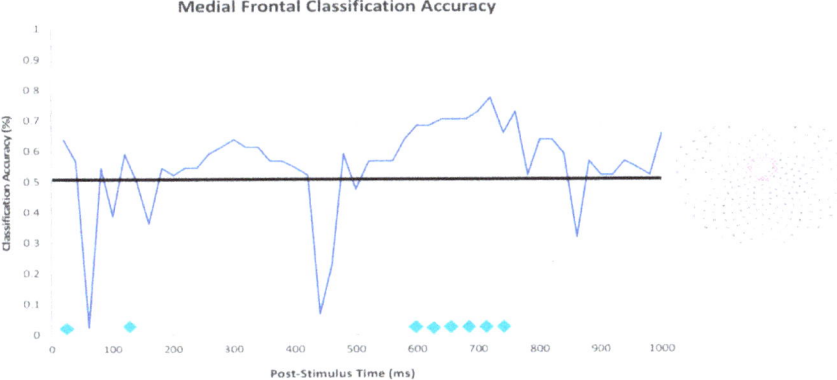

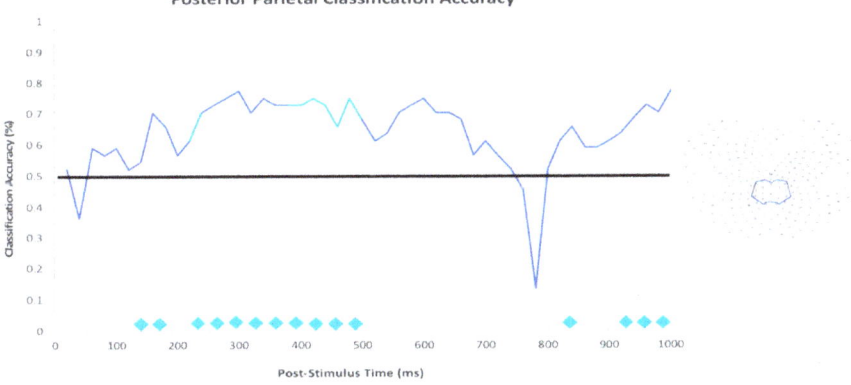

Figure 18. Region-based classification accuracy over time and correlated with behavioral performance. Top: Classification accuracy for the left-frontal electrode montage. Classification accuracy peaks between 400 and 700 ms. During this timeslot, classification is positively correlated with performance. Middle: Classification accuracy for the medial frontal electrode montage. Accuracy peaks between 600 and 750 ms after stimulus onset and does not correlate with behavior in any way. Bottom: Classification accuracy for the posterior parietal electrode montage. Accuracy peaks the earliest in this region, occurring between 220–500 ms. Interestingly, the classification accuracy is negatively correlated with behavioral performance within this window.

We were also interested in whether different neural strategies employed for the two types of trials—as evidenced by better SVM differentiation between neural patterns that are associated with each trial type—are beneficial to performance. Thus, we ran an exploratory analysis using a Pearson's correlation between the SVM classification accuracy and the behavioral performance on the categorization task of each subject. In Figure 18, the trajectory lines are color-coded red or cyan corresponding to timepoints where the SVM classification accuracy was significantly correlated with behavioral performance below a threshold of $p = 0.05$. The timepoints that are highlighted in red indicate that the SVM classification accuracy was positively correlated with behavioral performance, and those in cyan were negatively correlated with performance. The classification accuracy of the medial prefrontal region did not significantly predict behavioral outcome at virtually any timepoint. In contrast, the left frontal region, which is the location of the left LIAN component, was positively correlated with behavior throughout its classification peak. One interpretation of this finding is that the ability to flexibly employ different strategies best matching the current demands may optimize performance overall. Unexpectedly, the classification accuracy of the posterior parietal region was negatively correlated with behavior in several timepoints between 220 and 500 ms. One interpretation of this finding is that the shift away from verbalizable rule-based strategies itself requires executive resources and, thus, excessively differential allocation of resources at this topology and timepoints might make it difficult to continue learning beyond explicit rule-application [50]. Of all the regions, the right frontal area (the location of the right LIAN) was responsible for the very latest classification accuracy peak, occurring between 800 and 1000 ms. The classification accuracy in this region did not significantly correlate with behavior within this window. The three occipital areas along with the two parietal areas failed to demonstrate consistent windows of reliable classification accuracy.

4. Discussion

4.1. fMRI Pilot Experiment

The main goal of this pilot experiment was to determine the extent to which people engage multiple memory systems during a single categorization task. In line with past literature, the results showed that once subjects acquired the formations in the task, rule-based and perceptual similarity categoriation strategies engaged separate neural systems. These two systems were also recruited during a test block where the subjects were forced to generalize the categorizations strategies that they developed during training. For the machine-learning analysis, regions in the superior and inferior parietal lobes, along with MOFC, fusiform, and IFG successfully dissociated between conditions in the task. This provided enough preliminary evidence to motivate the fully-powered dEEG experiment.

4.1.1. Univariate Analysis

The categories in this experiment were designed, such that they require the subjects to discover a counting rule to differentiate between two visually similar categories and utilize a perceptual similarity strategy to identify the members of a visually distinct category. Our subjects' performance on the generalization block supports the assumption that they would recruit the proper strategies. Specifically, they would not have been able to accurately categorize novel formations into the trained categories had they exclusively relied on declarative recall of individual formations.

The superior and inferior frontal gyri were more active during the categorization of visually similar trials when compared to visually distinct trials. These regions are a part of the working memory system, where it is inferred that they are responsible for orienting attention and establishing executive control [22,51–53]. In our experiment, the subjects focused their attention toward the players on the line of scrimmage, where they were required to count each player if the formation belonged to one of the two visually similar categories. This is due, in part, to the visually similar categories having low between-category variability, which requires the engagement of a rule-based system. The comparison of the visually distinct category to each of the visually similar categories has much greater between-category variability and, thus, do not require the use of the cognitively taxing rule-based system [54].

Interestingly, caudate nucleus, a region that is integral to rule application, did not reach a level of significance (although this is expected given the small sample size) for the rule-based condition during training. Instead, a cluster over the hippocampus had the highest level of activation during training—a region that is well-known for its role in declarative recall [55]. It is possible that subjects utilized the rule for a short period of time during training, but relied more on the declarative recall of the few relevant players, given that subjects only needed to attend to a single feature within each stimulus to perform categorization (the number of players on the line of scrimmage). However, when encountering novel formations in the generalization block that belong to the categories acquired during training, the subjects were forced into applying the counting rule and, thus, the strong presence of caudate nucleus during generalization could reflect a more consistent reliance on rule application.

In support of our hypothesis, the robust activation of the lateral occipital cortex was present for the visually distinct category when compared to the visually similar categories. This held true throughout training and extended into the generalization block. The lateral occipital cortex has been well-established as the main region governing perceptual similarity categorization [18–21]. Perceptual similarity categorization can be carried-out with minimal working memory resources and it is optimized for instances with low within-category similarity [21]. The absence of the working memory system when subjects viewed members of the visually distinct category further supports our conclusion that this category engages the perceptual similarity system.

4.1.2. Multi-Voxel Pattern Analysis

Our region-based MVPA showed that the lateral frontal and parietal regions provided the most reliable classification between the visually similar and visually distinct categories, as consistent with previous findings that rule-based categorization requires a higher degree of attentional resources. On the other hand, MVPA provides a more sensitive measure of these conditional effects. More specifically, MVPA provides an avenue for detecting more subtle differences between our conditions that lie within the activity patterns of single regions–information that is sometimes subtracted-out by traditional analyses [56]. These small activation patterns can potentially code for task-relevant information that is important to both memory systems in our experiment.

Frontoparietal regions are well-known for their importance to cognitive control; mainly selective attention to information that is relevant to the task [57,58]. However, non-human primate experiments have demonstrated that activity in the frontal and parietal regions is predictive of an array of different task-relevant features, such as representations of individual stimuli, rule selection, or response selection [59–61]. Follow-up studies in humans have shown similar dissociations between stimulus sets and rules using MVPA [62,63]. These task features are essential to the rule- *and* perceptual similarity-based systems. The successful dissociation between category structures while using MVPA over frontoparietal regions in our task supports these previous findings.

4.2. Experiment 2 (dEEG)

The primary objectives of this experiment were to further determine whether multiple memory systems are recruited in a single task and evaluate the time course under which these systems are recruited. The results showed that, once the participants acquired the task, clear differences in the Left LIAN, MFN, and P3b components were seen between our two conditions. Overall, the amplitude of each ERP that reflected a difference between the visually similar and visually distinct categories was largest for the similarity-based category. However, the amplitude for the right LIAN was larger for the visually similar categories, although this effect did not reach statistical significance. For the machine learning analysis, the classification accuracy peaked earliest in the posterior parietal region (the location of the P3b), but reliable classification could be performed while using additional electrode clusters, including the left prefrontal and medial prefrontal areas.

4.2.1. ERPs

The MFN amplitude in this experiment was larger for the visually distinct category, albeit the significance of this effect was only marginal. The moderate difference in amplitude between our categories support recent findings that suggest multiple categorization strategies—even those inferred to rely very little on the working memory system—need executive functions in order to select the memory system that is optimal for a task [50]. For stimuli that would benefit most from perceptual similarity, this requirement of effortful control would be very brief—commencing well before an action is committed [50]. The latency of the MFN (180–300 ms) corresponds to the initial orienting of attention in a visuomotor association task and, thus, we propose that the MFN in our task is indexing the controlled attention that is required to select the memory system best suited for categorizing the presented stimulus and does not depend on the optimal system needed to perform a task.

Like the MFN, the P3b in our experiment was larger for the visually distinct stimuli when compared to stimuli that required the application of an explicit rule. Our initial assumption for this component was that the amplitude should be largest for the visually similar categories based on the perceptual similarity literature, which typically describes the robust activation of posterior visual cortex (and no posterior corticolimbic areas) for the visually distinct category [18–20]. However, this would only be the case if the participants were exclusively relying on perceptual similarity to categorize members of the visually distinct category. High trial counts could result in subjects utilizing different systems to categorize formations in the visually distinct group as their performance improves. When we analyzed the strategies that subjects were using post-hoc, 89% of participants reported using an explicit counting rule or declarative recall for categorizing the visually distinct formations (68% of the total count being declarative recall and 21% counting rules), while only 11% reported using a perceptual similarity strategy. This theory satisfies the two-stage learning *and* multiple memory systems models, where the early stages of learning are marked by a reliance on a variety of strategies (that may rely on dissociable neural systems) to work toward a more routinized and automatic recall of declarative information. However, more studies are required that track changes in the P3b across training to further associate the amplitude of the P3b with specific categorization strategies. Theoretically, we would see changes in the P3b amplitude as participants progress throughout training and, in turn, that should mirror any changes in the strategy they were using for specific categories.

The amplitude of the left LIAN was the largest for the visually distinct condition, whereas the right LIAN was largest for the visually similar condition, although the latter effect did not reach statistical significance. The left/right conditional flip makes the interpretation of this component fairly difficult. At this time, we are unsure whether both components are interpretable on their own, or if the LIAN is a hemisphere-specific component and the effect observed on the contralateral side is a byproduct of volume conduction. Luu et al. (2007) found that the amplitude of the right LIAN decreased as subjects acquired the ability to perform spatial analyses in a visuomotor association task, but the amplitude of the component remained unchanged when the targets in the task were digits that evoked the phonological loop [39]. They also found that the amplitude of the left LIAN increased as the subjects acquired digit targets in their task, whereas the amplitude remained unchanged as they acquired the ability to perform spatial analyses. Motivated by the findings of their experiment, we drew an initial assumption that the amplitude of both the left and right LIAN should be largest for visually similar condition in the current experiment. As similarly discussed in our interpretation of the P3b, however, this would only be the case if the subjects exclusively relied on perceptual similarity analyses to categorize formations in the visually distinct category—similar to the spatial analyses that were performed in Luu et al. (2007) [39].

Given the vast majority of subjects in our experiment used rote learning to categorize the visually distinct condition instead of the hypothesized perceptual similarity, one interpretation of our findings is to view them as a contrast between declarative recall of individual stimuli (visually distinct category) and explicit rule application (visually similar categories). When viewed from this perspective, the location of the LIAN coincides with structures that are essential for both forms of analysis, such as the temporal lobe and inferior frontal gyrus (IFG) [64,65]. Based on the higher accuracy for the visually distinct category, our findings that the right LIAN was smaller for this category is in-line with meta-analytic findings that show a right hemisphere-specific reduction in anterior temporal and IFG activity with the development of expertise in visuomotor tasks [8]. We could be seeing right hemisphere-specific reductions in the attentional resources that are needed to categorize the visually distinct group of formations simply because our subjects are consistently at a more advanced stage of learning for this condition when compared to the visually similar condition. Our left LIAN results also become more interpretable through this lens. If our subjects are significantly more advanced at declaratively recalling the visually distinct formations, then we would expect the left LIAN to be larger for this condition based on the findings of Luu et al. (2007) [39]. The amplitude of the left LIAN linearly increased for digit targets in their visuomotor learning task, which theoretically engage the same explicit form of memory as both conditions in our experiment. Thus, the left LIAN differences seen in our study could be reflecting differences in expertise between our subject's ability to categorize the visually similar and visually distinct categories.

4.2.2. dEEG Machine Learning

Using machine learning, we were able to successfully dissociate between our two conditions when utilizing raw voltages distributed across the entire scalp. We were especially interested in the timepoint-by-timepoint classification to identify the earliest point at which we can differentiate between our conditions as subjects view a stimulus. In our study, the onset of a stable period of reliable dissociation was around 200 ms after stimulus onset, which coincides with the initial onset of the MFN ERP component. We interpret this early classification timepoint as reflecting the initial controlled attention required to select a memory system based on the stimulus being presented.

We ran a second machine learning analysis on only the voltages of single groups of electrodes in 20 ms intervals to understand which individual regions were driving the classification accuracy. Our results from this analysis showed that the medial prefrontal, left frontal, and posterior parietal regions collectively contributed to the earliest reliable classification point. fMRI studies using multi-voxel pattern analysis (MVPA) have consistently demonstrated that individual rules can be reliably decoded in frontal and parietal regions [32–34]. Our EEG decoding results expand on these findings by specifying that the pattern representations of these concepts coincide with the initial orientation of attention. Through sufficient trial and error learning, the context under which an action is learned in a visuomotor task becomes tied to each individual stimulus in the task [66]. We can assume that the initial conscious registration of a stimulus prompted a conditioned re-establishment of the explicit rules (the learning context) that would dictate their subsequent action selection since we only analyzed trials after our subjects had been sufficiently trained on the task. This theory could explain why the first pattern dissociation between our two categories happens around the earliest time that a person can explicitly orient attention.

4.3. Category Learning Strategies as a Function of Expertise

The theories of categorization that formed the basis for our experiments commonly discuss these memory systems individually. However, the results from our experiments indicate that multiple memory systems may develop alongside one another in a single task, alternating from trial-to-trial to meet task demands. The development of expertise within each system could happen independently, and they likely share the same end-goal of automating the attention process with extended training.

Palmeri (1997) made one of the first attempts at describing the time that it takes subjects to reach automaticity while using perceptual similarity versus rule-based categorization [67]. In one experiment, Palmeri had subjects categorize objects with high within-category similarity, whereas in a separate experiment had subjects categorize objects with high between-category similarity, which required the discovery of a rule. The results from these experiments demonstrated that subjects utilizing perceptual similarity reached automaticity notably faster than those that relied on rules. This led to the development of a new theory termed Exemplar-Based Random Walk (EBRW) which proposes that, when a probe is presented, exemplars stored in memory race to be retrieved with a speed that is proportional to their similarity to the probe. Each one of the retrieved exemplars drives a random walk until sufficient evidence is presented. Once enough evidence has been retrieved, a subject makes a response [68,69].

Computational models of EBRW allow for the reaction times to be sped up by increasing within-category similarity and increasing the number of exposures to an exemplar [67]. This would result in a shorter training period before subjects reach automaticity when categorizing visually similar exemplars. The model also accounts for a longer training period when the subjects are forced to rely more on the random walks or the evidence-gathering aspect of the process when the categories have low within-category similarity and/or high between-category similarity, which was the case for our visually similar categories. EBRW, when interpreted on a conceptual level, helps to explain how implicit and explicit forms of categorization are a simple function of expertise development. The different strategies are called upon, depending on the structure of a category being presented and they share the common function of serving as an intermediate strategy before transitioning to an automatic mode of operation. However, a potential shortcoming of EBRW is that it postulates a single, unitary memory system underlying performance, which does not align well with neuroscience evidence in favor of multiple category learning systems [15,70]. We propose that this theory be altered to accept these processes as the work of distinct memory systems. It is clear that future work is needed to develop new theories for how these distinct systems develop under learning conditions that may require more than one type of system to optimize performance.

4.4. Alternative Interpretations and Limitations

While we interpret the neurophysiological differences between categories to reflect the use of different categorization strategies, a key challenge to clear interpretation is that the conditions differ in difficulty. The subjects had an easier time recognizing and categorizing the visually distinct category, whereas it took longer to do the same for the visually similar categories. The current task and result can be alternatively framed in terms of the differences in the relative contribution of top down vs. bottom up processes during learning. Specifically, for the visually distinct categories, subjects could largely rely on bottom-up (stimulus-driven) signals. In contrast, the categorization of visually similar categories requires a greater involvement of top-down signal guiding attention to relevant details to implement an explicit counting rule. Relatedly, we can view our results from a general cognitive resources framework. As stated earlier, the two visually similar categories have a relatively small between-category variance, which would require more working memory resources to discern, and arguably engage, the rule-based categorization system. On the other hand, the between-category variance between each of the two visually similar categories as compared with the visually distinct category is much higher. In theory, making a distinction with high between-category variance should not be as cognitively taxing. The differences seen in our ERPs reflect the differential allocation of cognitive resources, and this difference has been argued to be controlled by dissociable memory systems [15,54].

Unfortunatley, a fundamental feature of naturalistic learning environments is that some deviation in individual learning strategy is expected. Although we make the argument that rule-based and perceptual simliarity-based judgements play an intermediate role on the path to declaritive recall and automazation, there is no clear way to determine whether the subjects switched their strategies with extended training in the current experiments. A future experiment is necessary to further explore the finer details of any inferred stategy shifts related to expertise.

5. Conclusions

A large number of studies have outlined the behavioral and neural processes that are associated with different methods of categorization. The overwhelming consensus amongst these studies is that different categorization strategies serve the purpose of making learning as efficient as possible under different learning conditions. These strategies rely on distinct memory systems. A common feature of category learning studies is that they use tasks that are designed to recruit these systems and strategies one at a time. Yet, real-world learning likely involves the ability to switch between memory systems, including different approaches to different stimuli within a seeming same task. Through the conducted experiment, we provided initial evidence that people can switch between memory systems to optimize performance in a single task. In addition, we determined the time course by which the brain shows dissociable neural signatures signifying the selection of these different memory systems.

Author Contributions: Conceptualization, K.K.M. and D.Z.; Methodology, K.K.M., D.Z., P.L. and D.T.; Formal analysis, K.K.M., D.Z., and P.L.; Investigation, K.K.M., D.Z., P.L., and D.T.; Resources, D.Z., and D.T.; Data curation, K.K.M. and D.Z.; Writing—original draft preparation, K.K.M.; Writing—review and editing, D.Z., P.L., and D.T.; visualization, K.K.M.; Supervision, K.K.M., and D.Z.; Project administration, K.K.M.; Funding acquisition, D.Z. and D.T. All authors have read and agreed to the published version of the manuscript.

Funding: This research received no external funding.

Conflicts of Interest: The authors declare no conflict of interest.

References

1. Bruner, J.; Goodnow, J.J.; Austin, G.A. *A Study of Thinking*; Science Editions: New York, NY, USA, 1967.
2. Schneider, W.; Shiffrin, R.M. Controlled and automatic human information processing: I. Detection, search, and attention. *Psychol. Rev.* **1977**, *84*, 1–66. [CrossRef]
3. Zeithamova, D.; Maddox, W.T. Dual task interference in perceptual category learning. *Mem. Cogn.* **2006**, *34*, 387–398. [CrossRef] [PubMed]
4. Knowlton, B.J.; Squire, L.R. The learning of categories: Parallel brain systems for item memory and category knowledge. *Science* **1993**, *262*, 1747–1749. [CrossRef] [PubMed]
5. Gabrieli, J.D.E. Cognitive neuroscience of human memory. *Annu. Rev. Psychol.* **1998**, *49*, 87–115. [CrossRef]
6. Smith, E.E.; Patalano, A.L.; Jonides, J. Alternative strategies of categorization. *Cognition* **1998**, *65*, 167–196. [CrossRef]
7. Casale, M.B.; Ashby, F.G. A role for the perceptual representation memory system in category learning. *Percept. Psychophys.* **2008**, *70*, 983–999. [CrossRef]
8. Chein, J.M.; Schneider, W. Neuroimaging studies of practice-related change: fMRI and meta-analytic evidence of a domain-general control network for learning. *Cogn. Brain Res.* **2005**, *25*, 607–623. [CrossRef]
9. Gabriel, M.; Burhans, L.; Talk, A.; Scalf, P. Cingulate cortex. In *Encyclopedia of the Human Brain*; Ramachandran, V.S., Ed.; Elsevier Science: Amsterdam, The Netherlands, 2002; pp. 775–791.
10. Schneider, G.E. Two visual systems. *Science* **1969**, *163*, 895–902. [CrossRef]
11. Ungerleider, L.G.; Mishkin, M. Two cortical visual systems. In *Analysis of Visual Behavior*; Ingle, D.J., Goodale, M.A., Mansfield, R.J.W., Eds.; MIT Press: Cambridge, MA, USA, 1982; pp. 549–586.
12. Keele, S.W.; Ivry, R.; Mayr, U.; Hazeltine, E.; Heuer, H. The cognitive and neural architecture of sequence representation. *Psychol. Rev.* **2003**, *110*, 316–339. [CrossRef]
13. Luu, P.; Jiang, Z.; Poulsen, C.; Mattson, C.; Smith, A.; Tucker, D.M. Learning and the development of contexts for action. *Front. Hum. Neurosci.* **2011**, *5*, 159. [CrossRef]
14. Kemler-Nelson, D.G. The effect of intention on what concepts are acquired. *J. Verbal Learn. Verbal Behav.* **1984**, *23*, 734–759. [CrossRef]
15. Ashby, F.G.; Alfonso-Reese, L.A.; Turken, A.U.; Waldron, E.M. A neuropsychological theory of multiple systems in category learning. *Psychol. Rev.* **1998**, *105*, 442–481. [CrossRef] [PubMed]
16. Rosch, E. Cognitive representations of semantic categories. *J. Exp. Psychol. Gen.* **1975**, *104*, 192–233. [CrossRef]
17. Rosch, E. *Principles of Categorization*; Lawrence Erlbaum Associates: Hillsdale, NJ, USA, 1978.
18. Aizenstein, H.J.; MacDonald, A.W.; Stenger, V.A.; Nebes, R.D.; Larson, J.K.; Ursu, S.; Carter, C.S. Complementary category learning systems identified using event-related functional mri. *J. Cogn. Neurosci.* **2000**, *12*, 977–987. [CrossRef] [PubMed]
19. Reber, P.J.; Stark, C.E.L.; Squire, L.R. Contrasting cortical activity associated with category memory and recognition memory. *Learn. Mem.* **1998**, *5*, 420–428. [PubMed]

20. Reber, P.J.; Squire, L.R. Intact learning of artificial grammars and intact category learning by patients with Parkinson's disease. *Behav. Neurosci.* **1999**, *113*, 235–242. [CrossRef] [PubMed]
21. Nosofsky, R.M. Attention, similarity, and the identification-categorization relationship. *J. Exp. Psychol. Gen.* **1986**, *115*, 39–57. [CrossRef]
22. Ashby, F.G.; Ell, S.W. The neurobiology of human category learning. *Trends Cogn. Sci.* **2001**, *5*, 204–210. [CrossRef]
23. Waldron, E.M.; Ashby, F.G. The effects of concurrent task interference on category learning: Evidence from multiple category learning systems. *Psychon. Bull. Rev.* **2001**, *8*, 168–176. [CrossRef]
24. Minda, J.P.; Miles, S.J. The influence of verbal and nonverbal processing on category learning. *Psychol. Learn. Motiv.* **2010**, *52*, 117–162.
25. Dale, A.M. Optimal experimental design for event-related mri. *Hum. Brain Mapp.* **1999**, *8*, 109–114. [CrossRef]
26. Jenkinson, M.; Beckmann, C.F.; Behrens, T.E.; Woolrich, M.W.; Smith, S.M. FSL. *NeuroImage* **2012**, *62*, 782–790. [CrossRef] [PubMed]
27. Worsley, K.J. Statistical analysis of activation images. In *Functional Mri: An Introduction to Methods*; Jezzard, P., Matthews, P.M., Smith, S.M., Eds.; Oxford University Press: New York, NY, USA, 2001; pp. 251–270.
28. Nomura, E.M.; Maddox, W.T.; Filoteo, J.V.; Ing, A.D.; Gitelman, D.R.; Parrish, T.B.; Mesulam, M.M.; Reber, P.J. Neural correlates of rule-based and information-integration visual category learning. *Cereb. Cortex* **2006**, *17*, 37–43. [CrossRef] [PubMed]
29. Norman, K.A.; Polyn, S.M.; Deltre, G.J.; Haxby, J.V. Beyond mind-reading: Multi-voxel pattern analysis of fMRI data. *Trends Cogn. Sci.* **2006**, *10*, 424–430. [CrossRef]
30. Dale, A.M.; Fischl, B.; Sereno, M.I. Cortical surface-based analysis. I. Segmentation and surface reconstruction. *NeuroImage* **1999**, *9*, 179–194. [CrossRef]
31. Fischl, B.; Salat, D.H.; Busa, E.; Albert, M.; Dieterich, M.; Haselgrove, C.; van der Kouwe, A.; Killiany, R.; Kennedy, D.; Klaveness, S.; et al. Whole brain segmentation: Automated labeling of neuroanatomical structures in the human brain. *Neuron* **2002**, *33*, 341–355. [CrossRef]
32. Woolgar, A.; Thompson, R.; Bor, D.; Duncan, J. Multi-voxel coding of stimuli, rules, and responses in human frontoparietal cortex. *NeuroImage* **2011**, *56*, 744–752. [CrossRef]
33. Reverberi, C.; Görgen, K.; Haynes, J.D. Compositionality of rule representations in human prefrontal cortex. *Cereb. Cortex* **2012**, *22*, 1237–1246. [CrossRef]
34. Nelissen, N.; Strokes, M.; Nobre, A.C.; Rushworth, M.F. Frontal and parietal cortical interactions with distributed visual representations during selection attention and action selection. *J. Neurosci.* **2013**, *33*, 16443–16458. [CrossRef]
35. Rissman, J.; Gazzaley, A.; D'Esposito, M. Measuring functional connectivity during distinct stages of a cognitive task. *NeuroImage* **2004**, *23*, 752–763. [CrossRef]
36. Avants, B.B.; Tustison, N.J.; Song, G.; Cook, P.A.; Klein, A.; Gee, J.C. A reproducible evaluation of ANTs similarity metric performance in brain image registration. *NeuroImage* **2011**, *54*, 2033–2044. [CrossRef] [PubMed]
37. Mur, M.; Bandettini, P.A.; Kriegeskorte, N. Revealing representational content with pattern-information fMRI—An introductory guide. *Soc. Cogn. Affect. Neurosci.* **2009**, *4*, 101–109. [CrossRef] [PubMed]
38. Esterman, M.; Tamber-Rosenau, B.J.; Chiu, Y.; Yantis, S. Avoiding non-independence in fMRI data analysis: Leave one subject out. *NeuroImage* **2010**, *50*, 572–576. [CrossRef] [PubMed]
39. Luu, P.; Tucker, D.M.; Stripling, R. Neural mechanisms for learning action in context. *Brain Res.* **2007**, *1179*, 89–105. [CrossRef]
40. Morgan, K.K.; Luu, P.; Tucker, D.M. Changes in p3b latency and amplitude reflect expertise acquisition in a football visuomotor learning task. *PLoS ONE* **2016**, *11*, e0154021. [CrossRef] [PubMed]
41. Bush, G.; Vogt, B.A.; Holmes, J.; Dale, A.M.; Greve, D.; Jenike, M.A.; Rosen, B.R. Dorsal anterior cingulate cortex: A role in reward-based decision making. *Proc. Natl. Acad. Sci. USA* **2002**, *99*, 523–528. [CrossRef] [PubMed]
42. Halgren, E.; Baudena, P.; Heit, G.; Clarke, J.M.; Marinkovic, K.; Chauvel, P. Spatio-temporal stages in face and word processing. 2. Depth-recorded potentials in the human frontal and Rolandic cortices. *J. Physiol.* **1994**, *88*, 51–80. [CrossRef]

43. Halgren, E.; Baudena, P.; Clarke, J.M.; Heit, G.; Liegeois, C.; Chauvel, P.; Musolino, A. Intracerebral potential to rare target and distractor auditory and visual stimuli. I. Superior temporal plane and parietal lobe. *Electroencephalogr. Clin. Neurophysiol.* **1995**, *94*, 191–220. [CrossRef]
44. Halgren, E.; Baudena, P.; Clarke, J.M.; Heit, G.; Marinkovic, K.; Devaux, B.; Vignal, J.P.; Biraben, A. Intracerebral potential to rare target and distractor auditory and visual stimuli. II. Medial, lateral, and posterior temporal lobe. *Electroencephalogr. Clin. Neurophysiol.* **1995**, *94*, 229–250. [CrossRef]
45. Baudena, P.; Halgren, E.; Heit, G.; Clarke, J.M. Intracerebral potentials to rare target and distractor auditory and visual stimuli. III. Frontal cortex. *Electroencephalogr. Clin. Neurophysiol.* **1995**, *94*, 251–264. [CrossRef]
46. Smith, M.E.; Halgren, E.; Sokolik, M.; Baudena, P.; Musolino, A.; Liegeois-Chauvel, C.; Chauvel, P. The intracranial topography of the p3 event-related potential elicited during auditory oddball. *Electroencephalogr. Clin. Neurophysiol.* **1990**, *76*, 235–248. [CrossRef]
47. Brankack, J.; Seidenbecher, T.; Muller-Gartner, H.W. Task-relevant late positive component in rats: Is it related to hippocampal theta rhythm? *Hippocampus* **1996**, *6*, 475–482. [CrossRef]
48. Shin, J. The interrelationship between movement and cognition: Theta rhythm and the p330 event-related potential. *Hippocampus* **2011**, *21*, 744–752. [CrossRef] [PubMed]
49. Kahana, M.J.; Seelig, D.; Madsen, J.R. Theta returns. *Curr. Opin. Neurobiol.* **2001**, *11*, 739–744. [CrossRef]
50. Miles, S.J.; Matsuki, K.; Minda, J.P. Continuous executive function disruption interferes with application of an information integration categorization strategy. *Atten. Percept. Psychophys.* **2014**, *76*, 1318–1334. [CrossRef]
51. Lombardi, W.J.; Andreason, P.J.; Sirocco, K.Y.; Rio, D.E.; Gross, R.E.; Umhau, J.C.; Hommer, D.W. Wisconsin card sorting test performance following head-injury: Dorsolateral fronto-striatal circuit activity predicts perseveration. *J. Exp. Neuropsychol.* **1999**, *21*, 2–16. [CrossRef]
52. Rao, S.M.; Bobholz, J.A.; Hammeke, T.A.; Tosen, A.C.; Woodley, S.J.; Cunningham, J.M.; Cox, R.W.; Stein, E.A.; Binder, J.R. Functional mri evidence for subcortical participation in conceptual reasoning skills. *Neuroreport* **1997**, *8*, 1987–1993. [CrossRef]
53. Rogers, R.D.; Andrews, T.C.; Grasby, P.M.; Brooks, D.J.; Robbins, T.W. Contrasting cortical and subcortical activations produced by attentional-set shifting and reversal learning in humans. *J. Cogn. Neurosci.* **2000**, *12*, 142–162. [CrossRef]
54. Ashby, F.G.; Paul, E.J.; Maddox, W.T. COVIS. In *Formal Approaches in Categorization*; Pothos, E.M., Wills, A.J., Eds.; Cambridge University Press: New York, NY, USA, 2011; pp. 65–87.
55. Eichenbaum, H. A cortical-hippocampal system for declarative memory. *Nat. Rev. Neurosci.* **2000**, *1*, 41–50. [CrossRef]
56. Haynes, J.D.; Rees, G. Decoding mental states from brain activity in humans. *Nat. Rev. Neurosci.* **2006**, *7*, 523–534. [CrossRef]
57. Desimone, R.; Duncan, J. Neural mechanisms of selective visual attention. *Annu. Rev. Neurosci.* **1995**, *18*, 193–222. [CrossRef] [PubMed]
58. Miller, E.K.; Cohen, J.D. An integrative theory of prefrontal cortex function. *Annu. Rev. Neurosci.* **2001**, *24*, 167–202. [CrossRef] [PubMed]
59. Asaad, W.F.; Rainer, G.; Miller, E.K. Neural activity in the primate prefrontal cortex during associative learning. *Neuron* **1998**, *21*, 1399–1407. [CrossRef]
60. Freedman, D.J.; Assad, J.A. Experience-dependent representation of visual categories in parietal cortex. *Nature* **2006**, *443*, 85–88. [CrossRef] [PubMed]
61. White, I.M.; Wise, S.P. Rule-dependent neuronal activity in the prefrontal cortex. *Exp. Brain Res.* **1999**, *126*, 315–335. [CrossRef] [PubMed]
62. Bode, S.; Haynes, J.D. Decoding sequential stages of task preparation in the human brain. *NeuroImage* **2009**, *45*, 606–613. [CrossRef] [PubMed]
63. Haynes, J.D.; Sakai, K.; Rees, G.; Gilbert, S.; Frith, C.; Passingham, R.E. Reading hidden intentions in the human brain. *Curr. Biol.* **2007**, *17*, 323–328. [CrossRef]
64. Toni, I.; Rammani, N.; Josephs, O.; Ashburner, J.; Passingham, R.E. Learning arbitrary visuomotor associations: Temporal dynamics of brain activity. *NeuroImage* **2001**, *14*, 1048–1057. [CrossRef]
65. Groll, M.J.; de Lange, F.P.; Verstraten, F.A.J.; Passingham, R.E.; Toni, I. Cerebral changes during performance of overlearned arbitrary visuomotor associations. *J. Neurosci.* **2006**, *26*, 117–125. [CrossRef]
66. Donchin, E.; Coles, M.G.H. Is the p300 component a manifestation of context updating? *Behav. Brain Sci.* **1988**, *11*, 357–374. [CrossRef]

67. Palmeri, T.J. Exemplar similarity and the development of automaticity. *J. Exp. Psychol. Learn. Mem. Cogn.* **1997**, *23*, 324–354. [CrossRef] [PubMed]
68. Nosofsky, R.M.; Palmeri, T.J.; McKinley, S.C. Rule-plus-exception model of classification learning. *Psychol. Rev.* **1994**, *101*, 53–79. [CrossRef] [PubMed]
69. Palmeri, T.J.; Nosofsky, R.M. Recognition memory for exceptions to the category rule. *J. Exp. Psychol. Learn. Mem. Cogn.* **1995**, *21*, 548–568. [CrossRef] [PubMed]
70. Zeithamova, D.; Maddox, W.T.; Schnyer, D.M. Dissociable prototype learning systems: Evidence from brain imaging and behavior. *J. Neurosci.* **2008**, *28*, 13194–13201. [CrossRef] [PubMed]

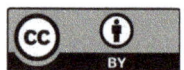
© 2020 by the authors. Licensee MDPI, Basel, Switzerland. This article is an open access article distributed under the terms and conditions of the Creative Commons Attribution (CC BY) license (http://creativecommons.org/licenses/by/4.0/).

MDPI
St. Alban-Anlage 66
4052 Basel
Switzerland
Tel. +41 61 683 77 34
Fax +41 61 302 89 18
www.mdpi.com

Brain Sciences Editorial Office
E-mail: brainsci@mdpi.com
www.mdpi.com/journal/brainsci